# Psychiatric Diagnosis

# Psychiatric Diagnosis
## A World Perspective

Edited by
Juan E. Mezzich   Yutaka Honda
Marianne C. Kastrup

Section on Classification, Diagnostic Assessment, and Nomenclature, World Psychiatric Association

With 16 Illustrations

Springer-Verlag
New York Berlin Heidelberg London Paris
Tokyo Hong Kong Barcelona Budapest

Juan E. Mezzich, M.D., Ph.D.
Professor of Psychiatry and
Epidemiology
University of Pittsburgh
Western Psychiatric Institute and Clinic
3811 O'Hara Street
Pittsburgh, PA 15213-2593 USA

Yutaka Honda, M.D., Ph.D.
Director, Seiwa Hospital
Neuropsychiatric Research Institute
Tokyo, Japan

Marianne C. Kastrup, M.D., Ph.D.
Associate Professor of Psychiatry
University of Copenhagen
Copenhagen, Denmark

Library of Congress Cataloging-in-Publication Data
Psychiatric diagnosis: a world perspective / edited on behalf of the Section on Classification, Diagnostic Assessment, and Nomenclature of the World Psychiatric Association by Juan E. Mezzich, Yutaka Honda, Marianne C. Kastrup.
p. cm.
Updated versions of papers presented at the International Symposium on Psychiatric Diagnosis, held in Tokyo in 1990.
Includes bibliographical references and index.
ISBN 0-387-94221-1.—ISBN 3-540-94221-1
1. Mental illness—Classification—Congresses. 2. Mental illness—Diagnosis—Congresses. 3. Psychiatry, Transcultural—Congresses.
I. Mezzich. Juan E. II. Honda, Y. (Yutaka), 1929.
III. Kastrup, M. IV. World Psychiatric Association. Section on Classification, Diagnostic Assessment, and Nomenclature.
V. International Symposium on Psychiatric Diagnosis (1990: Tokyo, Japan)
[DNLM: 1. Mental Disorders—diagnosis—congresses. 2. Mental Disorders—classification—congresses. 3. Cross-Cultural Comparison—congresses. WM 141 P97353 1990]
RC455.2.C4P77 1994
616.89075'09—dc20
DNLM/DLC
for Library of Congress 93-46006

Printed on acid-free paper.



Production coordinated by Chernow Editorial Services and managed by Henry Krell; manufacturing supervised by Gail Simon.
Typeset by Best-set Typesetter Ltd., Hong Kong.
Printed and bound by Edwards Brothers, Inc., Ann Arbor, MI.
Printed in the United States of America.

9 8 7 6 5 4 3 2 1

ISBN 0-387-94221-1 Springer-Verlag New York Berlin Heidelberg
ISBN 3-540-94221-1 Springer-Verlag Berlin Heidelberg New York

# Foreword

It can be said that the classical concepts of psychiatric diagnosis and classification were developed in France and Germany, as epitomized by the work of Emil Kraepelin. While trying to set basic nosological principles at home, Kraepelin traveled to Indonesia to explore the comparability of psychiatric morbidity. In his own way, he illustrated the tension between universality and diversity, which is central to our field.

A major actor in the modern evolution of diagnostic classification has been the World Health Organization (WHO), taking the post from bodies such as the International Statistical Institute, which actually initiated the decennial editions of the *International Classification of Diseases and Causes of Death*. Of seminal importance were the series of workshops on various forms of psychiatric pathology that the WHO organized between 1965 and 1975 in preparation for the ICD-9 classification of mental disorders.

In 1980, the American Psychiatric Association (which had been well known for endorsing a predominantly psychodynamic perspective) sent shock waves throughout the world with the publication of *Diagnostic and Statistical Manual of Mental Disorders*, 3rd edition (DSM-III). Soon its major innovations, for example, descriptive phenomenological emphasis, explicit diagnostic criteria, and multiaxial approach, were widely accorded great interest and significance.

More recently, the Section on Classification, Diagnostic Assessment, and Nomenclature of the World Psychiatric Association (WPA) has assumed a leading role in the discussion and coordination of international psychiatric diagnosis. While working with the WHO in the development and implementation of the 10th revision of the International Classification of Diseases and Health Related Problems (ICD-10), the WPA has fostered the consideration of regional and national perspectives. In addition to DSM-IV, there are now a number of national adaptations of the international classification, such as the Chinese Classification of Mental Disorders, Second Edition (CCMD-II) and the Japanese Clinical Modification of ICD-10.

Of considerable significance for this integration of diverse viewpoints in our field have been two major conferences organized by the WPA Classification Section. First, the International Conference on Psychiatric Classification: Unity and Diversity, held in Montreal in 1985, featured the presentation and wide discussion of the principles of ICD-10. In 1990, the International Symposium on Psychiatric Diagnosis held in Tokyo, which I had the honor to preside, reviewed the development of various components of the ICD-10 family of classifications within an international and transcultural framework. Updated versions of the symposium papers are now presented in this book.

The location as well as the content of the 1990 International Symposium recognized several contributions made by Japanese psychiatrists. For example, Morita described *shinkeishitsu* (a concept related to what would be later known as avoidant personality disorder) in the 1930s. Shimoda originated immodysthymic character as a premorbid personality of major depression in 1941, earlier than the *typus melancholicus* described by Tellenbach in Germany in 1961. As a third example, Mitsuta advanced on genetic grounds the concept of "atypical psychosis" in 1953, which can be contrasted to that presented by Leonhard in 1960.

I believe that every country or region has its own traditional perspectives on psychiatric classification, based on its particular culture. It is hoped that in the future, ICD-11 as well as DSM-V and other national adaptations may be able to integrate further those cultural characteristics, not only in the classification but also in the nomenclature and diagnostic assessment of psychiatric problems.

Much progress has been made on international psychiatric diagnosis as documented in this volume. We expect that etiological research and catamnestic outcome studies will lead to further progress in our field.

Masaaki Kato
Emeritus Professor of Psychiatry
Tokyo Medical College
Former Director, National Institute of Mental Health
Japan

# Preface

The complexity of our world, highlighted by the fact that more than 80% of the planet's population (and presumably a similar proportion of all psychiatric patients) live in non-Western, traditional societies, makes a compelling point for a truly international psychiatry. Furthermore, it happens that psychiatric diagnosis, as the field's central concept and tool, has a remarkable international anchorage. In effect, each of the major advances in diagnostic theory and methods of recent times, represented pioneering contributions emerging from a range of geographical and cultural regions.

The current emphasis on phenomenological or descriptive approaches to nosology had important beginnings with the construction of symptoms as units of analysis of abnormal behavior in 19th century France (Berrios 1994). Clinical description, at a higher level of organization, was lastingly moved forward by the delineation of clinical evolution, also in France (Magnan and Sérieux 1893), and by the conceptualization of nosological entities in Germany (Kraepelin 1896, Leonhard 1957).

The need for greater clarity in the definition of mental disorders, which became crucial for empirical research, was cogently argued by the British psychiatrist Stengel (1959) on reflecting on the results of his international survey of classifications commissioned by the World Health Organization (WHO). The proposal of explicit diagnostic criteria or assignment rules was pioneered by Berner (1958) in Austria for the definition of psychoses, by the Chileans Horowitz and Marconi (1966) for the case of alcoholism in epidemiological studies, and, more recently, by Feighner et al (1972) in the United States for the research diagnosis of a group of 15 mental disorders.

Regarding the third major conceptual and methodological advance, the earliest multiaxial schemes were designed by Essen-Möller and Wohlfahrt (1947) in Sweden; and Lecomte, Damey, Delage et al (1947) in France, as a dichotomical assessment of syndrome and etiology; and shortly afterwards by Bilikiewicz (1951) in Poland and Leme Lopes (1954) in Brazil, proposing a triaxial formulation of clinical syndromes, personality, and etiopathogenic constellations. The first pertinent use of the term multiaxial involved an influential classification of child psychiatric conditions prepared in 1969 by experts from six countries (Rutter, Levobici, Eisenberg, Sneznevskij, Sadoun, Brooke, and Lin) under WHO's auspices. In addition to the about 20 published multiaxial systems originating in 11 different countries for general psychiatry (Mezzich 1988), there have been schemas for specific clinical conditions, such as the one developed by Kasahara and Kimura (1975) in Japan for depressed patients.

The advances in the standardization, precision, and thoroughness of psychiatric diagnosis mentioned above are being incipiently supplemented with attention to personalized or idiographic descriptive approaches. This promises not only to enhance our understanding of the case, but to make fuller and more effective use of the evolving range of therapeutic possibilities. One of the ideographic perspectives under recent development is a cultural formulation from the perspective of the patient's personal experience and primary reference group, and dealing with the patient's identity; the experiencing, reporting and interpretation of psychopathology, its context and impact; and the clinician–patient relationship (Mezzich et al, in press).

In an attempt to articulate key developments in the field, the Section on Classification, Diagnostic Assessment and Nomenclature of the World Psychiatric Association has prepared this volume. This is inscribed within the Section's ongoing efforts on international diagnosis, much of this focused on ICD-10, in close collaboration with the WHO (Sartorius 1988). The volume is built on presentations made at a major international conference presided over by Masaaki Kato in September 1991 in Tokyo, and later elaborated further by their authors.

The book is organized around five major themes, all among the most prominent ones in contemporary psychiatric diagnosis and international psychiatry. Part I deals with major regional perspectives, which make patent the richness of cultural and theoretical traditions and challenges from which current diagnostic systems are emerging and to which they have to be referred. Part II focuses on the 10th revision of the *International Classification of Diseases and Health-Related Problems* (ICD-10) and various aspects of its extensive field trials. In connection to ICD-10, not only an international language for the field is emerging, but also promising adaptations to local clinical reality. Part III discusses the experience and prospects for comprehensive diagnosis through the multiaxial model. Particular attention is paid to the triad of pathology, consequent disabilities, and contextual factors. Part IV reviews one of the basic objectives of psychiatric diagnosis, that is, treatment planning and organization of health services, pointing out how important is to consider both the individual patient and how society organizes itself for clinical care. Last, but not least, Part V examines the role and challenges of psychiatric diagnosis in primary health care. The topic is important not only because most psychiatric patients in both industrialized and traditional societies are seen first by general health professionals, but because of the opportunities primary care is increasingly perceived to offer for more integrated and effective health care. The Epilogue probes an universal approach to psychiatric diagnosis.

The editors of this volume, representing three continents, join a distinguished group of clinical scholars from Africa, Asia, Europe, North America, Latin America and Oceania, in expressing the hope that this work usefully illustrates the achievements of the field and will stimulate further work toward diagnostic systems that are historically informed, thoughtfully empirical, and concerned with the wholeness of the patient.

Juan E. Mezzich
Yutaka Honda
Marianne C. Kastrup

## References

Berner P (1958). *Psychiatrie in der Allgemeinpraxis*. Paracelsus-Baihefte, Vienna.

Berrios GE (1994). The history of descriptive psychopathology. In JE Mezzich, MR Jorge, IM Salloum (eds), *Psychiatric Epidemiology: Assessment Concepts and Methods*. Johns Hopkins University Press, Baltimore, MD.

Bilikiewiwicz I (1951). Proba ukladu nosograficznego etioepigenetycznego w psychiatrii. *Neurologia i Neurochirurgia Polska* 1:68–78.

Essen-Möller E, Wohlfahrt S (1947). Suggestions for the amendment of the official Swedish classification of mental disorders. *Acta Psychiatrica Scandinavica* 47:551–555 (suppl).

Feighner JP, Robins E, Guze SB, et al (1972). Diagnostic criteria for use in psychiatric research. *Archives of General Psychiatry* 26:57–63.

Horowitz J, Marconi J (1966). El problema de las definiciones en el campo de la salud mental: Definiciones aplicables en estudios epidemiológicos. *Boletín de la Oficina Sanitaria Panamericana* 60:300–309.

Kasahara Y, Kimura B (1975). Zur Klassifizierung der depressiven Zustände. *Psychiatria et Neurologia Japonica* 77:715–735.

Kraepelin E (1986). Der psychologische Versuch in der Psychiatrie. *Psychologische Arbeiten* 1:1–91.

Lecomte M, Damey A, Delage E, et al (1947). Essai d'une statistique synoptique de médicine psychiatrique. *Techniques Hospitalières* 18:5–8.

Leonhard K (1957). *Afteilung der endogenen Psychosen*. Akademie, Berlin.

Leme-Lopes J (1954). *As Dimensoes do Diagnóstico Psiquiátrico*. Agir, Rio de Janeiro.

Magnan V, Sérieux P (1893). *Le délire chronique à evolution systématique*. Gauthier Villars/Georges Masson, Paris.

Mezzich JE (1988). On developing a psychiatric multiaxial schema for ICD-10. *British Journal of Psychiatry* 152:38–43 (suppl 1).

Mezzich JE, Kleinman A, Fabrega H, Parron D (in press). *Culture and Psychiatric Diagnosis*. American Psychiatric Press, Washington, DC.

Rutter M, Lebovici S, Eisenberg L, Sneznevskij AV, Sadoun R, Brooke E, Lin T-Y (1969). A triaxial classification of mental disorders in childhood. *Journal of Child Psychology and Psychiatry* 10:41–61.
Stengel E: Classification of mental disorders (1959). *Bulletin of the World Health Organization* 21:601–663.

# Contents

**Part II. ICD-10 Field Studies**

# Contributors

**Saburo Anzai, MD**
Director
Kanagawaken Psychiatric Clinic
Kanagawaken, Japan

**Kunihiko Asai, MD**
Medical Director
Asai Hospital
Togane City, Chiba Prefecture, Japan

**Enrique Bernal, MD**
Psychiatrist
Instituto Nacional de Salud Mental
Lima, Peru

**Ayo Binitie, MD**
Professor of Mental Health
University of Benin
Benin City, Nigeria

**Gilles Chaillet, MD**
Psychiatrist
Centre Hospitalier de Luxembourg
Luxembourg, Luxembourg

**John E. Cooper, BM, DPM**
Emeritus Professor of Psychiatry
University of Nottingham
Nottingham, United Kingdom

**Wendy Davis, MEd**
Editorial Coordinator, DSM-IV
American Psychiatric Association
Washington, DC, USA

**Satoko Ezoe, MD**
Neuropsychiatry Department
Keio University
Tokyo, Japan

**Horacio Fabrega, MD**
Professor of Psychiatry and Anthropology
University of Pittsburgh
Pittsburgh, Pennsylvania, USA

**Michael First, MD**
Assistant Professor of Clinical Psychiatry
Columbia University
New York, New York, USA

**Allen Frances, MD**
Professor and Head, Department of Psychiatry
Duke University
Durham, North Carolina, USA

**Akira Fujinawa, MD**
Director, National Center of Neurology and Psychiatry
Chiba, Japan

**Willa Hall, MA**
Research Associate, DSM-IV
Columbia University
New York, New York, USA

**Koichi Hanada, MD**
Associate Professor of Psychiatry
Shiga University of Medical Science
Japan

**Hanfried H. Helmchen, MD**
Professor of Psychiatry
Freien Universität Berlin
Berlin, Germany

**Yutaka Honda, MD, PhD**
Director, Neuropsychiatric Research Institute
Seiwa Hospital
Tokyo, Japan

**Felix Attah Johnson, MD**
Chief of Psychiatry
Hospital of the University of Papua New Guinea
Boroko, Papua New Guinea

**Miguel R. Jorge, MD, PhD**
Chairman, Department of Psychiatry
Escola Paulista de Medicina
São Paulo, Brazil

**Yomishi Kasahara, MD**
Professor and Chairman
Department of Psychiatry
Nagoya University
Nagoya, Japan

**Marianne C. Kastrup, MD, PhD**
Associate Professor of Psychiatry
University of Copenhagen
Copenhagen, Denmark

**Nobukatsu Katoh, MD**
Tokyo Metropoplitan Matsuzawa Hospital
Tokyo, Japan

**Heinz Katschnig, MD**
Professor and Head, Department of Psychiatry
Universität Wien
and
Director, Ludwig Boltzmann Institute for Social Psychiatry
Vienna, Austria

**Toshinori Kitamura, MD**
Chief, Sect. Mental Health for the Elderly
National Institute of Mental Health
Chiba, Japan

**Myriam Kline, MS**
Focussed Field Trials Coordinator, DSM-IV
Columbia University
New York, New York, USA

**Tsukasa Koyama, MD**
Department of Psychiatry
Hokkaido University
Sapporo, Japan

**Talya Landmann, MD**
Psychiatrist
Instituto Nacional de Salud Mental
Lima, Peru

**H.Y. Lee, MD**
Professor of Psychiatry
Yonsei University
Seoul, Republic of Korea

**Juan J. Lopez-Ibor, MD**
Director, Lopez-Ibor Clinic
Professor of Psychiatry
Universidad Complutense
Madrid, Spain

**Pedro Makabe, MD**
Psychiatrist
Instituto Nacional de Salud Mental
Lima, Peru

**Kelly McKinney, MA**
Research Associate, DSM-IV
Columbia University
New York, New York, USA

**Juan E. Mezzich, MD, PhD**
Professor of Psychiatry and Epidemiology
University of Pittsburgh
Pittsburgh, Pennsylvania, USA
and
Honorary Professor
Universidad Peruana Cayetano Heredia
Lima, Peru

**Katsumasa Miyasato, MD**
Department of Neuropsychiatry
Hamamatsu University
Hamamatsu, Japan

**Peter V. Morozov, MD**
Head, Department of Research, Planning and Coordination
National Mental Health Research Center
Moscow, USSR

**R. Srinivasa Murthy, MD**
Chairman, Department of Psychiatry
National Institute of Mental Health and Neurosciences
Bangalore, India

**Yoshibumi Nakane, MD**
Professor and Head, Department of Psychiatry
Nagasaki University
Nagasaki, Japan

**Masahisa Nishizono, MD**
Department of Psychiatry
Fukuoka University
Fukuoka, Japan

**Yoshiro Ohkubo, MD**
Department of Neuropsychiatry
Nagasaki University
Nagasaki, Japan

**Yuji Okazaki, MD**
Assistant Professor of Psychiatry
Nagasaki University
Nagasaki, Japan

**Keigo Okonogi, MD**
Professor of Neuropsychiatry
Keio University
Tokyo, Japan

**Yutaka Ono, MD**
Clinical Assistant, Department of Neuropsychiatry
Keio University, Japan

**Harold Pincus, MD**
Deputy Medical Director
American Psychiatric Association
Washington, DC, USA

**Charles B. Pull, MD**
Professor of Psychiatry
Centre Hospitalier de Luxembourg
Luxembourg, Luxembourg

**Bou-Yong Rhi, MD**
Professor of Psychiatry
Seoul National University
Seoul, Republic of Korea

**Nina Rosenthal, BS**
Research Associate, DSM-IV
Columbia University
New York, New York, USA

**Javier E. Saavedra, MD**
Head, Diagnosis and Evaluation Unit
Instituto Nacional de Salud Mental
and
Assistant Professor of Psychiatry
Universidad Peruana Cayetano Heredia
Lima, Peru

**Norman Sartorius, MD, PhD**
President Elect
World Psychiatric Association
and
Director, Division of Mental Health
World Health Organization
and
Professor of Psychiatry
University of Geneva
Geneva, Switzerland

**Yucun Shen, MD**
Director, Mental Health Institute
Beijing Medical University
Beijing, People's Republic of China

**Helen Stayna, MA**
Research Associate, DSM-IV
Columbia University
New York, New York, USA

**Erik Strömgren, MD**
Professor of Psychiatry
Aarhus University
Risskov, Denmark

**Ryo Takahashi, MD**
Department of Neuropsychiatry
Tokyo Medical and Dental University
Tokyo, Japan

**Saburo Takahashi, MD**
Professor and Chairman, Department of Psychiatry
Shiga University of Medical Science
Shiga, Japan

**Tooru Takahashi, MD**
National Institute of Mental Health
Chiba, Japan

**Fredy Vásquez, MD**
Psychiatrist
Instituto Nacional de Salud Mental
Lima, Peru

**Dante E. Warthon, MD**
Director
Hospital Victor Larco Herrera
Lima, Peru

**Thomas Widiger, PhD**
Professor of Psychology
University of Kentucky
Lexington, Kentucky, USA

**Narendra N. Wig, MD**
Regional Advisor in Mental Health
World Health Organization
Alexandria, Egypt

**Itaru Yamashita, MD**
Professor and Chairman, Department of Psychiatry and Neurology
Hokkaido University
Sapporo, Japan

**Kosuke Yamazaki, MD**
Professor of Psychiatry and Behavioral Science
Tokai University
Kanagawaken, Japan

**He Qin Yan, MD**
Director, Shanghai Mental Health Center
Shanghai, People's Republic of China

# Part I
# Regional Perspectives on Psychiatric Diagnosis

# 1
# An Overview of Cross-Cultural and National Issues in Psychiatric Classification

Narendra N. Wig

In this chapter, critical issues in psychiatric classification related to national and cross-cultural points of view are discussed. It may be relevant at the start to mention the author's psychiatric background: After training in the United Kingdom and United States, the author spent most of his clinical years in India, and for the last 6 years has been working with the World Health Organization in the eastern Mediterranean region. Hence, it is quite likely that his observations are influenced by experience in the countries of the Third World. In a way, this may be good because the majority of the mentally ill of the world live in these countries, and their point of view often is not well represented in the world fora of psychiatric classification.

The last decade has been one of the most exciting periods ever in psychiatric classification. The appearence of the *Diagnostic and Statistical Manual of Mental Disorders*, 3rd edition (DSM-III) in 1980 was like a breath of fresh air, breaking away from many old concepts and traditions. Its focus on operational definitions, multiaxial format, and innovative regrouping of categories had worldwide appeal. A large number of psychiatrists in many countries who had never before bothered about psychiatric diagnosis and classification suddenly found themselves interested in this field. The appearence of DSM-III was soon followed by the preparation for the World Health Organization's *International Classification of Diseases*, 10th revision (ICD-10), which was approved by the World Health Assembly in May 1990. The preparation for ICD-10 was a massive international operation, the like of which has perhaps never been undertaken before in psychiatric history. More than 700 psychiatrists in nearly 200 centers in over 50 countries in every region of the world were involved in its preparation and in a series of field trials to test the suitability of the new ICD-10 draft in different settings using different language versions. Many national psychiatric associations, through the good offices of the World Psychiatric Association, were also actively involved in this process. This resurgence of interest in psychiatric diagnosis and classification across the globe has brought us face to face with a number of issues that are important at the national level and also have significant cross-cultural implications. The following four areas deserve discussion.

## Psychiatric Conditions Seen in Daily Practice But Not Well Represented in International Classifications

Although the ICD-10 is being implemented as the official classification in most countries of the world and psychiatrists in many countries are using the ICD-10 or the DSM-III, "private" national systems of classification are still used by practicing psychiatrists in many countries. Some of these classifications (eg, those used in France, Scandinavia, and Germany) continue to have an influence in countries traditionally linked with them in scientific and educational endeavors. This situation resulted in two types of problems.

1. In some countries of Europe, some of the psychiatric disorders that are so easy to understand and to describe in the national classifications do not have an exact equivalent in the international classification. Examples are conditions like bouffée délirante or chronic interpretive delusional psychosis in French psychiatry or psychogenic psychosis in Scandinavian psychiatry, which were difficult to accommodate within the rubrics of ICD-8 or ICD-9. This problem has now been partly solved with the emergence of defined operational criteria and efforts at developing "crosswalks" among national classifications as well as between them and ICD-10.

2. The problem is much more complex in non-European countries. In the developed countries of Europe, the majority of psychiatric patients generally fit into the existing national and international classification, probably because these classifications originated in these countries and were based on initial observations made on those populations. In contrast, in Asia, Africa, and Latin America, there is often wide divergence between what is described in European and North American classifications and what is seen in the actual practice of psychiatry within the health services of these countries. Examples of such difficulties are many and have been well documented in recent years (Wig 1983, Wig et al 1985, Wig 1990). These include occurrence of large numbers of cases of acute psychotic disorders that do not fit well within schizophrenia or manic depressive psychosis concepts, or large number of cases of ill-defined somatic complaints that do not appear to be related to organic pathology but also do not easily fit into the conventional neurotic categories of ICD-

8 or ICD-9. Similarly, there are major difficulties in the application of the classification of psychiatric disorders of childhood as well as that of personality disorders. Also, there is major controversy about the status of the so-called culture-bound syndromes that have been reported from many non-Western cultures and that defy the conventional categories of existing psychiatric classifications.

Fortunately, this problem has also been significantly reduced in non-European countries due to the use of defined operational criteria for classification and to WHO's efforts at extensive consultation with experts from many countries when preparing the draft of ICD-10. From the available evidence of ICD-10 field trials, it seems that there is likely to be much wider acceptance of ICD-10 in developing countries than there was of ICD-8 or ICD-9. However, these problems cannot be adequately resolved until adequate and reliable data are produced by psychiatrists working in developing countries themselves.

## Role of Culture in Psychiatric Diagnosis and Classification

A second issue is the controversy over the role of culture in the development of psychopathology. The central point remains largely unresolved. Does the essential nature of psychiatric illness differ from culture to culture, or is the central core of psychiatric illness the same across countries, and the role of sociocultural factors only pathoplastic? And if the latter is true, is the impact of sociocultural factors the same across the spectrum of psychiatric disorders from organic brain conditions and functional psychosis to personality and stress-related disorders?

The past few decades brought a wide acceptance of the position that psychiatry is like other branches of medicine and that the essential nature of psychiatric disorders is similar all over the world. However, there are many dissenting voices. In recent years, a strong alternative position has been taken by the advocates of New Cross-Cultural Psychiatry, which has developed under the influence of social anthropology (Littlewood 1990, Kleinman 1977). This school doubts the so-called universality of psychiatric phenomenon and has argued that "psychiatry at present lacks any rigorous theory for dealing with the dialectical interplay of biology and human society or for examining the relationship between psychopathologies and its own procedures of research and practice" (Littlewood 1990). Indirectly, this view casts doubt on the whole approach of structured interviews and defined operational criteria on the grounds that the methods are as biased as the phenomenon they are supposed to study, and thus these methods of conventional cross-cultural psychiatry cannot establish the validity of these phenomenon.

This formulation appears very tempting to those who have had long experience studying the psychiatric phenomenon in non-European cultures. This writer has worked almost all his life in developing countries, and he can well empathize with this view, and recall his own frustrations in trying to fit observations on psychopathology into "Western" models of psychiatric classification. However, caution must be exercised vis-à-vis the inherent contradictions and negative consequences of such an approach.

In some ways, this approach is reminiscent of the psychoanalytic thought in the earlier part of this century when it was claimed that every individual is unique and her or his life experience is unique, thus categorization of human experience into psychiatric diagnoses is largely irrelevant. We have now seen how this approach retarded progress in psychiatry and delayed our understanding of important similarities in psychopathology in all patients. We are now confronted with a similarly drastic position about the "uniqueness" of each culture and subculture and there is a danger that this approach will obscure similarities among psychiatric problems in different lands. I think we have to strike some kind of a balance between these two very important dimensions. The advocates of the new cross-cultural psychiatry have performed an important service by drawing our attention to the limitations of our present-day methods of cross-cultural comparisons, which are generally based on Western assumptions. Although the scientific method may be universal, the topics chosen for scientific study, and the particular instrumentation, are determined by scientists, who are themselves prone to personal and cultural bias like any other groups of human beings. Yet without some degree of generalization and categorization, it is very difficult to proceed in modern science.

Psychiatry is an applied science and the ultimate test is its ability to help those who are suffering from psychiatric disorders. Hence, it is equally important to know how effective the practitioners of modern psychiatry have been in understanding the psychiatric phenomenon in their own countries and how successful they have been in helping their own patients with the currently available knowledge of psychopathology, classification, and treatment. Judged by this criteria, modern psychiatry is not doing badly in the non-European cultures of Asia, Africa and Latin America. The number of psychiatrists and psychiatric services are rapidly expanding all over the world. More and more patients and their relatives are coming forward, both in urban and rural areas, to seek help from the newly opened psychiatric services. In general, the population of these countries have supported psychiatric services, but people are also intelligent enough to know for which conditions modern treatment is effective and for which conditions it is not. For example, while working in the remote rural societies in India, Pakistan, Iran, Sudan, or Yemen, we found that for the treatment of epilepsy, psychosis, severe depression, and acute anxiety, the people trust the modern services and seek help in large numbers. However, for dissociative or somatoform disorders, or for antisocial personality, however interesting our theories might be, the people are not so convinced that our modern psychiatric treatment is of much help and often seek traditional healers.

In this context, the example of Japan is perhaps very relevant to the countries outside Europe and North America. In this century, Japan has been remarkable in effectively mastering Western science and technology while still holding on to a great extent to its own culture and traditions. Hence, it is very important for other countries to know Japanese experience in the field of modern psychiatric services, particularly in the use of psychiatric diagnosis and classification. Unfortunately, there has so far been very little information available in the international literature on this topic.

By and large, those trained in modern psychiatry have been able to work effectively in non-European cultures, recognizing that there are psychiatric syndromes that are frequent in some cultures but rare in others. For example, it was possible to find patients who fit the concept of schizophrenia in all countries participating in the well-known WHO study on schizophrenia (Sartorius 1986), although there were also large numbers of atypical cases of schizophrenia and acute psychotic disorders. Depression, which early European psychiatrists thought was uncommon in the countries of Asia and Africa, is now regularly and frequently diagnosed in psychiatric clinics all over the world by local psychiatrists.

We also need to understand and appreciate that the local psychiatrist using a present-day psychiatric classification and making the diagnoses of depressive episode or acute stress reaction is not oblivious to the cultural dimension in understanding and managing that patient. Culture-specific symptoms are often interpreted by the psychiatrist and the treatment or advice takes sociocultural factors into account. To abandon diagnosis and otherwise effective treatment techniques simply because they have not been crafted in the same culture may be a disservice to the patients at hand.

## *Culture-Bound Syndrome*

There is a common debate among psychiatrists in Third World countries regarding the place of the culture-bound syndromes in modern psychiatric classification. Some have favored grouping them separately, while others have favored integrating them into existing rubrics of psychiatric classification. In my view, it would be better to integrate various culture-bound syndromes into the existing international classification but have separate codes for national needs. Culture influences all aspects of health and illness, and thus affects all psychiatric syndromes. There are likely to be cultural differences in the clinical presentation of a case of anxiety, depression, or schizophrenia seen in England, Japan, or India. The stronger the roots of patients in their culture, the more likely such variations become. Therefore, it seems artificial to separate out a few conditions like Koro, Latah, or Amok for special consideration as culture-bound syndromes.

Although these culture-bound syndromes are of great academic interest for our understanding of the role of culture and illness, from the public health point of view the crucial questions are: How common are such culture-bound syndromes in the existing health services of a country? Will their separation into separate diagnostic categories help in the better management of these cases in the country's health services? Judged by these criteria, there are relatively few conditions that require separate coding.

It is not in the interest of the psychiatrists from Third World countries to demand the separation of all culture-bound syndromes into a separate classification group: This will only tend to increase the isolation of Third World psychiatry. It is more important that separation of such a condition is considered necessary for research or for clinical management that it be possible to do so within the existing framework of the international classification. However, the national and international classifications should, at all times remain compatible with each other.

## Issues Related to Future Research

As evidenced by the popularity of DSM-III and ICD-10, we have perhaps for the first time reached a stage in psychiatric classification when there is some kind of general consensus on the broad categories of psychiatric classification and the empirical criteria for diagnoses. This is no doubt a great achievement, but we have now also to think of the future. Perhaps too much agreement is not good for psychiatry. Science thrives on controversy and differences of positions. We are all aware that at present our basis of psychiatric diagnoses and their groupings is arbitrary and likely to change with the increase in knowledge about etiology. Meanwhile, new ideas and new hypotheses must be generated and tested.

The following approaches deserve priority consideration in our future research in classification.

1. The research diagnostic criteria of the present international classification ICD-10 needs to be tested widely, particularly in Asia, Africa, and Latin America. Simple studies can be undertaken using detailed clinical examination by structured interviews on a series of a particular group (eg, acute psychotic disorders, somatoform disorders, or dissociative disorders) to assess how satisfactorily the new classification works. The

reliability and goodness-of-fit of particular sets of diagnoses can be assessed in longitudinal studies of patient cohorts.

2. The multiaxial classification approach offers new avenues for international study. Work on the multiaxial system may help identify concepts useful in different cultural settings.

3. The cultural dimension in psychiatric classification is most important for non-European cultures (ie, the countries of Asia and Africa), thus more studies need to be organized in these countries. We have a paradoxical situation: Research occurs least in the cultural settings in which cultural influences seem to be most important in psychiatric classification (ie, in the traditional rural and tribal societies of the developing countries). This is a challenge for the international scientific community. The exciting areas of work in psychiatric classification are now in different cultural settings in the countries of the Third World, and we need international collaboration to carry out this enormous task.

Here again, the experience from Japan appears very relevant for the countries from non-Western cultures. Unfortunately, so far there have been very few collaborative studies between Japan and the developing countries in the field of psychiatric diagnosis and classification. It should be useful that in the future more Japanese academic centers are to be involved in such collaboration.

4. In psychiatric classification we have moved forward by adopting empirical criteria for diagnosis. In psychiatric research, we could be moving a step forward if we could simplify psychiatric terms and define them empirically in a neutral way as far as possible, without carrying along the load of philosophical controversies associated with some of the terms in nineteenth-century Europe.

The rich philosophical heritage of other cultures—Chinese, Japanese, Indian, or Arabic—is not reflected in the terminology used in psychiatry today. Modern science and psychiatry have a history which cannot be ignored and psychiatric language is part of that history. However, using simpler less controversial psychiatric terms may greatly help in communication among mental health specialists all over the world and extend this way the benefit of modern psychiatry. The World Psychiatric Association in collaboration with the World Health Organization should take up the task of preparing such simplified lexicon.

## Users of Psychiatric Classification

The last issue involves the users of psychiatric classification. Its traditional users (ie, psychiatrists working in psychiatric hospitals) are now gradually being outnumbered by psychiatrists in general hospitals and in private practice, primary-care physicians, and other groups of mental health professionals. More and more countries in Asia and Africa are trying to develop national programs of mental health using existing general health physicians to deliver mental health services. Psychiatric classification is also an important part of both undergraduate and postgraduate medical education, thus many other medical specialists like neurologists, pediatricians, and internists would also be using a psychiatric classification.

One of the important challenges in developing countries is how to ensure that psychiatric classification becomes an integral part of various mental health training programmes and that it is used properly in health services to improve patient care and generate adequate and reliable data. While in academic centers we quarrel about the appropriate subgroupings up to the fifth and sixth digits, it is sad to note that, in many settings, recording is not reliable even at the three-digit level!

Psychiatry has made great progress during the past 100 years. However, it seems that most of the great advances (eg, psychoanalysis, behavior therapy, even most of the newer psychopharmacological compounds) have largely benefited the richer strata of human society. Very little of the benefit of modern psychiatry has so far reached the large, poorer components of the population. We hope that the new international psychiatric classification will be able to improve the service to all segments of society across the world.

## *References*

Kleinman A (1977). Depression, somatization, and the new "cross-cultural psychiatry." *Social Science and Medicine* 11:3–10.

Littlewood R (1990). From categories to contexts: A decade of the new "cross-cultural psychiatry." *British Journal of Psychiatry* 156:308–327.

Sartorius N, Jablensky A, Korten A, et al (1986). Early manifestations and first contact incidence of schizophrenia in different cultures. *Psychological Medicine* 16:909–928.

Wig NN (1983). DSM-III—Its strength and weaknesses: A perspective from the Third World. In RL Spitzer, IBW Williams, AE Skodol (eds), *International Perspectives on DSM-III.* American Psychiatric Press Inc, Washington, DC.

Wig NN, Setyonegoro K, Shen YC, Sell H (1985). Problems of psychiatric diagnosis and classification in the Third World. *Excerpta Medical* 669:50–60.

Wig NN (1990). The Third World perspective on psychiatric diagnosis and classification, pp 181–210. In N Sartorius, A Jablensky, et al (eds), *Sources and Traditions of Classification in Psychiatry.* Hogrefe & Huber, Toronto.

# 2 DSM-IV and International Communication in Psychiatric Diagnosis

ALLEN FRANCES, HAROLD PINCUS, THOMAS WIDIGER, MICHAEL FIRST, WENDY DAVIS, WILLA HALL, KELLY MCKINNEY, AND HELEN STAYNA

The *Diagnostic and Statistical Manual of Mental Disorders*, 4th edition (DSM-IV) will be published in 1994 at about the time of the international implementation of *International Classification of Diseases*, 10th revision (ICD-10). This timing was chosen to facilitate mutual influence and increased compatibility between DSM-IV and ICD-10. There have been several formal conferences and numerous informal discussions between the workers on ICD-10 and on DSM-IV and these have resulted in many changes, improving both systems and bringing them closer together (Frances et al 1989).

The purpose of this chapter is to consider the ways in which DSM-IV may facilitate international communication in psychiatric diagnosis. We begin with a review of the historical relationship between the development of the DSM and ICD systems. Next, we outline the three-stage method (literature review, data reanalysis, and field trials) that is being used in the preparation of DSM-IV and its special emphasis on empirical support and generalizability to the widest diversity of settings. We then discuss the ways in which DSM-IV and ICD-10 will be more similar to each other than were their predecessors, but also the reasons for the remaining differences between the systems. Finally, we discuss the relationship of DSM-IV to ICD-10, to other national systems, and to international communication in psychiatric research, education, and clinical practice.

## Historical Context

The initial impetus in the United States for a system of classifying the mental disorders was purely statistical. The first official "nomenclature" in the United States could be said to be the 1840 census recording of the frequency of "idiocy/insanity" (Spitzer and Williams 1985, Sprock and Blashfield 1984). In the 1880 census, seven categories were distinguished (mania, melancholia, monomania, paresis, dementia, dipsomania, and epilepsy). In 1917, the Committee on Statistics of the American Psychiatric Association (APA) formulated a plan for uniform statistics across mental hospitals that was adopted in 1923 by the Bureau of the Census. This system devoted more attention to clinical utility but was still primarily a statistical classification (APA 1952). The APA subsequently collaborated with the New York Academy of Medicine to develop a nationally acceptable nomenclature that would be incorporated within the first edition of the American Medical Association's *Standard Classified Nomenclature of Disease* (APA 1933). This nomenclature was designed primarily for chronic psychiatric inpatients. To meet the needs of World War II service personnal and veterans who presented with problems (psychophysiological, personality, and acute disorders) that were not represented in the *Standard*, a much broader nomenclature was developed by the US Army and modified by the Veterans Administration.

More or less simultaneously, the World Health Organization (WHO) published the sixth edition of the ICD which, for the first time, provided a section on the mental disorders (Kramer 1988). ICD-6 included ten categories for psychoses, nine for psychoneuroses, and seven for disorders of character, behavior, and intelligence. The APA Committee on Nomenclature and Statistics developed a variant of the ICD-6 (which was itself influenced heavily by the US Veterans Administration nomenclature) for use within the United States. This was published in 1952 as the first edition of the DSM. ICD-7, published in 1955, was quite similar to ICD-6.

In part because of the lack of widespread acceptance of the mental disorder taxonomy contained in ICD-6 and ICD-7, the WHO sponsored a comprehensive review of diagnostic issues conducted by the British psychiatrist Stengel. He was charged with considering the existing nomenclatures and the advisability of conducting a revision toward ICD-8. Stengel's report provided a remarkably helpful overview of diagnostic issues and can be credited with having inspired many of the recent advances in diagnostic methodology (Stengel 1959). Stengel discussed the possibly conflicting goals of a nomenclature that would be used for statistical reporting, research, and clinical purposes. He noted the difficulty in separating description from theory and stated, "This requirement of neutrality in the controversies between various schools of thought imposes considerable limitations on an international classification" (p 618). He indicated the need for explicit definitions as a means of promoting reliable clinical diagnoses: "It will . . . be advisable not to recommend any such system for adoption without a glossary containing definitions and detailed instructions" (p 617). He discussed the recent critique of psychiatric nomenclatures by the philosopher of science,

Hempel (1961), and agreed that "a glossary with operational definitions of the various categories would have to be available" (Stengel 1959, p 618).

Not surprisingly, the next rounds of diagnostic revisions (DSM-II and ICD-8) did not follow Stengel's recommendations to any great degree. The WHO sponsored the development of ICD-8, with approval in 1966 and implementation in 1968. In 1965, the APA appointed a Committee on Nomenclature and Statistics to prepare a DSM-II based on ICD-8, with adjustments for usage within the United States. DSM-II was published in 1968, in coordination with the ICD-8 (APA 1968). Although DSM-II included a number of improvements over DSM-I, the suggestions by Stengel and Hempel regarding operational criteria were still too far ahead of their time.

As had been the case for DSM-I and DSM-II, the development of DSM-III was coordinated with the development of the next version of the ICD. ICD-9 was published in 1975, with implementation in 1978. Work began on DSM-III in 1974, with publication in 1980 (APA 1980). DSM-III introduced methodological innovations based on the earlier recommendations of Hempel (1961) and Stengel (1959) for explicit, descriptive criteria and a neutrality with respect to theoretical orientation. This effort was further stimulated and facilitated by the empirical work of Feighner et al (1972) and Spitzer et al (1978) on the construction and validation of explicit diagnostic criteria and semistructured interviews (Spitzer et al 1980).

DSM-III also included the additional innovation of a multiaxial assessment that had been proposed originally by the Swedish psychiatrists Essen-Möller and Wohlfahrt (1947). Essen-Möller suggested that the classification of disorders should occur along two separate axes, one for description of symptomatology and the other for etiology (1961). Rutter and his colleagues provided one of the earliest and most influential recommendations for separate axes to indicate the clinical syndrome, specific delays in development, intellectual level, physical conditions, and abnormal psychosocial situations (Rutter et al 1969, Rutter et al 1975). A variety of the other multiaxial systems were subsequently developed (Mezzich 1979, Strauss 1975, Williams 1985), but the final DSM-III formulation was quite close to the proposal by Rutter.

Although these two important methodological innovations introduced by DSM-III—the provision of diagnostic criteria and of the multiaxial system—had long international currency, they were not included in ICD-9 largely because the primary function of this international system has been the classification of morbidity in the collection of basic health statistics. In contrast, DSM-III was developed to provide a medical nomenclature for clinicians and researchers. Experience with DSM-III had uncovered a number of instances in which the criteria were not entirely clear, were inconsistent across categories, or were internally inconsistent. Therefore, in 1983 the APA appointed a Work Group to Revise DSM-III to make relatively minor revisions and corrections that led to DSM-III-R in 1987 (APA 1987).

Our major thrust in the development of DSM-IV is to maximize the impact of clinical research on any revisions that are implemented. Because DSM-III and DSM-III-R stimulated substantial research on the mental disorders, DSM-IV can rely less than these did on the consensus of experts, and instead, will be more comprehensively informed by empirical data (Frances et al 1990). The tenth edition of the ICD is scheduled for implementation in 1993 (Sartorius 1988). As has been the case for the simultaneous and coordinated appearance of DSM-I to DSM-III and ICD-6 to ICD-9, the APA is proceeding with DSM-IV on a time schedule that will allow it to remain coordinated with ICD-10. This also provides an opportunity to increase the compatibility and congruency of the two nomenclatures (Frances et al 1989, Kramer 1988).

The preparations of ICD-10 and DSM-IV have been closely coordinated with one another, with much mutual influence between systems. The clinical and research drafts of ICD-10 have been thoroughly reviewed by the DSM-IV Work Groups and have suggested important topics for DSM-IV literature reviews and data reanalyses. The ICD-10 criteria sets are included as alternatives to be compared with DSM-III, DSM-III-R and suggested DSM-IV criteria sets in extensive field testing that are being sponsored by the US National Institute of Mental Health. The ICD-10 is thus likely to influence the specific definitions of a number of DSM-IV categories and has suggested several new categories that are being given careful consideration by the DSM-IV Task Force.

In turn, the DSM-IV Task Force has made a number of suggestions that have been included in successive iterations of each of the versions of ICD-10. The most important result of this effort has been the simplification of the definitions in the ICD-10 short glossary to ensure that they are not overly specific and pseudo-precise. The success of this effort will make it easier for national systems of diagnosis to achieve code and to construct equivalence with ICD-10 while allowing for those differences in the specific criteria that seem necessary and appropriate. The DSM-IV Task Force has also made many specific terminological and definitional suggestions that have been included in the ICD-10 clinical and research criteria.

## Methods of Preparing DSM-IV

The Task Force on DSM-IV was appointed in May of 1988. It has 21 members, most of whom also chair a Work Group. There are 13 Work Groups, each of which is responsible for conducting a systematic empirical review that will result in the diagnostic criteria and accompanying text for a specific group of DSM-IV disorders. Each Work Group draws on the expertise of between 50 and 100 advisors, including many international advisors. There is also an International Advisory Board consisting of members drawn from around the world. The emphasis on empirical review and the large number and diversity of advisors is meant to ensure that DSM-IV will be applicable in the wide variety of settings in which it will be used.

Work on the development of DSM-IV has been divided into three separate steps. Initially, each Work Group considered each of the diagnostic categories within its purview and agreed on a series of issues requiring review and resolution in DSM-IV. Issues included problems with some aspect of the DSM-III or the DSM-III-R definitions, differences between the DSM system and the ICD-10, important developments in the research literature, input from clinical perspectives, and other specific issues that had been identified by advisors (Frances et al 1989, Frances et al 1990, Frances et al 1991). In the first step of empirical review, the Work Groups conducted 150 extensive literature reviews applying a uniform, systematic, and detailed methodology (Widiger et al 1990). Initial drafts of literature reviews have been circulated to advisors for their comment. Suggestions and additional data that advisors share with members of the Work Groups are incorporated into the successive drafts of these literature reviews, which are now nearing their final draft. The literature reviews are useful in developing options for possible alternative resolutions of these issues (ie, whether to maintain or revise DSM-III-R criteria in developing draft criteria for DSM-IV). The literature reviews will be published as the first volume of the DSM-IV *Sourcebook* to document the empirical data on which decisions have been based.

Although many issues have been satisfactorily answered by reviews of the available published literature, other questions have required reanalyses of previously collected, but unpublished or incompletely analyzed, data sets. Approximately, 50 reanalytic projects have been undertaken to address particular diagnostic issues clarified through the literature reviews. In some instances, data reanalysis has been used to generate empirically derived criteria sets for consideration in DSM-IV. (The reanalysis of unpublished data sets has been made possible by a grant from the John D. and Catherine T. MacArthur Foundation.) For each issue, a variety of sites, including many international sites, have participated in the reanalysis of existing data sets. This will help to ensure the generalizability and cross-cultural utility of the decisions made in DSM-IV.

There are some issues that cannot be completely resolved by literature reviews and unpublished data analysis. It is also important to test the implications of possible changes in DSM-IV through field trials. We have selected 11 such issues that will be the focus of field testing sponsored by the US National Institute of Mental Health. These field trials will be the most carefully designed and monitored of any field trials conducted to date. We are also pleased that several of the field trials include extensive international participation. The field trials will compare DSM-III, DSM-III-R, ICD-10, and proposed DSM-IV criteria items in terms of their impact on reliability, prevalence, performance characteristics, and validity. This will allow the DSM-IV Task Force to choose optimal criteria sets that will be most compatible with DSM-III-R and ICD-10 and will provide data upon which to base empirical crosswalks among systems.

We have convened several conferences to explore ways in which to ensure the cross-cultural applicability of DSM-IV. DSM-IV must be internationally and cross-culturally relevant even for use just within the United States. We will devote a section of the DSM-IV text specifically to noting the particular manifestations of the various disorders that may be emphasized in different cultural settings. We are also reviewing and discussing the methods of classifying the so-called culture-bound syndromes within the DSM-IV diagnostic system. We are making frequent presentations on DSM-IV at international meetings to solicit comments and suggestions and have received extensive commentary and data from our international advisors. The DSM-IV *Options Book* was available in mid-1991 and was distributed widely to the international psychiatric community for additional comment.

## Differences Between DSM-IV and ICD-10

We now outline the ways in which DSM-IV and ICD-10 approaches will remain different and indicate the reasons for these differences.

The most fundamental difference between the systems is that ICD-10 will come in many formats. The basic ICD-10 Chapter F, Mental and Behavioral Disorders, lists the codes and names of the disorders and provides a two- or three-sentence glossary description of each disorder. The basic form of Chapter F constitutes the official ICD-10 classification designed to ensure construct compatibility among the national systems in use around the world. In addition, WHO will introduce for the first time a number of additional separate products that may be used in conjunction with Chapter F. These include the "clinical descriptions and diagnostic guidelines" (an expanded description of each of the diagnostic categories in the ICD short glossary which is very similar in format to the "essential features" section of the DSM-III-R); "diagnostic criteria for research" (specific criteria for each of the diagnostic categories in the ICD-10 short glossary, very similar to criteria included for each disorder in the DSM-III-R); "multiaxial presentation of ICD-10"; "multiaxial classification of mental disorders in childhood and adolescence"; "clinical description and diagnostic guidelines for use in primary health care"; and "crosswalks," which will include cross-references between ICD-10 and major national classifications.

Clinicians and researchers in the area of mental disorders will have the option of using one or more of these extra ICD-10 volumes in much the same way that they use the DSM. These are clinical, educational, and research tools that go beyond the primary role of ICD-10 of providing an official code and glossary that can be used across national systems. ICD-10's approach in this area has the advantage of making it possible for clinicians and researchers to use only those products of relevance to them. The ICD-10 approach provides differing levels of detail and allows for simplicity in situations that demand fast, if imprecise, diagnosis.

However, there are also serious disadvantages in the ICD-10 decision to provide multiple formats. The many different volumes are cumbersome. The ICD-10 clinical criteria are in many instances themselves quite complex and are not always totally consistent with the ICD-10 research criteria. The major problem resulting from the separate ICD-10 formats is that these promote disparities in how clinical and research diagnoses are made, and thus increase the difficulty in generalizing the results of clinical research to clinical practice. It is the conviction of the DSM-IV Task Force that the bridging of the clinical/research interface is likely to be one of the major challenges facing psychiatry during the next several decades. For this reason, DSM-IV will continue to have one set of criteria intended for use in clinical, research, and educational settings. We realize that some of the DSM-III-R criteria sets may currently be too complicated for convenient use in clinical and educational settings and are attempting to find empirically supported ways of simplifying these without reducing research utility or changing the definition of caseness. Diagnostic criteria for each disorder in the DSM-IV will be accompanied by a series of text sections that will include information on each of the disorders under the following categories: diagnostic features; associated features and disorders; age-related features; cross-cultural features; onset and course; complications; familial pattern; differential diagnosis; relationship of DSM-IV to other diagnostic systems; predisposing factors; and impairment.

A second basic difference between ICD-10 and DSM-IV has to do with how the multiaxial system will be approached. ICD-10 will place all of the diagnoses included in the DSM-IV Axes I, II, and III on just one axis. The ICD-10 rationale for collapsing Axes I, II, and III is partly based on the theoretical argument that, at the boundaries, the disorders covered in each of these axes merge imperceptibly with one another. Indeed, there is no infallible or sharp boundary separating the clinical syndromes in psychiatry versus the personality disorders or versus the other medical disorders listed on DSM-IV's Axis III. An even more compelling reason for the ICD-10 decision is practicality—the concern that separate multiaxial listing of Axes I, II, and III would be too cumbersome in many settings in which simplicity is a high priority. Although the DSM-IV Task Force is mindful of these theoretical and practical concerns occasioned by the separation of the axes, we feel that it remains greatly advantageous to retain a more specific version of the multiaxial system. The provision of separate Axes II for personality disorders and Axis III for other medical disorders has focused attention on these (otherwise all too often missed) aspects of diagnosis and provides a well-accepted and lucid way of reporting findings.

The third major difference between ICD-10 and DSM-IV has to do with the degree to which systematic review of the empirical evidence has informed the development of each system. Because of its timing and method of development, ICD-10 (like DSM-III and DSM-III-R) has depended on expert consensus as the means of formulating criteria and has tested these with field trials that have focused primarily on goodness-of-fit and reliability. The major innovations of DSM-IV will not be in any of its text or criteria, but rather, in its much greater reliance on empirical review in developing the diagnostic system and in much more rigorous field testing. This reflects an expectable evolution of the authority used in establishing diagnostic systems, from the influential professor to the consensus of experts and finally, to the empirical evidence. Undoubtedly, future systems will rely even more on evidence and even less on unsupported opinion.

The final differences between ICD-10 and DSM-IV have to do with some of the definitions of the various disorders (ie, the items included and the thresholds chosen). As indicated above, ICD-10 and DSM-IV are, with very few exceptions, equivalent in their constructs but often differ in the specific diagnostic criteria they suggest. The reasons for these differences include: (1) the fact that ICD has separate clinical and research criteria (which also differ between themselves); (2) the somewhat different constituencies and purposes served by the ICD and DSM systems; (3) the need in DSM-IV to reduce disruptions with its predecessors and therefore to remain as compatible as possible with DSM-III and DSM-III-R; (4) the greater reliance on empirical evidence in DSM-IV; and (5) differences in historical traditions, the people responsible, and the timing of preparation of the two systems.

## DSM-IV and International Communication

What is the likely role to be played by DSM-IV in promoting what has become a rapidly expanding and deepening international communication among psychiatrists (as well as other mental health professionals)? It is certainly too early to predict how this will or should evolve. Many outcomes are possible and these may all occur in one or another part of the world, given the heterogeneity of uses, settings, traditions, and professional, institutional, and governmental relationships that influence in what diagnostic language psychiatrists are best able to communicate with one another.

DSM-III has made a number of positive contributions to international communication. The use of DSM-III helped to make psychiatric diagnosis much more interesting and clinically relevant than had been the case with DSM-II and ICD-9. It provided a uniform set of diagnostic criteria that could be translated, both linguistically and clinically, across cultural settings. DSM-III-R has been translated into nine languages and has been widely used to promote international clinical research, training, and practice. DSM-III and DSM-III-R have become the basic mode in which clinical research findings have been reported in studies conducted and reported all over the world.

In DSM-IV we have endeavored to build upon this tradition in a number of ways: (1) DSM-IV will be totally compatible with the ICD-10 system and will have a section in the text explaining the relationship of DSM-IV to other diagnostic systems including the ICD-10. Moreover, we are endeavoring to improve the user friendliness of the DSM-IV by simplifying and clarifying its language and revising those criteria sets whose contents have been most cumbersome and obscure. (2) Translations of DSM-IV will be clinically and idiomatically correct and will include culturally relevant examples. (3) International advisors to DSM-IV are participating in all of the stages of empirical review to ensure the accuracy, comprehensiveness, and generalizability of criteria for DSM-IV. (4) We have scheduled a series of discussions on the DSM-IV at international meetings and to ensure that international users of the DSM are apprised of and involved in the process of developing DSM-IV. Draft criteria of the DSM-IV will be widely circulated to international audiences. (5) There will be a new section of text in DSM-IV entitled Cross-Cultural Features that will systematically consider each diagnostic category and differences in the manifestation of symptons across cultures. (6) A guideline for cultural formulation to supplement the standardized diagnostic ratings will be included in the appendix. The National Institute of Mental Health (NIMH) has sponsored conferences on these issues in 1991 and 1993 (Mezzich et al, in press).

## Conclusion

DSM-IV will appear in 1994, coordinated with the international implementation of ICD-10. DSM-IV uses the ICD-10 codes and will be completely compatible with ICD-10 short glossary definitions, but will differ from the supplementary ICD-10 products in several ways. DSM-IV will continue to have one set of criteria for clinical paractice, education, and research. It will continue to provide a separate Axis II for the diagnosis of personality disorders and an Axis III for the diagnosis of other medical disorders. DSM-IV also differs from ICD-10 (and DSM-III and DSM-III-R) in its emphasis on empirical support and documentation.

We are currently revising the literature reviews, completing the data reanalyses, and conducting the field trials that are providing the data necessary to make decisions that will shape DSM-IV. A DSM-IV *Options Book* outlining the possible decisions for DSM-IV and a DSM-IV *Diagnostic Criteria Draft* have been available for criticism and suggestions.

The careful steps used in preparing the DSM-IV make it likely that it will be the most up-to-date, empirically sound, and useful system for clinical, training, and research purposes. We must recognize, however, that the momentous strides being made in our scientific understanding of mental disorders are, unfortunately, still at a stage too formative to have had any pervasive impact on the system of classification. Soon we will move beyond a psychiatric classification that resides almost exclusively at the descriptive level of organization. The next generation of diagnostic systems will undoubtedly be informed by a deeper understanding of pathogenesis as the basis for organizing the classification and making specific decisions. The best possible descriptive system of classification is needed now to facilitate the research necessary to enlarge our understanding of psychopathology—research that is often limited precisely by the limitations of the diagnostic system.

Our advice to clinical researchers is to cast a broad net in their assessment of symptoms. Often, perhaps usually, the items that are finally included in the DSM-IV or the ICD-10 criteria sets are only marginally more diagnostically efficient than were any number of alternative possible items (which are often listed among the associated features section of the DSM-IV text). Progress in diagnosis requires that researchers not restrict themselves to the narrow band of criteria included in any one system, but rather determine the predictive validity of a wide spectrum of possible psychopathological items and their combinations. Moreover, researchers will want the flexibility to assess and report their findings in relationship to more than one diagnostic system.

It is very fortunate that the ICD and DSM systems have achieved equivalence in coding and constructs and differ only in the specific wording of criteria and the degree to which the systems have tapped the available empirical evidence. Communication between workers on ICD-10 and workers on DSM-IV has greatly improved both systems. Communication between them should be relatively convenient during the next 10 to 15 years in which both will be in wide use.

Author notes: The opinions expressed herein are those of the authors and do not necessarily represent the position of the American Psychiatric Association and its Task Force on DSM-IV.

*Acknowledgment.* We wish to acknowledge the very special efforts of N Sartorious, JE Cooper, D Regier, M Sabshin, JE Mezzich, RL Spitzer, and JA Costa e Silva in promoting communication and compatibility between DSM-IV and ICD-10. We also thank the DSM-IV Task Force, its International Advisors, and the many hundreds of people who have shared so generously of their time and ideas. The work described here is funded through NIMH grant #1 P01 NH47200–01 and a grant from the John C and Catherine T MacArthur Foundation.

## *References*

American Psychiatric Association (1933). Notes and comments: Revised nomenclature of mental disorders. *American Journal of Psychiatry* 90:1369–1376.

American Psychiatric Association (1952). *Diagnostic and Statistical Manual of Mental Disorders*. American Psychiatric Association, Washington, DC.

American Psychiatric Association (1968). *Diagnostic and Statistical Manual of Mental Disorders* (2nd ed). American Psychiatric Association, Washington, DC.

American Psychiatric Association (1980). *Diagnostic and Statistical Manual of Mental Disorders* (3rd ed). American Psychiatric Association, Washington, DC.

American Psychiatric Association (1987). *Diagnostic and Statistical Manual of Mental Disorders* (3rd ed, rev). American Psychiatric Association, Washington, DC.

Essen-Möller E (1961). On the classification of mental disorders. *Acta Psychiatrica Scandinavica* 37:119–126.

Essen-Möller E, Wohlfahrt S (1947). Suggestions for the amendment of the official Swedish classification of mental disorders. *Acta Psychiatrica et Neurologica Scandinavica* 47:551–555 (suppl).

Feighner J, Robins E, Guze S, Woodruff R, Winokur G, Munoz R (1972). Diagnostic criteria for use in psychiatric research. *Archives of General Psychiatry* 26:57–63.

Frances A, Widiger TA, Pincus HA (1989). The development of DSM-IV. *Archives of General Psychiatry* 46:373–375.

Frances A, Pincus HA, Widiger TA, Davis WW, First MB (1990). DSM-IV: Work in progress. *American Journal of Psychiatry* 147:1439–1448.

Frances A, Widiger TA, First M, Pincus HA, Tilly S, Miele G, Davis WW (1991). DSM-IV: Toward a more empirical diagnostic system. *Canadian Psychology* 32(2):174–176.

Hempel C (1961). Introduction to problems of taxonomy, pp 3–22. In J Zubin (ed), *Field Studies in the Mental Disorders*. Grune & Stratton, New York.

Kramer M (1988). Historical roots and structural bases in the International Classification of Diseases. In J Mezzich, M von Cranach (eds), *International Classification of Psychiatry: Unity and Diversity*. Cambridge University Press, New York.

Mezzich JE (1979). Patterns and issues in multiaxial psychiatric diagnosis. *Psychological Medicine* 9:125–137.

Mezzich JE, Kleinman A, Fabrega H, Parron D (eds) (in press). *Culture and Psychiatric Diagnosis*. American Psychiatric Press, Washington, DC.

Rutter M, Lebovici S, Eisenberg L, Sneznevskij A, Sadoun R, Brooke E, Lin T (1969). A tri-axial classification of mental disorders in childhood. *Journal of Child Psychology, Psychiatry, and Related Disciplines* 10:41–61.

Rutter M, Shaffer D, Shepherd M (1975). *A Multi-Axial Classification of Child Psychiatric Disorders*. World Health Organization, Geneva, Switzerland.

Sartorius N (1988). International perspectives of psychiatric classification. *British Journal of Psychiatry* 152:9–14 (suppl 1).

Spitzer R, Endicott J, Robins E (1978). Research diagnostic criteria: Rationale and reliability. *Archives of General Psychiatry* 35:773–782.

Spitzer R, Williams J (1985). Classification of mental disorders, pp 591–613. In H Kaplan, B Sadock (eds), *Comprehensive Textbook of Psychiatry* (vol 1, ed 4), Williams & Wilkins, Baltimore, MD.

Spitzer R, Williams J, Skodol A (1980). DSM-III: The major achievements and an overview. *American Journal of Psychiatry* 137:151–164.

Sprock J, Blashfield R (1984). Classification and nosology, pp 289–307. In M Hersen, A Kazdin, A Bellack (eds), *The Clinical Psychology Handbook*, Pergamon, New York.

Stengel E (1959). Classification of mental disorders. *Bulletin of the World Health Organization* 21:601–663.

Strauss J (1975). A comprehensive approach to psychiatric diagnosis. *American Journal of Psychiatry* 132:1193–1197.

Widiger TA, Frances A, Pincus HA, Davis W (1990). DSM-IV literature reviews: rationale, process, and limitations. *Journal of Psychopathology and Behavioral Assessment* 12:189–202.

Williams J (1985). The multiaxial systems of DSM-III: Where did it come from and where should it go? I. Its origins and critiques. *American Journal of Psychiatry* 42:175–180.

# 3
# The Nosological Views of French-Speaking Psychiatry

Charles B. Pull and Gilles Chaillet

French psychiatric nosology began with Pinel at the end of the 18th century and is the result of a long historical process. The present nosological tradition rests largely on a movement that developed at the end of the 19th century. Between 1890 and World War I, Magnan constructed a nosological system that borrowed elements from Esquirol's syndromic tradition, Bayle's medical model, and Morel's theoretical concept of degeneration. Afterwards, attempts to integrate Kraepelinian nosology with Magnan's system led to compromises, most obvious in the field of delusional disorders. In particular, acute and transient psychotic disorders, called bouffées délirantes, and a large part of chronic delusional states were retained outside of dementia praecox. These developments have been described in detail by Pichot (1982).

Up until recently, French psychiatrists have remained strongly attached to traditional French nosology. The French attitude regarding the World Health Organization's *International Classification of Diseases* (ICD) has been characteristic in this respect. Neither ICD-8 nor ICD-9 have been officially accepted in France. The attachment to tradition has led to the production of an official French classification for statistical purposes (INSERM 1969). Although attempts were made for the INSERM classification to be compatible with the ICD, the French classification did not abandon any of the specific French concepts that had been developed at the turn of the century.

The situation has changed considerably during the last decade. The publication of the third edition of the *Diagnostic and Statistical Manual of Mental Disorders* (DSM-III) and the development of the 10th revision of the ICD (ICD-10) have not gone unnoticed. With regard to the radically new approach to diagnosis and classification in the new systems, the French classification now appears outdated and obsolete. The present chapter gives an account of the current state of the traditional French system, and of the reaction of French psychiatrists to DSM-III and ICD-10, and attempts to predict the future of diagnostic classification in France.

## The Official French Classification

The current official French Classification of Mental Disorders was published in 1969 by the *Institut National de la Santé et de la Recherche Médicale* (INSERM). Up until now, the system has had to be used for the annual statistics of public psychiatric hospitals in France. It was developed by a committee, in collaboration with a number of major groups of French experts. It is consistent with traditional French nosology and reflects, to a large extent, the mainstream of French psychiatric opinion in the 1960s. It continues to provide the basis for French textbooks of psychiatry and for the teaching of psychiatry in French universities.

With the exception of a few categories, which reflect the peculiarities of French nosology, the content of the classification is essentially compatible with other traditional systems, in particular with ICD-9. The main classification criterion is the division between neurosis and psychosis, most obvious in the differentiation of manic and depressive psychoses and of nonpsychotic depressive states (neurotic depression and depressive reaction). Additional classification criteria are based on established and theoretical etiological factors, symptomatology, and course of illness. Major peculiarities are to be found almost exclusively in the definition of schizophrenia.

The INSERM classification is a simple nomenclature. It lists 20 names of categories, with up to 10 names for subcategories. It is not accompanied by a glossary or by any other information to guide the clinician in its use. There has been no attempt up to now to revise the 1968 edition, and as such, the classification does not include any of the recent developments that have been incorporated in the more recent systems.

## Empirical French Diagnostic Criteria

During the 1980s, there were two attempts to develop specified diagnostic criteria for some of the categories of the INSERM classification: the first was for schizophrenia, acute delusional disorders, and chronic delusional disorders; the second was for psychotic depression and nonpsychotic depressive states.

In traditional French nosology, schizophrenia is defined as a chronic disorder, whereas the acute and transitory delusional states are classified in a separate category. In addition, a large part of the chronic delusional states are also classified outside of schizophrenia. The traditional French nosology of mood disorders is based on the classical endogenous versus psychogenic dichotomy. The term psychotic is used instead of endogenous, and nonpsychotic instead of psychogenic.

The attempt to develop diagnostic criteria for schizophrenia and other psychotic disorders was based on the results of an empirical investigation (Pull et al 1987). Eighty-nine French clinicians selected five cases among patients who had been diagnosed as presenting either chronic schizophrenia, acute delusional disorder, or chronic delusional disorder. For each patient, the clinicians assessed the presence or absence of 70 criteria included in a diagnostic checklist, the List of Integrated Criteria for the Evaluation of Taxonomy in nonaffective psychotic disorders (LICET-S) (Pull et al 1981).

French diagnostic criteria for depression were obtained in a second empirical investigation (Pull et al 1988). Fifty French clinicians selected five cases among patients who had been diagnosed as presenting either a psychotic depression or a nonpsychotic depressive state. For each patient, the participants assessed the presence or absence of 100 criteria contained in another diagnostic checklist, the List of Integrated Criteria for the Evaluation of Taxonomy in depressive disorders (LICET-D-100) (Pull et al 1984).

In terms of the categories under discussion, the description of cases provided through LICET-S and LICET-D was of a quite remarkable homogeneity. The results were highly consistent in age of onset, duration, symptom pattern, and exclusions. In addition, the data consisted of easily identifiable behavioral signs and symptoms. As such, the major elements required to construct diagnostic criteria could be elucidated and integrated into diagnostic algorithms.

The final diagnostic criteria are "empirical" inasmuch as they have been derived from the assessment of actual patients. They are "French" inasmuch as they are based on data obtained from representative samples of French psychiatrists. They have high face validity in that they correspond to (and in fact simply translate) French diagnostic practices in the fields investigated. They have satisfactory discriminative validity in that they "correctly" reclassify a majority of patients (ie, achieve agreement with clinical diagnosis in more than three cases of four).

The French position concerning acute and transitory psychotic disorders clearly emerges from the definition of bouffée délirante, which is presented in Table 3.1.

The French position on how to differentiate between psychotic depression and nonpsychotic depressive states rests upon a diagnostic index, which is presented in Table 3.2.

The results of the two investigations are interesting in that they provide evidence that (1) traditional French concepts can be defined by explicit diagnostic criteria; (2) the meaning of those concepts can be described without ambiguity, using a terminology that is understood anywhere in the world; (3) the concepts can be correlated with quite similar concepts in other nosologies; (4) the French position is in line with the latest

TABLE 3.1. French empirical criteria for *bouffée délirante*.

A. Delusional ideas characterized by each of the following:
   1. A sudden onset of less than 48 hours
   2. A multiplicity of themes and delusional "mechanisms" (polymorphous delusions)
   3. A lack of organization on a single prominent theme or a series of related themes
B. Emotional turmoil without disorientation in time or place, characterized by at least three of the following:
   1. Sudden changes from one emotional reaction to another (eg, from anxiety to anger)
   2. Sudden changes from one dysphoric mood to another (eg, from euphoria to depression)
   3. Sudden changes from one type of psychomotor behavior to another (eg, from agitation to prostration)
   4. Depersonalization: impairment in perception or awareness of the self and/or derealization; impairment in perception or awareness of the outside world
   5. Hallucinations or unusual perceptions of any kind
C. Disappearance of the pathological manifestations in A and B and complete restitution to the premorbid state in less than 2 months
D. Absence of any previous psychiatric disorders other than possibly one or more *bouffées délirantes*
E. Not due to an organic brain disorder, alcoholism, or drug abuse
F. Not due to a manic or depressive psychosis

Clinical forms: authentic *bouffée délirante* of the Magnan type
1. Meets the criteria for *bouffée délirante*
2. No obvious stress prior to the onset of the symptoms

Reactive *bouffée délirante*
1. Meets the criteria for *bouffée délirante*
2. Presence of an obvious stress prior to the onset of the symptoms

TABLE 3.2. Diagnostic index for psychotic vs nonpsychotic depression.

1. Distinct quality of depressive mood (ie, the depressed mood is experienced as being distinctly different from the kind of feelings experienced following the death of a loved one)
2. Lack of reactivity to usually pleasurable stimuli
3. Social withdrawal
4. Feelings of inadequacy or loss of self-esteem
5. Feelings of worthlessness, self-reproach, or excessive or inappropriate guilt
6. Recurrent thoughts of death, suicidal ideation, wishes to be dead, or suicide attempt
7. Marked psychomotor agitation or retardation
8. Early morning awakening (at least 2 hours before usual time of awakening)
9. The depression is regularly worse in the morning
10. Delusions or hallucinations
11. Previous episodes of "psychotic" depression
12. Previous episodes of mania
13. Tearfulness or crying
14. Psychosocial stressors (judged to have been significant contributors to the development or exacerbation of the current episode)
15. Superimposed on a personality disorder
16. Superimposed on a preexisting nonpsychotic mental disorder

Note. Criteria 1 to 12 are given a weight of +1; criteria 13 to 16 are given a weight of −1; criteria that are absent are scored 0; a score of 5 or more leads to a diagnosis of psychotic depression; a score of 4 or less leads to a diagnosis of nonpsychotic depression.

developments in some areas and identical to positions that have only recently been questioned elsewhere.

The diagnostic criteria for bouffée délirante are to a large extent similar to criteria for acute polymorphic psychotic disorder in ICD-10 and to criteria for schizophreniform disorder in DSM-III-R. As such, the French definition can be viewed as a specific national attempt to differentiate acute and transitory psychotic states from schizophrenia. In regard to the diagnostic index for depression, the French definition is quite similar to other definitions that have been provided over the years to differentiate between endogenous and nonendogenous depression. However, the dichotomy itself has been the object of major controversy in recent years, and as such, the validity of the French definition must be questioned as well.

## The Diagnostic and Statistical Manual of Mental Disorders

The French translation of DSM-III was published 3 years after its original publication in the United States. In his introduction to the French translation, Pichot considered DSM-III to be a major event in psychiatric nosology, comparable to the publication of the sixth edition of *Kraepelin's Handbook* in 1896. A French translation of DSM-III-R (American Psychiatric Association, 1989) has also appeared.

The translation team did not encounter any major difficulties, with the exception of certain terms that have different meanings in French and in English (a typical example is paranoid), and of certain concepts that were unknown in France at the beginning of the 1980s (like panic disorder, which is at present used routinely). The most important difficulties had to do not so much with the literal translation as with the style used in the DSMs. The multiple repetitions of certain terms, which corresponds to a deliberate attitude of the American authors, is contrary to "good French," which does not allow too many repetitions.

DSM-III and DSM-III-R have become immediate best-sellers in France. The two editions have stirred extraordinary interest among French psychiatrists, and given rise to much discussion and controversy. On the whole, and despite whatever reservations French clinicians may have had or still have concerning the DSMs, the fact that they constitute major accomplishments has never been questioned. The DSMs have been extensively referenced in scientific publications and used in scientific investigations. Two factors have undoubtedly contributed to use of the DSMs in France. First, pharmaceutical companies have requested that they be used in drug trials to facilitate acceptance of results in the United States. Second, French investigators wish to publish their results in journals that appear in the United States, and consequently have used the DSMs to enhance understanding of their work by American readers.

However, this does not mean, that DSM-III and DSM-III-R have become universally accepted in France or that French psychiatrists have shed their reservations toward a classification that they continue to view as typically American. In a survey, Pichot et al (1983) have elucidated the major negative reactions to DSM-III. French clinicians have objected that DSM-III was not as generally atheoretical with regard to etiology as its authors claimed. Many of the diagnostic inclusion and exclusion criteria have been criticized for being largely arbitrary. Use of five different axes has almost consistently been found unfeasible. Although it has been recognized that explicit diagnostic criteria enhance the interrater reliabilty of psychiatric diagnosis, it has also been pointed out that even perfect interrater reliability is no proof of validity at all.

The publication of DSM-III-R has given rise to renewed major controversy, owing to the fact that most of the changes that were introduced in the revision relied not on empirical data but on decisions made by committees.

In 1983, Pichot and coworkers predicted that whatever the ultimate interest the classification might awaken, the likelihood of its official adoption was practically nil in France, but that the classification would probably be used in parallel with other systems. Up until now, this prediction has held true. Neither DSM-III nor DSM-III-R have replaced the INSERM classification, which still is the only official French classification in psychiatry. On the other hand, hardly any recent research protocol has omitted inclusion of DSM criteria, in parallel or even without consideration for the INSERM classification.

## The 10th Revision of the *International Classication of Diseases*

As stated earlier, neither the eighth nor the ninth edition of the *International Classification of Diseases* has been officially accepted in France. In fact, they have hardly ever been used by French clinicians at all. In the 1960s and 1970s, the major reason for this was undoubtedly a strong attachment to traditional French nosology. Attachment to tradition is, however, probably insufficient to explain neglect of the ICD in the 1980s. ICD-9 was a traditional system that had resulted from a number of compromises between diverging schools of nosology and continued to be based on the classical dichotomy between psychosis and neurosis; it neither presented any major innovation in comparison with the previous edition, nor included any of the nosological developments that had appeared in the 1970s (eg, explicit diagnostic criteria for defining diagnostic categories). As such, ICD-9 simply did not represent an interesting alternative to the traditional French system. Attention shifted to the radically new approach taken in DSM-III.

The situation has changed with the circulation of the successive drafts of ICD-10. Renamed as Mental and Behavioural Disorders, Including Disorders of Psychological Development, the ICD-10 chapter dealing with mental disorders differs substantially from previous editions in both content and form. The number of categories has been increased from 30 to 100. Disorders are no longer classified along the psychotic–neurotic dichotomy, but arranged in groups according to major common themes or descriptive similarities. For example, all of the mood disorders are now included in the same chapter.

One particular feature of the new classification is that it is presented in a number of different versions, differing only in the amount of information provided for making diagnoses: a glossary version similar in length and format to the glossary in ICD-9, a version of clinical descriptions and diagnostic guidelines, a set of diagnostic criteria for research, a simplified version for use in primary care, and a multiaspect system for the description of patients and their disorders.

The successive drafts of the different versions have been translated into French as soon as they were available in English. The translators, many of whom had participated in the translation of the DSMs, did not encounter any major difficulty in their work. In fact, the problems with translation were similar to the ones that have been mentioned for the translation of the DSMs.

The successive drafts of ICD-10 have been received very positively in France (Pull et al 1991). The radically new approach taken in the classification has stirred considerable interest and discussion. Major satisfaction has been expressed in particular with regard to the following innovations in ICD-10: (1) the clear structure of the classification, which allows easy identification of disorders and code numbers; (2) the availability of different versions for different purposes; (3) the description of acute polymorphic psychotic disorder, which is identical with the definition of bouffée délirante. Reservations towards ICD-10 are by and large identical to those that have been mentioned for DSM-III and DSM-III-R. It is interesting to note that, although most French clinicians have found the use of five axes unfeasible with the DSMs, they favor multiaxial use in the ICD.

Ten centers from French-speaking countries participated in the international field trial with the 1987 draft of the clinical descriptions and diagnostic guidelines, which was to answer the following questions: (1) Does the classification cover the diagnoses that are made in practice? (2) Is the classification acceptable and easy to use for clinicians and researchers? (3) Can clinicians using the classification achieve acceptable levels of agreement in the categorization of their diagnoses?

The results of the field trial were most encouraging. French clinicians found that the clinical descriptions were adequate and that they could easily identify an ICD-10 category for most patients; they reached good agreement on most categories and found that the classification was by and large easy to use.

The tests of the ICD-10 Diagnostic Criteria for Research started during 1991. More than 30 centers from French-speaking countries have asked to partipate in these field trials.

## Structured Diagnostic Interviews

Three structured diagnostic instruments for the assessment of mental disorders in ICD-10 and DSM-III-R: The Composite International Diagnostic Interview (CIDI) (Robins et al 1988), the Schedules for Clinical Assessment in Neuropsychiatry (SCAN) (Wing et al 1990) and the International Personality Disorder Examination (IPDE) (Loranger et al [in press]) have been translated into French under the direction of the first author and have been extensively field-tested in French-speaking countries. Official WHO training centers have been set up in Luxembourg (for all three instruments) and in France (Paris, for the CIDI, Strasbourg, for the SCAN).

## Conclusion

On the eve of the third millennium, psychiatrists throughout the world are coming close to using a common language in the field of diagnosis and classification. With the exception of DSM-III and DSM-III-R, which have achieved international fame and are used in many countries for research on psychiatric disorders, national classifications are disappearing.

For the time being, the 1969 edition of the French classification of mental disorders, INSERM, still is the only official psychiatric classification in France. However, the INSERM classification is regarded by many French clinicians as outdated and obsolete, and considered an obstacle for international understanding. There has so far been no attempt to update the system. Attempts to construct diagnostic criteria have been limited to only a few categories and will not be continued for the rest of the classification. On the whole, the INSERM classification is a system of the past, and its image will probably disappear in the years to come.

The publication of DSM-III, DSM-III-R, and the successive drafts of ICD-10 have opened new perspectives in the field of psychiatric classification and diagnosis, and are viewed increasingly by French clinicians as possible alternatives to their own classification system. The DSMs are already widely used in research settings in France and the drafts of ICD-

10 have been received quite well. The ICD (World Health Organization 1992a) is the official international classification of diseases and, as such, could be adopted for official use as well as for research purposes in France (World Health Organization 1992b). It is highly probable, however, that French researchers will continue to use DSM-III-R and the forthcoming DSM-IV in tandem with whatever diagnostic system may be adopted officially in the years to come.

## References

American Psychiatric Association (1980). *Diagnostic and Statistical Manual of Mental Disorders* (3rd ed). American Psychiatric Association, Washington, DC.

American Psychiatric Association (Pichot P et al, trans) (1983). *DSM-III: Manuel diagnostique et statistique des troubles mentaux*. Masson, Paris.

American Psychiatric Association (1987). *Diagnostic and Statistical Manual of Mental Disorders* (3rd ed, rev). American Psychiatric Association, Washington, DC.

American Psychiatric Association (Pichot P et al, trans) (1989). *DSM-III-R: Manuel diagnostique et statistique des troubles mentaux*. Masson, Paris.

Institut National de la Santé et de la Recherche Médicale (INSERM), Section Psychiatrie (1969). *Classification française des troubles mentaux. Bulletin de l'Institut National de la Santé et de la Recherche Médicale* 24 (suppl 2).

Loranger AW, Hirschfeld RMA, Sartorius N, Regier DA. The WHO/ADAMHA International Pilot Study of Personality Disorders. *Journal of Personality Disorders* (in press).

Pichot P (1982). The diagnosis and classification of mental disorders in French-speaking countries: Background, current views and comparison with other nomenclatures. *Psychological Medicine* 12:475–492.

Pichot P, Guelfi JD, Kroll J (1983). French perspectives on DSM-III, p 155. In RL Spitzer, JBW Williams, AE Skodol (eds), *International Perspectives on DSM-III*. American Psychiatric Press, Washington, DC.

Pull CB (1991). Field trials with the 1987 draft of ICD-10 "Clinical Descriptions and Diagnostic Guidelines" in French-speaking countries. Technical Report, Centre Hospitalier de Luxembourg.

Pull CB, Pull MC, Pichot P (1981). LICET-S: Une liste intégrée des critères d'Évaluation Taxinomiques pour les psychoses non-affectives. *Journal de Psychiatrie Biologique et Thérapeutique* 1:33–37.

Pull CB, Pull MC, Pichot P (1984). LICET-D-100: Une approche nouvelle du diagnostic des dépressions. *Annales Médico-Psychologiques* 142:831–847.

Pull CB, Pull MC, Pichot P (1987). Des critères empiriques français pour les psychoses III. Algorithmes et arbres de décision. *L'Encéphale* XIII:59–66.

Pull CB, Pull MC, Pichot P (1988). French diagnostic criteria for depression. *Psychiatry and Psychobiology* 3:321–328.

Robins LN, Wing JK, Wittchen HU, Helzer JE, Babor TF, Burke J, Farmer A, Jablensky A, Pickens R, Regier DA, Sartorius N, Towle LH (1988). The Composite International Diagnostic Interview. *Archives of General Psychiatry* 45:1069–1077.

Wing JK, Babor T, Brugha T, Burke J, Cooper JE, Giel R, Jablensky A, Regier D, Sartorius N (1990). SCAN: Schedules for Clinical Assessment in Neuropsychiatry. *Archives of General Psychiatry* 47:589–593.

World Health Organization (1978). *Mental Disorders: Glossary and Guide to Their Classification in Accordance with the Ninth Revision of the International Classification of Diseases*. World Health Organization, Geneva, Switzerland.

World Health Organization (1992a). *International Classification of Diseases (10th rev), Chapter V(F): Mental and Behavioral Disorders, including disorders of psychological development*. World Health Organization, Geneva, Switzerland.

World Health Organization (Pull CB et al, trans) (1992b). *Classification Internationale des Maladies (10 ième rév) Chapitre V(F): Troubles mentaux et comportementaux, y compris les troubles du développement psychologique*. OMS, Genève.

# 4
# Scandinavian Contributions to Psychiatric Nosology

Erik Strömgren

The populations of Scandinavian countries, or more precisely, of the Nordic countries of Europe—Denmark, Finland, Iceland, Norway, and Sweden—show many similarities anthropologically, socially, economically, politically, and culturally, and contact and exchange is quite extensive among them. This applies also to the field of psychiatry. There are nevertheless also many differences as well, and it is thus not possible to give a uniform view of Scandinavian perspectives on psychiatric classification. Many different viewpoints are also represented within each of the countries. There are, however, some concepts and viewpoints that can be said to be generally accepted within psychiatry in these Nordic countries. In the following, such concepts and viewpoints are stressed, partly on the basis of the extensive trials of *International Classification of Diseases*, 10th revision (ICD-10) that have taken place in Scandinavia during the last few years.

## General Experience

The ICD-8 (WHO 1967) was the first international classification to be accepted in the Nordic countries. The earlier editions of ICD showed great weaknesses in the chapter on mental disorders that was accepted by only five member countries of the United Nations. Until then, each of the Nordic countries had its own classification. An early interest was shown in multiaxial classifications and were advocated first by Essen-Möller and Wohlfahrt (1947) and later elaborated by Essen-Möller (1971), and Ottosson and Perris (1973). In Denmark, the Danish Psychiatric Association introduced a new classification in 1952 (Dickmeiss et al 1952) that was in fact biaxial—one axis regarding etiology, the other symptomatology. This classification worked quite well and was given up only because ICD-8 appeared, representing the first real chance of international acceptance of a psychiatric classification.

ICD-8 was, on the whole, well accepted in the Nordic countries, being quite compatible with the classifications in use in these countries. Therefore, it was seen as a complicating factor that ICD-9 (WHO 1977) appeared relatively soon after ICD-8 had been accepted. This had only recently been definitely incorporated in the daily work of psychiatrists and transition to a new classification was felt to be confusing. Therefore, many countries, among them the Nordic ones, chose not to accept ICD-9. On the other hand, those countries that in recent years had become members of the United Nations naturally chose ICD-9. Thus, after some years, the countries were divided between those using ICD-8 and those using ICD-9. This imposed great difficulties since in many chapters the classifications were incompatible to such a degree that the data processing equipment could not translate one into the other.

When the *Diagnostic and Statistic Manual of Mental Disorders*, 3rd edition (DSM-III) (American Psychiatric Association 1980) was published, it aroused considerable interest, especially because it used clearly defined operational diagnostic criteria and was multiaxial. On the other hand, many definitions differed from those prevalent in the Nordic countries. It was, therefore, hoped that ICD-10 might take over the new useful methodological principles of DSM-III and avoid its problematic items.

In the meantime, DSM-III and later DSM-III-R (American Psychiatric Association 1987) have been widely used in the Nordic countries. Many feel they are easier to use than ICD-8 and ICD-9 and many are impressed by the seemingly exact diagnostic criteria that, in addition, often seem to have a high reliability in clinical use. A number of clinics are using DSM-III or DSM-III-R instead of ICD and are intending to do so at least until ICD-10 has been adopted. It has been very much hoped that ICD-10 (WHO 1992) would comprise some of the advantages of DSM and avoid some of the disadvantages.

In many Scandinavian psychiatric departments, clinical field trials of the preliminary stages of ICD-10 have been performed (Bech 1990). Results of these field trials have influenced the further development of ICD-10. There is great satisfaction with the principle of detailed clinical diagnostic guidelines that, in some cases, seem more realistic than those applied in DSM-III.

It has been felt that it was a great improvement when the axes in DSM-III-R underwent a radical change that seemed to bring it much closer to practical applicability. It is hoped that the multiaxial principle will soon be included in ICD-10.

## Critical Aspects

There have been some quite definite criticisms of the general features of DSM-III, first of all with regard to the principle of making diagnoses on the basis of counting symptoms, for instance, making a diagnosis on the basis of presence of five out of nine possible symptoms. It is obvious that such nine symptoms cannot possibly be equivalent for a diagnosis of a particular disorder, and they should never be added to each other without the symptoms having been weighed beforehand on the basis of intensive research. This criticism seems especially relevant with regard to the diagnosis of depressive disorders in which a number of symptoms appear that may also appear in many other disorders, and that, nevertheless, are given the same counting value as those symptoms that are more or less specific to depression. This is an arguable form of pseudomathematics, which unfortunately seems to appeal to many psychiatrists who may feel that such procedures bring psychiatry closer to real science.

Simultaneously with the development of DSM-III, different systems of diagnostic criteria for research have come into existence, and in ICD-10 there are now also diagnostic criteria for research that are in some points different from the ordinary clinical guidelines. This may be confusing. An example can clearly show the problem: In the diagnostic guidelines for schizotypal disorder, in ICD-10, it is mentioned that "a history of schizophrenia in a first degree relative gives additional weight to the diagnosis." In the diagnostic criteria for research, this qualification is omitted, which is certainly fortunate since its presence would have made the diagnosis inapplicable for research in the genetics of schizotypal disorder. As a result, we have two different definitions of schizotypal disorder, which may comprise two different groups of individuals. This example illustrates that the term diagnostic criteria for research is inadequate and may be misleading. No such criteria can be adequate for all kinds of research, and for some, the criteria may be directly hazardous. Unfortunately, this seems not to be understood by all those who are applying such criteria. This is a basic, general kind of criticism. There is, of course, also criticism specifically from a Scandinavian perspective. One shall be mentioned because it is of great importance for daily clinical work in the Nordic countries. It concerns the placement of cases of "psychogenic" or reactive psychoses in the classifications. This concept is widely used in the Nordic countries, comprising a great fraction of the psychoses, and to psychiatrists in these countries it is felt to be indispensable. It seemed logical to divide psychoses into two main groups according to their etiology: those that have a known cause, and those that do not have one, and then to subdivide the first group into three subgroups, namely those with organic, those with psychological, and those with mixed causation. Thus the psychogenic psychoses fit in as an evident and indispensable group. The natural history of the reactive psychoses is characteristic in that the course is practically always favorable. Table 4.1 gives a view of the main forms of reactive psychoses as they are usually diagnosed in the Nordic countries.

For the reactive psychoses, there were adequate classes in ICD-8 as well as in ICD-9. Naturally (and unfortunately) this subclass was not used in countries where psychiatrists are not familiar with the concept of

TABLE 4.1. Reactive (psychogenic) psychoses.

1. Emotional syndromes
   A. Depressions
   B. Excitations
   C. Emotional paralysis
2. Syndromes with disturbance of consciousness
   A. Delirious states
   B. Dissociative states, twilight states, fugues
3. Paranoid (delusional) states
   A. Sensitive delusions of reference
   B. Litigious paranoia
   C. Incarceration psychoses
   D. Delusional psychoses in the deaf
   E. Delusional psychoses in other forms of sensory deprivation
   F. Psychoses following linguistic isolation
   G. Induced psychoses

reactive psychosis, or do not approve of it. International statistical comparisons could thus not be made in a reliable way. Nevertheless, it was useful that schools of psychiatry for which the concept is important had the possibility of using it in their daily work. Unfortunately, a coherent presentation of the concept does not exist in either DSM-III, DSM-III-R, or ICD-10. In these classifications, the Nordic concept is spread over a large number of classes and subclasses. The following two tables (Tables 4.2 and 4.3) illustrate this situation. They show where the psychogenic psychoses can be found in DSM-III-R and in ICD-10, respectively. It is understandable that Nordic psychiatrists and psychiatrists from many other countries who also use the concept of reactive psychosis have difficulties when they try to find adequate categories for the subforms of this group.

However, a great fraction of reactive psychoses have some possibilities for being placed in ICD-10 and DSM-III. But in ICD-10 there is practi-

TABLE 4.2. Where are the "reactive psychoses" in DSM-III-R?

| | |
|---|---|
| 295.40, | Schizophreniform disorder |
| 297.10, | Delusional (paranoid) disorder |
| 298.80, | Brief reactive disorder |
| 295.70, | Schizoaffective disorder |
| 297.30, | Induced psychotic disorder |
| 298.90, | Atypical psychosis |
| 296, | Mood disorders |
| 309.89, | Post-traumatic stress disorder |
| 300.14, | Multiple personality disorder |
| 300.13, | Psychogenic fugue |

TABLE 4.3. Where are the "reactive psychoses" in ICD-10?

| | |
|---|---|
| F22.0, | Delusional disorder |
| F23.X1, | Acute and transient psychotic disorders (subgroups with associated acute stress) |
| F25, | Schizoaffective disorder |
| F38, | Other single affective episode |
| F43.0, | Acute stress reaction |
| F44.0, | Dissociative amnesia |
| F44.1, | Dissociative fugue |
| F44.2, | Dissociative stupor |
| F44.3, | Trance and possession disorders |

cally no possibility of placing the largest subgroup among the reactive psychoses, namely the psychogenic depressive psychosis. In contrast, in the new group, acute and transient psychotic disorders, it can, for each case, be stated whether it has arisen in connection with severe stress or not. But this group only comprises two of the subgroups of reactive psychoses, namely those connected with disturbance of consciousness and with delusional cases, whereas the psychotic depressions of reactive nature cannot be found here. In the sections on depression, any distinction between psychogenic and endogenous depression is impossible.

These problems seem to make it impossible to create automatic conversion keys not only for the Scandinavian classifications to ICD-10 and DSM-III-R (and vice versa) but also between the relevant sections of ICD-8 and ICD-9, on the one hand, and ICD-10 and DSM-III-R, on the other.

The consequence of these problems will no doubt be that in Nordic countries special modifications of ICD-10 will have to be made before it can be generally applied in these countries.

Problems like those mentioned here do not, of course invalidate international classifications in general; they are necessary and valuable, if not ideal, tools for comparative epidemiological work. ICD-10 and DSM-III-R are probably the best international classifications that until now have come into existence. But it should not be forgotten that there are limitations to their applicability within psychiatry. They are indispensable and useful for many, but certainly not for all purposes within descriptive psychiatry.

## Conclusion

ICD-8 and ICD-9, like most national classifications, were influenced to a high degree by nosological concepts, whereas ICD-10 and DSM-III-R are mainly based on symptoms and course. This difference greatly invalidates the compatibility between the two groups of classifications. As an illustration of these problems, the placement of the group of reactive psychoses is presented. In many countries, among them the Scandinavian ones, this group comprises a great part of the psychoses. It is regarded as a nosological concept based on etiological considerations and, as such, it has found a natural location within ICD-8 and ICD-9. However, since the group is symptomatologically heterogeneous it is spread over a great number of classes in ICD-10 and DSM-III-R, which imposes difficulties in crosswalks between the newer and the older classifications.

## *References*

American Psychiatric Association (1980). *Diagnostic and Statistical Manual of Mental Disorders* (3rd ed). American Psychiatric Association, Washington, DC.

American Psychiatric Association (1987). *Diagnostic and Statistical Manual of Mental Disorders* (3rd ed, rev). American Psychiatric Association, Washington, DC.

Bech P (1990). Diagnostic and classification tradition of mental disorders in the 20th century in Scandinavia, pp 153–169. In N Sartorious, A Jablensky, DA Regier, JD Burke, RMA Hirschfeld (eds), *Sources and Traditions of Classification in Psychiatry*. Hogrefe & Huber, Toronto.

Dickmeiss P, Lunn V, Strömgren E, Svendsen BB (1952). Diagnoseliste med Kommentarer. *Nordisk Psykiatrisk Medlemsblad* 6:277–295 (English version in Stengel [1959]).

Essen-Möller E (1971). Suggestions for further improvement of the international classification of mental disorders. *Psychological Medicine* 1:308–311.

Essen-Möller E, Wohlfahrt S (1947). Suggestions for the amendment of the official Swedish classification of mental disorders. *Acta Psychiatrica et Neurologica* 47:551–555 (suppl).

Ottoson JO, Perris C (1973). Multidimensional classification of mental disorders. *Psychiological Medicine* 3:238–243.

World Health Organization (1967). *Manual of the International Statistical Classification of Diseases* (8th Rev). World Health Organization, Geneva.

World Health Organization (1977). *Manual of the International Statistical Classification of Diseases* (9th Rev). World Health Organization, Geneva.

World Health Organization (1992). *ICD-10 Classification of Mental and Behavioral Disorders*. World Health Organization, Geneva.

# 5
# Perspectives on the Use of International Diagnostic Systems in the USSR

Peter V. Morozov

The classification and the diagnosis of mental disorders are among the most important and vital problems of present-day psychiatry. Although there have been numerous revisions of the international classification of diseases over the past 100 years, this process has been especially active during the last 20 years, particularly regarding mental disorders. This may have been partly due to progress in biomedical research and rapid development in the fields of genetics, psychoimmunology, epidemiology, and psychopharmacology. This last field has helped to achieve considerable success not only in the therapy of mental disorders, but also to change the image of psychiatry and its concern for both inpatients and outpatients. Also contributing to interest in psychiatric classification have been pathomorphosic-related changes in the course and symptoms of mental disorders, and the observation of subclinical manifestations of various disorders.

The ever-growing number of psychosocial factors derived from industrial and urban development also greatly influence the emergence of mental disorders, bearing as well on psychiatric classification and societal concerns on the very notion of mental disorder and reflected in the appearance of the so-called "antipsychiatry movement."

The development of national mental health programs across the world would be nearly impossible without sound research methodology, within which concepts of diagnosis and classification have a central place, together with information on therapy, rehabilitation, and epidemiology. The need for adequate tools of systematization and communication at various levels of care (primary health care, large medical institutions, clinicians, researchers) prompted the World Health Organization to undertake a decade-long effort toward the preparation of *International Classification of Diseases*, 10th revision (ICD-10) and its chapter on mental disorders (WHO 1992).

With regard to the prospects of using ICD-10 in a particular country, one should note peculiarities in the development of national classification and elucidate the factors influencing this process. This should enhance efforts to adjust ICD-10 to local realities.

The views that follow derive from a survey conducted on the classification of mental diseases among leading experts residing in the United States, Canada, Great Britain, West Germany, Switzerland, Austria, France, Denmark, Sweden, Norway, Finland, and Iceland, as well as from information obtained by the author through visits to psychiatric institutions of these countries and interviews with their directions.

## Comparative International Views

The currently existing psychiatric classifications reflect a number of factors with particular historical roots and inscribed within a specific social and economic framework, including ethnic and cultural forces and the scientific, organizational, and legal underpinnings of psychiatric care in a given country.

This point is considered next before proceeding to the discussion of Soviet psychiatry.

The emergence of Kraepelin's nosological concept (Kraepelin 1896), fundamental to general psychopathology, and other important contributions of classical German psychiatry were closely associated with an upsurge in social and economic developments in Germany at the time of Bismarck. A network of psychiatric hospitals and university clinics were created at the time, which opened up new prospects for outpatient care and follow-up studies. Nosological contributions were also facilitated by the traditional German concern with systematization (eg, Schneider 1950) and the long-standing ties between medical and philosophic disciplines in German-speaking countries.

The approach of the French psychiatric school, based on excellent observations on psychopathology, symptoms, and syndromes, had interesting and potent origins (eg, Magnan and Serieux 1893). It was a long time before the French psychiatric legislation elaborated by Esquirol (1838) was revised. The early social insurance system for patients did not promote outpatient care, and as a result, did not facilitate long-term dynamic treatment. Thus, despite the introduction of a sectoral psychiatric system in France, generations of psychiatrists studied patients predominantly in cross-sectional terms, thereby stimulating the development of syndromatic approaches and, in this way, affecting the formulation of classification concepts.

The British psychiatric school is characterized by the absence of its own classification system, and has tended to use few and relatively simple diagnostic terms, which reflects the traditionally independent and skeptical attitude of the British workers towards complex diagnostic schemes lacking sufficiently clear ethiopathogenetic and clinical grounds. British psychiatrists, however, were among the first to devise and to use various psychopathology rating scales (eg, Hamilton 1959, 1967), that are indispensable in clinical, psychopharmacological, and epidemiological research. They also have made conspicuous contributions to the successive revisions of the International Classification of Diseases.

Typical of Scandinavian psychiatry is a contextualized and personalized approach to patients reflecting the prevailing social system in the Nordic countries, as well as specific cultural traditions. This approach influenced to a great extent the views of Scandinavian scientists on the effect of external factors and generated the notion of the so-termed reactive or psychogenic psychoses (Wimmer 1916). These were emphasized as a result of a reduction in the scope of the concepts of schizophrenia and manic-depressive psychoses and of extending the third intermediate group of functional psychoses. The traditional interest for medical statistics in those countries also stimulated the development of scientific approaches to the creation and application of classification principles.

Rapid development of outpatient network, deinstitutionalization, and adequate social security available to the mentally ill have stimulated the attempts of Scandinavian psychiatrists to develop new classification systems based on multiaxial approaches (eg, Essen-Möller and Wohlfahrt 1947, Ottosson and Perris 1973).

The American psychiatric school, which was formed much later than those in Europe, incorporated a number of features from different psychiatric traditions of the Old World. That is probably why it is in many ways so diverse and eclectic. In the 1960s and 1970s, closer ties developed between psychiatry and general medicine, outpatient counseling networks expanded, and more funding was allocated for research, including epidemiological, clinical, and biological studies. These processes seem to have contributed to the DSM-III's (American Psychiatric Association 1980) use of a descriptive approach, specific diagnostic criteria, and a multiaxial diagnostic schema, which are further developed in the DSM-IV (American Psychiatric Association 1994).

A study of the conceptualization of Chapter V of ICD-10 (WHO 1992) suggests that their main architects borrowed several principles of DSM-III and went along somewhat "atheoretical" lines, resulting in an eclectic classification model. The intention of the ICD-10 Work Group to develop a uniform assessment of mental disorders using an anosological method seems to push psychiatry back to the stage of syndromological approaches.

## Russian and Soviet Psychiatry

Russian psychiatry took shape in the late 19th and early 20th century and was influenced by classical German psychiatry and the French psychopathological school. This was due not only to the traditional ties of Russia with those countries, but also to the development of outpatient services (dispensaries) that facilitated long-term and dynamic study of the patients.

It should be noted that Russian and Soviet psychiatry has tended to be biologically oriented and that scientists in that part of the world proceeded from nosological principles in the classification of mental disorders. Consideration of these facts should make it clear that changes in such concepts and systems cannot be easily and smoothly obtained.

The development of the concept of endogenous diseases by the Snezhnevsky (1990) school and research (clinical, biological, epidemiological, and pathopsychological studies) conducted within this framework were not always accompanied by adequate social guarantees for the protection of the interests of the mentally ill. This problem came to the forefront during the relatively recent years of *perestroika* and necessitated a number of reforms. It should be noted, however, that along with the reinvigoration of the mental health law adopted during the first years of the Soviet state, the National Association of the Psychiatrists of the USSR made the decision in the past decade to work toward the development and eventual use of Chapter V of ICD-10.

Understandably, limitations in knowledge about the nature of mental disorders makes it difficult for researchers to eliminate cumbersome terminology and develop better classifications of mental disorders. Further progress in the study of the etiology and pathogenesis of mental disorders may alleviate the difficulties derived from the formulation of disorders on almost exclusively phenomenological grounds.

## Contributions to the Perspectives on ICD-10

Besides the legal and social factors that may facilitate the successful introduction of ICD-10 in our land, it should be noted that Soviet psychiatrists participated in the preparation of the Chapter on Mental Disorders of the new classification. All this has happened in the context of an increase of the health care budget and certain changes in the structure of the psychiatric services. For example, psychiatric and narcological dispensaries have been separated, psychoneurologist's consulting rooms have been opened in district outpatient clinics, and the principle of voluntary hospitalization and a registration has been introduced. Structural changes in the outpatient clinics, and their reorganization into district mental health centers, may further stimulate the implementation of the new classification in actual clinical practice.

Despite the prevalence of the descriptive clinical method in the works of our psychiatrists and a certain lag in research methodology (especially regarding standardized assessment of patients and computerized processing of the data), studies within the framework of WHO projects, as well as epidemiological investigations carried out since the early 1960s in the Institute of Psychiatry (more recently the National Mental Health Research Center) of the USSR Academy of Medical Sciences, represent significant advances.

An interesting clinical data base has been developed from service to an area of 1 million people (three districts of Moscow). As part of this, 7500 schizophrenic patients have been thoroughly studied. Use of this clinical information opens up new possibilities for conducting research within the framework of ICD-10.

Soviet psychiatrists have considered different axes for a comprehensive evaluation of psychiatric patients since the beginning of the 1960s. These include psychiatric syndrome, personality structure, social and demographic description, occupational adjustment and capabilities, illness course, and psychosocial stress. It is noteworthy that etiopathogenesis is not on this list. Most of the parameters cited here are seen from a dynamic point of view that increases the value of the clinical material.

It may be possible to adjust these clinical data to ICD-10 parameters, despite its complexity. This would help to make this material comparable to data obtained by scientists in other countries and open up new horizons for international cooperation on the diagnosis and classification of mental disorders.

The adoption of the syndromatic approach for the diagnosis for mental disorders is another promising decision. Despite our traditional nosological principles, the relatively "atheoretical" nature of ICD-10 seems to be justified. The syndromatic approach, through which the diagnostic process is simplified, appears to be helpful for promoting diagnostic reliability. This is essential for international research, especially biological and epidemiological studies. The Soviet psychiatric experience in various WHO multicenter projects has been a vivid proof of this. Reliability exercises carried out in the National Mental Health Research Center with patients experiencing endogenous pathology have yielded positive results. Thus, it appears that the postponement of nosological principles has led to improvement in the instrumentation for clinical research which, in turn, may promote research on the etiology of mental disorders. In this context, ICD-10 opens up new prospects for psychiatry in our land and across the world.

## Conclusion

In consideration of the differences existing between ICD-10 and Soviet national classification concepts, it should be emphasized that a minimally adapted version of ICD-9 (WHO 1977) has been officially used in this country as has been the case in most other countries. Thus, the main transitional difficulties to be experienced in implementing the new international classification lie in the differences between ICD-9 and ICD-10.

However, it should be mentioned that the diagnosis of schizophrenia in ICD-10 is narrower due to the exclusion of slow-progressive forms and acute delusional conditions with mild personality changes. These conditions are listed in ICD-10 under the rubrics of schizotypal personality disorder and transient psychotic disorders. Also helpful is the fact that ICD-10 enables the coding of illness course under the fifth character of the diagnostic code, which should facilitate adherence to international standards and expand the informative impact of the diagnosis. ICD-10 is more detailed than previous revisions and requires fewer additions for national usage.

Soviet psychiatrists are aware of the fact that the structure of Chapter V of ICD-10 is open for future improvement, and most appear prepared to participate fully in this work and contribute in this way to the well-being of our patients and the advancement of the field.

## References

American Psychiatric Association (1980). *Diagnostic and Statistical Manual of Mental Disorders* (3rd ed). American Psychiatric Association, Washington, DC.

American Psychiatric Association (1993). *DSM-IV Diagnostic Criteria Draft.* American Psychiatric Association, Washington, DC.

Esquirol E (1838). *Des maladies mentales.* J-B Baillière, Paris.

Essen-Möller E, Wohlfahrt S (1947). Suggestions for the amendment of the Swedish classification of psychiatric disorders. *Acta Psychiatrica Scandinavica* 47:551–555 (suppl).

Hamilton M (1959). The assessment of anxiety states by ratings. *British Journal of Psychology* 32:50–55.

Hamilton M (1967). Development of a rating scale for primary depressive illness. *British Journal of Social and Clinical Psychology* 6:278–296.

Kraepelin E (1896). *Psychiatrie Ein Lehrbuch für Studeriende und Ärzte.* 5 Auflage. Abel, Leipzig.

Magnan V, Sérieux P (1893). *Le délire chronique à évolution systématique.* Gauthier Villars, Paris.

Ottosson JO, Perris C (1973). Multidimensional classification of mental disorders. *Psychological Medicine* 3:238–243.

Schneider K (1950). *Klinische Psychopathologie.* Thieme Verlag, Stuttgart.

Sneznerskij AV (1990). On the forms of development in mental disorders. In N Sartorius, A Jablensky, DA Regier, JD Burke, RMA Hirschfeld (eds), *Sources and Traditions of Classification in Psychiatry.* Hogrefe & Huber, Toronto.

World Health Organization (1977). *International Classification of Diseases* (9th rev). World Health Organization, Geneva.

World Health Organization (1992). *International Classification of Diseases and Health Related Problems* (10th rev). World Health Organization, Geneva.

Wimmer A (1916). Psykogene Sindssygdomsformer. In A Wimmer (ed), *St Hans Hospital 1816–1915.* G.E.C. Gads Forlag, Copenhagen.

# 6
# Latin American Contributions to Psychiatric Nosology and Classification

MIGUEL R. JORGE AND JUAN E. MEZZICH

If we consider the complexity of human behavior and its pathology, the principles and methods of diagnosis and classification in psychiatry require creativity and solid judgment as well as applicability in the setting in which they will be used. In recent years, growing international concern has been reflected in a large number of papers related to classification systems (eg, Sartorius 1988, Frances et al 1989, Mezzich 1989).

The present chapter is aimed at discussing Latin American contributions to psychiatric nosology and classification. The approach used involved computerized and manual searches of the literature available as well as data informally collected by both authors through personal contacts in Latin America and other countries.

It is important to note that some interesting studies presented at national and regional Latin American meetings are never published. Further complicating accessibility to sources, Latin American journals and books are not uniformly available in other countries. Consequently, the origins of the authors of this report (Brazil and Peru, respectively) have to be taken into account and may be reflected in the greater number of references included from these two countries.

The information collected was organized into the following broad topics: psychopathological description, theoretical considerations on the nature of psychopathology, epidemiological studies, and the architecture and contextualization of classification systems.

## Psychopathological Description

The most prominent textbook of psychiatry from Latin America is perhaps Honorio Delgado's *Curso de Psiquiatría* (1953). The Peruvian professor organized with clarity and concision psychopathologic description through syndromes and illness, which led to the adoption of this book in many undergraduate medical courses and residency programs in South America.

More recently, the Pan American Health Organization (PAHO) sponsored the edition of the textbook *Psiquiatría*, edited by Vidal and Alarcón (1986) for Latin American students. This book is the first attempt at producing a broadly based Latin American textbook of psychiatry, with more than 50 Latin American authors residing in 11 countries across the Americas.

The collection of papers published in Brazil by Carol Sonenreich represents a substantial analysis of contemporary psychopathology based on the author's experience heading a major clinical facility (eg, Sonenreich 1977, Sonenreich and Estevão 1984, Sonenreich and Teixeira 1971, Sonenreich et al 1971, Sonenreich et al 1984, Sonenreich et al 1986).

Another remarkable work came from Chile (Horwitz and Marconi 1966), also under the auspices of the PAHO, reflecting the necessity of systematization in diagnostic definitions. This paper, aimed at the formulation of morbid entities in objective and operational terms, is contemporary to the development of explicit diagnostic criteria by Berner (1969) and precedes the work of Feighner et al (1972), all considered as fundamental contributions to modern diagnostic methodology.

It is also important to note the description of native "psychiatric syndromes." Their clear and culturally contextualized definitions provide means for their identification and differential diagnosis. Among these are *susto* (Rubel 1964) or *espanto* (León 1963), and the *mal de ojo* (León and Climent 1968), as well as the description of syndromes induced by psychoactive substances (Rotondo 1943, Jeri 1978, Nizama 1979) and interesting reports by Calderon, Castellanos, and Llinas, all quoted by Roselli (1968, 1970).

## Theoretical Considerations on the Nature of Psychopathology

The pioneer work of Carlos Alberto Seguín (1946, 1956) from Peru conceptualizing mental illness in relation to stress was used and discussed in later international works (eg, Dohrenwend 1975, Kendell 1975, Kasl 1984, Brown and Harris 1989).

Horacio Fabrega, professor of psychiatry and anthropology at the University of Pittsburgh (USA) proposed an ethnomedical model to understand disease and how society deals with it (Fabrega 1975). This model integrates neurobiology, personal experience, and cultural context, transcending traditional biomedical reductionism. This topic was also usefully approached by Javier Mariátegui (1978, 1980).

Furthermore, this author (Mariátegui 1985) published a penetrating analysis of the use and abuse of alcohol in ancient Peru. He described the socially sanctioned, ceremonial use of the *chicha*, a corn-based alcoholic beverage. With the arrival of Iberian conquerors and the rupture of traditional psychopolitical and sociocultural controls, many forms of problematic behavior and self-destructive toxic use appeared among native people. This analysis constitutes a promising ethnohistorical model to understand the development and expression of mental pathologies.

Another disciplinary perspective with substantial nosographic implications is transcultural psychiatry, which constitutes one of the most important and original Latin American contributions to world psychiatry. José Angel Bustamante, professor of psychiatry at the University of Havana (Cuba), inagurated this field of study. In his *Psiquiatría Transcultural*, he and anthropologist A. Santa Cruz defined the field in terms of two basic concerns: one quantitative and directed to measurable differences (related to epidemiology), and the other qualitative, examining the variance of mental disorders in different cultures (related to clinical-anthropological inquiries) (Bustamante and Santa Cruz 1975).

A related disciplinary contribution from Latin America is folkloric psychiatry, a field in which popular notions from many regions of the world are structurally organized. This theme has been presented by Latin Americans at world congresses of psychiatry and other scientific meetings over the past 30 years (Bustamante 1961, Rogler and Hollingshead 1961, Alvarado 1965, Adis Castro and Hernandez-Ureña 1967, Bastide 1967, Seguín 1971, Rubim de Pinhio, personal communication), and has its high point in the volume *Psiquiatría Folklórica* (Seguín 1979).

## Epidemiological Studies

Epidemiology is one of the basic sciences of psychiatry and an important tool for the development and refinement of diagnostic systems. Latin American contributions in this field are quite prominent.

Caravedo, Rotondo, and Mariátegui (1963) edited *Estudios de Psiquiatría Social en el Perú* in which they organized a group of research reports from Peruvian urban and rural areas documenting existing psychiatric morbidity and the integrative value for mental health of traditional forms of collaborative work, familial bonds, and mutual help among compatriots and relatives.

Two other books (Mariátegui and Adis Castro 1970, Roselli 1970) constitute important collections of papers, not only showing the great interest of Latin American authors in this field but also the perceived necessity to understand the distribution of mental health problems in the community and their relations to cultural patterns and specific ways of life.

In the field of alcohol and drugs there is a notable book by Horwitz, Marconi, and Adis Castro, *Epidemiología del Alcoholismo en America Latina* (1967), and the investigations directed by Juan Marconi in Chile (eg, Marconi 1955, 1967) and Jandira Masur in Brazil (eg, Masur et al 1980, Masur and Monteiro 1983, Jorge and Masur 1985, Masur and Jorge 1986). Also noteworthy are the studies of de la Fuente and Campillo-Serrano (1977) describing patterns of alcohol and drug abuse in Mexico; of Carvalho et al (1987) on illicit drug consumption in Brazil, and of Carlini-Cotrim and Carlini (1988) describing the prevalence of drug use among Brazilian children and adolescents from low socioeconomic backgrounds.

Also important is the classification of the epidemiologic approach and its interface with the clinic for psychiatric case definition offered by Almeida (1989), professor of preventive medicine in Salvador, Bahia, and by Mari (eg, Mari et al 1988, Sen, Wilkinson, and Mari 1987), professor of psychiatry in Saõ Paulo.

Several other empirical studies have been conducted in Latin America, reflecting a diversity of interests in various countries. The best-known studies of mental disorder prevalence in Latin America are those by Horwitz (1958), Rotondo et al (1963), León (1967), Moya et al (1969), Bachini et al (1970), Bermann (1970), Cabildo (1970), Marconi and Muñoz (1970), Mariátegui et al (1970), Tarnopolski et al (1977), Gonzalez (1978), di Marco (1982), Almeida et al (1983), Tellez-Carrasco (1983), Aszkenazi and Casullo (1984), Medina-Mora (1985), and Llanos (1989).

Some epidemiological studies in the region involved the primary care setting. One exponent in this area is Busnello, professor of psychiatry in Brazil, with notable work on recording health problems triaxially (physical, psychological, and social components of primary health care contacts [eg, Busnello 1982, 1986, Busnello et al 1983, 1985]). Other studies in Brazil (Mari 1987), Colombia (Harding et al 1985) have documented the distribution of psychiatric disorders in primary care settings in this part of the world.

A particularly interesting epidemiological study in primary care was carried out by Bruno Lima and collaborators (eg, Lima et al 1987). They studied the psychological consequences in 200 victims of a volcanic eruption that destroyed a small town in Colombia, and concluded that the high prevalence of emotional distress following major disasters in developing countries supports the need to deliver mental health care through primary level services.

Also worthy of mention is the participation of Latin American researchers in broad epidemiologic studies. Carlos León, from Colombia, was a site director in the World Health Organization (WHO) International Pilot Study of Schizophrenia (León 1976, León 1986, World Health Organization, 1973). This project not only described the schizophrenic syndrome in nine different places across the world but demonstrated in a prospective study a better prognosis for Third World patients such as those from Cali, Colombia. Climent, also from Colombia, and Busnello, from Brazil, were involved in the WHO Collaborative Study on Strategies for Extending Mental Health Care, which was designed to develop and evaluate alternative and low-cost methods of mental health (including training methods) in seven developing countries (eg, Giel et al 1981). Another Latin American contribution under this broad epidemiological perspective was the study of Latin American populations in the US National Institute of Mental Health (NIMH) Epidemiological Catchment Area (ECA) project during the past decade. This participation involved the Spanish translations of the Diagnostic Interview Schedule (DIS) (Karno et al 1983) and its use in Spanish-speaking populations in Los Angeles (Karno et al 1987). The same instrument (the DIS) was used in Puerto Rico (Bravo, et al 1987, Canino et al 1987) and the results obtained were discussed from a transcultural perspective by Canino et al (1988).

Among the conceptual approaches to epidemiological psychiatry, it is important to note the contributions of Carlos León (1985). He analyzed the diagnosis and classification of mental disorders under an epidemiological perspective and identified the following obstacles for the development of the field:

> a deeply ingrained egotistical or "territorial" attitude of authors of particular systems which does not tolerate any criticism or attempts at improvement . . . a collective sense of chauvinism or insularity which gives members of a given cultural or ethnic group the feeling that they, and only they, are correct in their notions and perceptions, and that theirs is the "right" way of seeing or doing things, whereas others, "foreigners" or "outsiders", are necessarily in the wrong [way] . . . a tendency in some quarters to immoderate use of technology as a panacea for solving all problems and as a versatile tool for the hasty assembly of products which are then claimed to be scientifically sound, clear and complete. Alternative ways of doing things are summarily dismissed as old-fashioned or obsolete; it is as if technology is an adequate substitute for careful thinking and unhurried observation.

## Classification Systems

Dario Curiel, professor of social medicine at the Central University of Caracas, created in 1954 in Venezuela one of the first World Health Organization (WHO) Collaborative Centers for the Classification of Diseases (Puffer 1964). The center was an international model with a remarkable impact in the regional training of specialized professionals and in the formulation of the 8th revision of the International Classification of Diseases (ICD) (World Health Organization 1967), the first one with a massive presence of Latin American contributors.

José Leme Lopes (1954), professor of psychiatry in Rio de Janeiro, published in Brazil an innovative book presenting a diagnostic schema involving three axes: syndrome, premorbid personality, and etiologic constellation. The multiaxial diagnostic model was first proposed by Essen-Möller and Wohlfahrt (1947) in Sweden and Bilikiewicz (1951) in Poland, and constitutes one of the¨undamental perspectives of contemporary psychiatric diagnosis (Mezzich 1985).

Also with regard to the general structure of a classification system, José Lucena (1963), professor of psychiatry in Recife (Brazil), published a proposal to consider systematically etiology, symptomatology, and course when classifying mental diseases.

Carlos Acosta, professor of psychiatry at the University of Havana, published with collaborators the *Second Cuban Glossary of the International Classification of Diseases* (Acosta-Nodal et al 1983). This work, prepared in collaboration with hundreds of adult and child psychiatrists, contains a detailed analysis of the *International Classification of Diseases*, 9th revision (ICD-9) Chapter V (World Health Organization 1977) from the perspective of Cuban clinical reality, building on experience obtained with the *First Cuban Glossary*. Most of the modifications involved the necessity of including new diagnostic entities, subcategories, or qualifying terms.

Also in 1983, Renato Alarcón, a Peruvian psychiatrist and professor at the University of Alabama (USA), published a balanced analysis of the (*Diagnostic and Statistical Manual of Mental Disorders*, 3rd edition (DSM-III) (American Psychiatric Association 1980) from a Latin American perspective. Alarcón noted that the phenomenological descriptive approach taken by the DSM-III has enjoyed a long and prestigious tradition in the region but considered that "what is lacking in the system is the explicit recognition of psychocultural categories and cultural criteria to aid in the identification of crucial categories and in the description of clusters of symptoms" (Alarcón 1983). He also pointed out substantial cross-cultural limitations in the personality disorders section, and the formulation of axes IV (typology and severity of stressors) and V (level of adaptive functioning). Recently, an empirical study comparing the distributions of DSM-III diagnoses in North and South American clinical samples was published by Sogi et al (1989).

From 1985 to 1987, the World Psychiatric Association (WPA) consulted by mail its national member societies regarding ICD-10 proposals, under a collaborative agreement established with WHO. Thirty WPA member societies answered the consultation at one or more points, six of them from Latin America (Argentina, Brazil, Colombia, Mexico, Peru, Venezuela). The main recommendations for advancing ICD-10, on which Latin American societies agreed with those from the rest of the world, included the adoption of a multiaxial diagnostic scheme and enhancing compatibility between the new system and the realities of different countries, cultures, and settings (including primary care and general hospital services), through worldwide field-trial validation studies (Mezzich

1990). These suggestions were accepted by WHO, and field trials have been mounted in many countries.

# Conclusion

Despite socioeconomic and technological limitations, Latin America has made significant contributions to psychiatric nosology. A key feature has been the contextualization of diagnosis, from historical and socio-environmental perspectives. This probably reflects the deep concern with historical roots in Latin American culture as well as the less-than-super-specialized, more general nature of psychiatric practice in the region.

## *References*

Acosta-Nodal C, Mignagaray R, Nogueira G, Duarte FD, Magriñat JM (1983). *Segundo Glosario Cubano de la Novena Clasificación Internacional de Enfermedades Psiquiátricas.* Editorial Científico-Técnica, La Habana.

Adis Castro C, Hernández Ureña RA (1967). Causas de enfermedad mental; conceptos populares. *Revista Interamericana de Psicologia* 1:297–312.

Alarcón RD (1983). A Latin-American perspective on DSM-III. *American Journal of Psychiatry* 140:102–105.

Almeida N (1989). *Epidemiologia Sem Números: Uma Introdução Crítica à Ciência Epidemiológica.* Campus, Rio de Janeiro.

Almeida N, Santana V, Coutinho D, et al (1983). Prevalência de desordens mentais em uma área industrial da região metropolitana de Salvador. Aspectos metodológicos e achados preliminares. *Universitas* 32:59–72.

Alvarado JM (1965). Supersticiones y mitos en la psiquiatria indigena de Bolivia. *Acta Psiquiátrica y Psicológica de América Latina* 11:24–35.

American Psychiatric Association (1980). *Diagnostic and Statistical Manual of Mental Disorders* (3rd ed). Washington, DC, American Psychiatric Association.

Aszkenazi M, Casullo MM (1984). Factores socioculturales y presencia de psicopatologias en poblaciones de distintas localidades argentinas. *Acta Psiquiátrica y Psicológica de América Latina* 30:11–20.

Bachini O, Zabala D, Murguia D, Tobler C, Pupo H, Vaghi D, Seigal J (1970). Estudios epidemiológicos en psiquiatria en el Uruguay. In H Roselli (ed), *Psiquiatria en la América Latina*, Tercer Mundo, Bogotá.

Bastide R (1967). *Les Amériques noires: Les civilisations africaines dans le Nouveau Monde.* Editions Payot, Paris.

Bermann S (1970). Problemas actuales de la epidemiologia psiquiátrica en América Latina. In H Roselli (ed), *Psiquiatria en la América Latina.* Tercer Mundo, Bogotá.

Berner P (1969). Der lebensabend der paranoiker. *Wien Zeitschrift Nervenheilkunde* 27:115–161.

Bilikiewicz T (1951). Proba ukladu nozograficznego etioepigenetycznego w psychiatri. *Neurologia I neurochirurgia Polska* 1:68–78.

Bravo M, Canino G, Bird H (1987). El DIS en español: Su tradución y adaptación en Puerto Rico. *Acta Psiquiátrica y Psicológica de América Latina* 33:27–42.

Brown GW, Harris TO (1989). *Life Events and Illness*. Guilford Press, New York.
Busnello E (1982). A mechanism for recording and reporting physical and psychosocial components of health in a community health system in Porto Alegre, Brazil. In M Lipkin, K Kupka (eds), *Psychosocial Factors Affecting Health*. Praeger, New York.
Busnello E (1986). A register based on family records and priority cards. In GHMM Ten Horn, R Giel, WH Gulbinat, JH Henderson (eds), *Psychiatric Case Registers in Public Health*. Elsevier, Amsterdam.
Busnello E, Lima BR, Bertolote JM (1985). Psychosocial issues related to the classification of mental health problems in a community programme in Brazil. In A Jablensky (ed), *Mental Disorders; Alcohol- and Drug-Related Problems. International Perspectives on Their Diagnosis and Classification*, International Congress Series 669. Excerpta Medica/Elsevier, New York.
Busnello E, Lima BR, Bertolote JM, Gomes R, Wildt M (1983). O estudo conjunto da OMS sobre o registro triaxial dos problemas de saúde. Comunicação preliminar. *Jornal Brasileiro de Psiquiatria* 32:151–154.
Bustamante JA (1961). Importancia del folklore en la psiquiatria. In *Proceedings of the III World Congress of Psychiatry*. World Psychiatric Association, Toronto.
Bustamante JA, Santa Cruz A (1975). *Psiquiatría Transcultural*. Editorial CientíficoTécnica, La Habana.
Cabildo HA (1970). Investigación epidemiológica en Mexico. In J Mariátegui, G Adis Castro (eds), *Estudios sobre Epidemiologia Psiquiátrica en América Latina*. Acta, Buenos Aires.
Canino GJ, Bird HR, Shrout PE, Rubio-Stipec M, Bravo M, Martinez R, Sesman M, Guevara LM (1987). The prevalence of specific psychiatric disorders in Puerto Rico. *Archives of General Psychiatry* 44:251–259.
Canino GJ, Rubio-Stipec M, Bravo M (1988). La clasificación diagnóstica psiquiátrica en estudios epidemiológicos transculturales. *Acta Psiquiátrica y Psicológica de América Latina* 34:251–259.
Caravedo B, Rotondo H, Mariátegui J (1963). *Estudios de Psiquiatría Social en el Perú*. Ediciones del Sol, Lima.
Carlini-Cotrim BH, Carlini EA (1988). The use of solvents and other drugs among children and adolescents from a low socioeconomic background: A study in São Paulo, Brazil. *International Journal of the Addictions* 23: 1145–1156.
Carvalho JA, Almeida N, Rego R, Santana V (1987). Prevalência do consumo de drogas ilícitas em uma amostra populacional de Salvador, Bahia. *Revista ABP-APAL* 9:131–139.
de la Fuente R, Campillo-Serrano C (1977). Alcoholism and drug abuse in Mexico. In B Rutledge, EK Fulton (eds), *International Collaboration: Problems and Opportunities*, Addiction Research Foundation, Toronto.
Delgado H (1953). *Curso de Psiquiatría*. Imprenta Santa Maria, Lima.
di Marco G (1982). Prevalencia de desórdenes mentales en el área metropolitana de la República Argentina. *Acta Psiquiátrica y Psicológica de América Latina* 28:93–102.
Dohrenwend BP (1975). Sociocultural and socio-psychological factors in the genesis of mental disorders. *Journal of Health and Social Behavior* 16:365–392.

Essen-Möller E, Wohlfahrt S (1947). Suggestions for the amendment of the official Swedish classification of mental disorders. *Acta Psychiatrica Scandinavica* 47:551–555 (suppl).

Fabrega H (1975). The need for an ethnomedical science. *Science* 189:969–975.

Feighner JP, Robins E, Guze SB, Woodruff RA, Winokur G, Muñoz R (1972). Diagnostic criteria for use in psychiatric research. *Archives of General Psychiatry* 26:57–63.

Frances AJ, Widiger TA, Pincus HA (1989). The development of DSM-IV. *Archives of General Psychiatry* 46:373–375.

Giel R, Busnello E, Climent CE, Elhakim ASED, Ibrahim HHA, Ladrido-Ignacio, Wig NN (1981). The classification of psychiatric disorder. A reliability study in the WHO collaborative study on strategies for extending mental health care. *Acta Psychiatrica Scandinavica* 63:61–74.

Gonzalez M (1978). Epidemiologia de los transtornos mentales en Bogotá. Primera etapa. *Acta Psiquiátrica y Psicológica de América Latina* 24:93–95.

Harding TW, de Arango MV, Baltazar J, Climent CE, Ibrahim HHA, Ladrido-Ignacio L, Murthy RS, Wig NN (1985). Mental disorders in primary health care: A study of their frequency and diagnosis in four developing countries. *Psychological Medicine* 10:231–241.

Horwitz J (1958). Investigaciones epidemiologicas acerca de la morbilidad mental en Chile. *Revista del Servicio Nacional de Salud* 3:277–291.

Horwitz J, Marconi J (1966). El problema de las definiciones en el campo de la salud mental. Definiciones aplicables en estudios epidemiologicos. *Boletin de la Oficina Sanitaria Panamericana* 60:300–309.

Horwitz J, Marconi J, Adis Castro G (1967). *Epidemiología del Alcoholismo en América Latina.* Acta, Buenos Aires.

Jeri R (1978). El síndrome de la pasta de cocaína. *Revista de la Sanidad del Ministerio del Interior* 39:1–18.

Jorge MR, Masur J (1985). An attempt to improve the identification of alcohol-dependent patients in a teaching general hospital. *Drug and Alcohol Dependence* 16:67–73.

Kasl SV (1984). Stress and health. *Annual Review of Public Health* 5:319–341.

Kendell RE (1975). *The Role of Diagnosis in Psychiatry*. Blackwell, Oxford.

Leme Lopes J (1954). *As Dimensões do Diagnóstico Psiquiátrico*. Agir, Rio de Janeiro.

León CA (1963). El "espanto": sus implicaciones psiquiatricas. *Acta Psiquiátrica y Psicológica de América Latina* 9:207–217.

León CA (1967). Prevalencia de transtornos mentales en un sector urbano de Cali. *Revista Colombiana de Psiquiatria* 2:24–36.

León CA (1976). El Estudio Piloto Internacional sobre Esquizofrenia: sus implicaciones para la América Latina. *Acta Psiquiátrica y Psicológica de América Latina* 22:167–183.

León CA (1985). Epidemiological perspective on the diagnosis and classification of mental disorders: an overview. In A Jablensky (ed), *Mental Disorders; Alcohol- and Drug-Related Problems. International Perspectives on Their Diagnosis and Classification*, International Congress Series 669. Excerpta Medica/Elsevier, New York.

León CA (1986). Curso clinico y evolucion de la esquizofrenia en Cali. Un estudio de seguimiento de diez años. *Acta Psiquiátrica y Psicológica de América Latina* 32:85–136.

León CA, Climent CE (1968). Anotaciones sobre el ojo en Cali. *Acta Psiquiátrica y Psicológica de América Latina* 14:23–34.

Lima BR, Pai S, Santacruz H, Lozano J, Luna J (1987). Screening for the psychological consequences of a major disaster in a developing country: Armero, Colombia. *Acta Psychiatrica Scandinavica* 76:561–567.

Llanos R (1989). Ethnopsychiatric systems in different cultural areas of Peru. In *Proceedings of the VIII World Congress of Psychiatry*. World Psychiatric Association, Athens.

Lucena JC (1963). Contribuição à classificação brasileira de doenças mentais. *Neurobiologia* 26:10–22.

Marconi J (1955). A survey on the prevalence of alcoholism among the adult population of a suburb of Santiago. *Quarterly Journal of Studies on Alcohol* 16:428–446.

Marconi J (1967). El alcoholismo en Chile. In J Horwitz, J Marconi, G Adis Castro (eds), *Epidemiologia del Alcoholismo en América Latina.* Acta, Buenos Aires.

Marconi J, Muñoz L (1970). Visión general de la investigación epidemiológica en salud mental en Chile. In H Roselli (ed), *Psiquiatria en la América Latina.* Tercer Mundo, Bogotá.

Mari JJ (1987). Psychiatric morbidity in three primary medical care clinics in the city of São Paulo. Issues on the mental health of the urban poor. *Social Psychiatry* 22:129–138.

Mari JJ, Sen B, Cheng T (1988). Case definition and case identification in cross-cultural perspectives. In P Williams, G Wilkinson, K Rawsley (eds), *Scientific Approaches in Epidemiological and Social Psychiatry—Essays in Honour of Michael Shepherd.* Tavistock Publications, London.

Mariátegui J (1978). Ecologia y psiquiatria. *Acta Psiquiátrica y Psicológica de América Latina* 24:101–108.

Mariátegui J (1985). Concepción del hombre y alcoholismo en el antiguo Peru. *Acta Psiquiátrica y Psicológica de América Latina* 31:253–267.

Mariátegui J, Adis Castro G (1970). *Epidemiologia Psiquiátrica en América Latina.* Acta, Buenos Aires.

Mariátegui J, Alva V, de Leon O (1970). Prevalencia de desórdenes mentales en un distrito urbano de Lima. In H Roselli (ed), *Psiquiátria en al América Latina.* Tercer Mundo, Bogotá.

Mariátegui J, Valdizán H (1980). La psiquiatria comparativa y la medicina folklorica. *Acta Psiquiatrica y Psicológica de América Latina* 26:96–196.

Masur J, Cunha JM, Zwicker AP, Laranjeira RR, Knobel E, Sustovich DR, Lopes AC (1980). Prevalência de pacientes com indicadores de alcoolismo internados em uma enfermaria de clínica geral. Relevância de forma de detecção. *Acta Psiquiátrica y Psicológica de América Latina* 26:125–130.

Masur J, Jorge MR (1986). Dados relacionados a bebidas alcoólicas e alcoolismo no Brasil: uma revisão. *Revista ABP-APAL* 8:157–165, 1986.

Masur J, Monteiro MG (1983). Validation of the "CAGE" alcoholism screening test in a Brazilian psychiatric inpatient hospital setting. *Brazilian Journal of Medical and Biological Research* 16:215–218.

Medina-Mora ME, Padilla GP, Mas CC, Ezban BM, Caraveo AJ, Campillo SC, Corona J (1985). Prevalencia de transtornos mentales y factores de riesgo en una población de práctica médica general. *Acta Psiquiátrica y Psicológica de América Latina* 31:53–61.

Mezzich JE (1985). Multiaxial diagnostic systems in psychiatry. In HI Kaplan, BJ Sadock (eds), *Comprehensive Textbook of Psychiatry*, 4th ed. Williams & Wilkins, Baltimore.

Mezzich JE (1989). International diagnostic systems and Latin-American contributions and issues. *British Journal of Psychiatry* 154:84–90 (suppl 4).

Mezzich JE (1990). The World Psychiatric Association and the development of ICD-10. In CN Stefanis, CR Soldatos, AD Rabavilas (eds), *Proceedings of the VIII World Congress of Psychiatry*. Elsevier, Amsterdam.

Moya L, Marconi J, Horwitz J, Muñoz L, Bahamondes A, Saint Jean (1969). Estudios de prevalencia de desordenes mentales en al area norte de Santiago de Chile. *Acta Psiquiátrica y Psicológica de América Latina* 15:137–148.

Nizama M (1979). Síndrome de pasta basica de cocaína. Fenomenologia clínica, historia natural y descripción de la subcultura. *Revista de Neuropsiquiatria* 42:114–134; 185–208.

Puffer RR (1964). Los primeros diez años del Centro Latinoamericano de la Classificación de Enfermedades. *Boletin de la Oficina Sanitaria Panamericana* 57:218–229.

Rogler LH, Hollingshead A (1961). The Puerto Rican spiritualist as a psychiatrist. *American Journal of Sociology* 67:17–21.

Roselli H (1968). *Historia de la Psiquiatria en Colombia*, vol I. Editorial Horizontes, Bogotá.

Roselli H (1970). *Psiquiatria en la América Latina*. Tercer Mundo, Bogotá.

Rotondo H (1943). Fenomenologia de la intoxicación mescalínica y análisis del pensamiento en su decurso. *Revista de Neuropsiquiatria* 6:58–142.

Rotondo H, Aliaga LP, Garcia Pacheco C (1963). Estudios de morbilidad psiquiátrica en la población urbana de Mendoncita. In B Caravedo, H Rotondo, J Mariátegui (eds), *Estudios de Psiquiatria Social en el Peru*. Ediciones del Sol, Lima.

Rubel AJ (1964). The epidemiology of a folk illness: Susto in Hispanic America. *Ethnology* 3:268–283.

Sartorius N (1988). International perspectives of psychiatric classification. *British Journal of Psychiatry* 152:9–14 (suppl 1).

Seguin CA (1946). The concept of disease. *Psychosomatic Medicine* 8:252–257.

Seguin CA (1956). Migration and psychosomatic disadaptation. *Psychosomatic Medicine* 13:404–409.

Seguin CA (1971). Conceptos basicos en la psiquiatria folklorica. In *Proceedings of the VI World Congress of Psychiatry*. World Psychiatric Association, Ciudad del Mexico.

Seguin CA (1979). *Psiquiatria Folklórica*. Ediciones Errmar, Lima.

Sen B, Wilkinson G, Mari J (1987). Psychiatric morbidity in primary health care. A two-stage screening procedure in developing countries: Choice of instruments and cost-effectiveness. *British Journal of Psychiatry* 151:33–38.

Sogi C, Warthon D, Mezzich JE, Valverde J, Saavedra-Castillo A, Ahn CW (1989). Comparative distributions of DSM-III diagnoses in North and South American clinical samples. *British Journal of Psychiatry* 164:91–95 (suppl 4).

Sonenreich C (1977). *Esquizofrenia*. Editora Manole, São Paulo.
Sonenreich C, Bassit W, Estevão G (1984). Psicopatologia no idoso. *Temas* 27:127–157.
Sonenreich C, Estevão G (1984). Das fobias. *Temas* 28–29:19–52.
Sonenreich C, Eva AC, Signorini J, Martins C (1971). Observações psicopatológicas sobre 100 casos de focos temporais. *Revista Brasileira de Psiquiatria* 5:91–100.
Sonenreich C, Estevão G, Ribeiro LC, Falivene JA (1986). Depressões: um conceito. *Revista ABP-APAL* 8:43–48.
Sonenreich C, Teixeira AF (1971). *Estudos sobre Histeria*. IAMSPE, São Paulo.
Tarnopolski A, Caetano R, Levav I, del Olmo G (1977). Prevalence of psychiatric morbidity in an industrial suburb of Buenos Aires. *Social Psychiatry* 12:75–88.
Téllez-Carrasco PJ (1983). Psicopatologia transcultural de los delirios en Venezuela. In *Proceedings of the VII World Congress of Psychiatry*. World Psychiatric Association, Vienna.
Vidal G, Alarcón RD (1986). *Psiquiatria*. Editorial Médica Panamericana, Buenos Aires.
World Health Organization (1967). *Manual of the International Statistical Classification of Diseases, Injuries and Causes of Death* (8th rev). World Health Organization, Geneva.
World Health Organization (1973). *Report of the International Pilot Study of Schizophrenia*. World Health Organization, Geneva.
World Health Organization (1977). *International Classification of Diseases: Manual of the International Statistical Classification of Diseases, Injuries and Causes of Death* (9th rev). World Health Organization, Geneva.

# 7
# African Perspectives on Mental Disorder

FELIX ATTAH JOHNSON

In Africa as in Europe, North America, South America, Asia, and Oceania, the advantages of diagnostic classification of psychiatric disorders include: (1) a means of communication and of ordering clinical material, (2) the management, treatment, and care of patients, (3) prognosis, and (4) the great scientific interest found in discrepancies in the classification, which may form the basis for asking further relevant clinical and research questions. It seems impossible to speak of a single African viewpoint because the continent contains a broad range of cultures. The Ga, the Masai, and the Kikuyu, for example, are as different in their specific ceremonies and customs as the Bantus are from the Belgians. Yet in sub-Saharan black Africa the different cultures do share a consciousness of the world. They have in common a characteristic perception of life and death that makes it possible to describe their overriding philosophy. The character and effectiveness of medicine for the mind and the body always and everywhere depend on the culture in which the medicine is practiced. In the West, healing is often considered to be a private matter between patient and therapist. In Africa, healing is an integral part of society and religion, a matter in which the whole community is involved. To understand African psychiatry and psychotherapy one must understand African thought and its social roots (Lambo 1974). For the African, the original concept of nature includes simultaneously the physical world and the social environment of both the living and the dead, together with the metaphysical forces of the universe. This concept is fundamental to a grasp of traditional African medicine in all its dimensions (Ampofo and Johnson-Ramauld 1978).

Indeed, the original African concept of disease is not merely of something resulting from a malfunction in this or that organ or of a lesion therein, whether spontaneous or provoked by some physical cause, but essentially of a rupture of life's harmony, to be imputed either to a material cause, instinct with an "intangible force" or, directly to that intangible force itself. Therefore, it is regarded as necessary in traditional medical practice to confront the symptomatology and etiology of disease not only in the material but also in the immaterial world (Ampofo and Johnson-Ramauld 1978). In precolonial times, the traditional healer was alone in helping people solve their health problems. Nowadays, there is no doubt that 75%, or more, of the rural population has no available alternative to traditional healers. In both rural and urban areas, the majority of African people initially consult a traditional healer with their health problems, then a modern Western-trained physician, and finally, return to the traditional healer for a total healing or reconciliation with the community (Forster 1971, personal communication).

The preceding description is a summary of the African world view and socicultural environment into which European medicine and psychiatry were gradually introduced during the late 19th century and early 20th century. The vast majority of African psychiatrists have been trained in Western Europe, specifically in the United Kingdom and France. The pioneering African psychiatrists and the acknowledged great teachers of the theory and practice of psychiatry include Lambo and Asuni (Nigeria), Bani Forster (The Gambia and Ghana), Tijani El-Mahi and Baasher (The Sudan), Allen German and Muhanji (Uganda), Collomb and Diop (Senegal), Mustapha and Muya (Kenya), Swift and Rugeyamu (Tanzania), Bruno Claver (La Côte D'Ivoire), and Amarguaye, Adomakoh and Sikarnartey (Ghana). These early pioneers brought with them to sub-Saharan black Africa the classification systems that they had learned in London, Edinburgh, or Paris and passed them on to their undergraduate medical students and postgraduate trainee-psychiatrists. Binitie (1988, p 66) states: "The influence of Kraepelin on the classification of psychiatric disorders, as well as the modifications made by Eugene Bleuler, are still evident in Nigerian psychiatry. In actual day-to-day practice, however, many psychiatrists have found that pathoplastic factors influence psychiatric diagnosis, so that many classically described syndromes show much variation when applied to live patients in the Nigerian setting." This statement is applicable to all sub-Saharan black African countries that have modern psychiatric services. Binitie (1988) also raises the highly pertinent question: What combination of genes and environment in an African setting contributes to the clinical picture hitherto regarded as classical? In an attempt to answer this complex question, he continues with the example of "the peculiarities of depression in Africans." He further illustrates the complexity of the original question with the following statement: "The example that we have given represents an exercise in appraising African culture by using a European yardstick. The converse experience of appraising European culture by means of an African yardstick has rarely occurred" (Binitie 1988, p 65). The present author considers this a challenge to contemporary African psychiatrists.

The majority of African psychiatrists support the view that culture is pathoplastic rather than pathogenic in terms of the influence of culture on

TABLE 7.1. The major groups of disorders in ICD-9, Chapter V.

| | |
|---|---|
| 1. | Dementias and confusional states |
| 2. | Psychoses due to drugs and alcohol |
| 3. | Other organic psychotic conditions |
| 4. | Schizophrenic psychoses |
| 5. | Affective psychoses |
| 6. | Paranoid and other nonorganic psychoses |
| 7. | Psychoses of childhood |
| 8. | Neurotic disorders |
| 9. | Personality disorders |
| 10. | Sexual deviations and disorders |
| 11. | Alcohol and drug dependence and abuse |
| 12. | Physiological malfunctions arising from mental factors |
| 13. | Special and other syndromes |
| 14. | Acute stress and adjustment reactions |
| 15. | Conduct disorders, and behavior and emotional disorders specific to or associated with childhood and adolescence |
| 16. | Mental retardation |

Adapted from Cooper 1988.

the diagnosis and classification of psychiatric disorders (Table 7.1). It is necessary to examine in detail the classification system commonly used by African psychiatrists to illustrate some of the pathoplastic effects of culture on the classical syndromes. "The matter in dispute in cross-cultural research is not the substantial prevalence of mental disorders in Africa. Rather, the literature shows that there is a need to clarify the nature and prognosis of somatization, depression and schizophrenia, and the prevalence of suicidal behavior and alcohol-related problems in comparison with their presentations and prevalence in the Western world. It seems to be in these nosological entities that psychiatric phenomenology in Africa differs somewhat from the situation in the West, and they therefore require some discussion" (Odejide et al 1989).

## Classification and Diagnosis of Psychiatric Disorders

What are some of the pathoplastic influences of African cultures on the classical psychiatric syndromes? Some controversial issues discussed are schizoaffective psychosis; manic-depressive psychosis, depressed type; acute transient psychosis; and brain fag syndrome.

### *Schizoaffective Psychosis*

The subcategories of schizophrenia—namely, simple, hebephrenic, paranoid, and catatonic—are diagnosed by African psychiatrists on the basis of the *International Classification of Diseases*, 9th revision (ICD-9) definitions of such categories. Most African psychiatrists have difficulty recognizing latent schizophrenia (ICD-9 Code 295.5), and thus seldom make that diagnosis. The subcategory, schizoaffective type (ICD-9 Code 295.7), is considered controversial by the majority of African psychiatrists: "Schizoaffective disorder has been a controversial diagnostic concept since its introduction in 1933 by Kasanin. Even today, there is still little consensus on whether it is an independent diagnostic disorder, a subtype of schizophrenia or affective disorder, or a borderline condition that falls somewhere along a continuum from schizophrenia to affective disorder" (Sprock 1988).

## *Manic-Depressive Psychosis, Depressed Type*

It is now generally agreed that depression is common among Africans. (Lambo 1960, Asuni 1972, Olatawura 1973, Ebie 1972, Binitie 1975a, Majodina and Johnson 1983, Johnson 1982/83, Johnson 1987). "Current workers are unanimous in agreeing that depressive illness, psychotic or otherwise, is common in Africa. Dispute persists, however, about the nature of symptoms" (German 1987). Patients were described by Field (1958) presenting with the classical symptoms of manic-depressive psychosis, depressed type, in the healing shrines of rural Ghana. "Difficulty in the diagnosis of depression in the African setting results from the pathoplastic effect of the culture-modifying symptoms, so that it is difficult to recognize the condition to be the same as that of the classical European affective syndrome. Instead, the African patient frequently exhibits many bodily complaints such as heat in the head or body, worms crawling all over the body, worms in the head, tightness of the head, or gas in the stomach. Such somatic complaints may so dominate the picture that the true nature and significance of the symptoms are lost" (Binitie 1988).

To develop cross-culturally applicable instruments for a standardized assessment of depressive states, and to evaluate the clinical and social characteristics of depressive patients seeking treatment in different cultures, WHO has coordinated a collaborative study with the participation of five research centres in Canada (Montréal), Iran (Teheran), Japan (Nagasaki, Tokyo) and Switzerland (Basel). A screening form and schedule for Standardized Assessment of Depressive Disorders (SADD) were designed, and proved to be reliable and easily applicable (Sartorius et al 1980). The study of characteristics of depression was continued by a follow-up investigation in which a follow-up version of the SADD was used.

Majodina and Johnson (1983) used the SADD instrument to study 50 depressed African patients in Accra (Ghana) and reported as follows: It is worth noting that the present findings are in some ways a definite departure from findings reported by earlier research workers in Africa. (1) There is a core of depressive symptomatology. This core was undoubtedly present in the sample under study and included the symptoms found in more than three-quarters of the patients. In this sample, anxiety and tension appear to be among the most frequent symptoms of depressive patients. (2) In terms of psychotic symptoms, delusions of any kind were infrequently reported and were present in between five and nine patients. No patient reported delusion of impoverishment. Hallucinations were present in 11 patients. (3) Feelings of guilt and self-reproach were present in 35%. This is in contrast to earlier reports of the rarity of this symptom in African patients. The majority of the patients were Christians. (4) Suicidal ideas were present in 16. (5) Hypochondriasis (not delusional) were present in 18. (6) Psychomotor agitation was found in 23; psychomotor retardation was reported in 36. (7) Somatic symptoms (other than feelings of pressure and pain, loss of appetite, change of body weight, and loss of libido) were present in 40. The most frequently reported somatic symptoms were headaches, burning sensations in the head, the sensation of heat all over the body, palpitations, joint pains, back and waist pain.

Ebie (1972) reported that of 25 patients diagnosed as suffering from depression, only one patient spontaneously complained of sadness of mood, directly, 17 of the 25 patients admitted complained of variation of mood. No patient reported spontaneously having diurnal tearfulness or feeling like crying, but 13 of the 25 patients admitted having this symptom when they were questioned directly about it. Ebie was able to demonstrate these core symptoms of depression because he spent adequate time to examine his patients. The following statement is an appropriate conclusion to this part of the discussion: "Might I suggest that, as regards the classification of depressive illness in African culture, Hamilton's triad of depressed mood, guilt and suicide should be modified to read depressed mood, projected guilt and suicide, and multiple bodily complaints?" (Binitie 1975b).

## *Paranoid State, Simple*

"A psychosis, acute or chronic, not classifiable as schizophrenia or affective psychosis, in which delusions, especially of being influenced, persecuted or treated in some special way, are the main symptoms. The delusions are of a fairly fixed, elaborate and systematized kind" (ICD-9, Code 297.0). African psychiatrists readily recognize this classical syndrome and base their diagnoses on the ICD-9 definition. In the illiterate and unsophisticated African patient in the rural areas, the paranoid delusions are usually projected on the environment (for example, influences by witchcraft and sorcery from enemies). On the other hand, in the educated and sophisticated African patient in the urban areas, the paranoid delusions are similar to those in Western patients (for example, influences from x-rays, electronic devices, or poisonous gas).

## Acute Transient Psychosis

Lambo (1960) referred to this syndrome as African periodic psychosis and observed: "In our experience many such cases are obscure and unclassifiable. The psychotic attacks are often transient, and the symptoms vague and ill defined in many cases. Criminal conduct may take place during one of these transient psychotic attacks, and when the patient is up for examination all symptoms of the psychosis may have disappeared. It is of importance that the mental disorder should be recognized, so that justice may not miscarry." These acute transient psychotic states constitute a controversial subject among African psychiatrists themselves. "This condition is especially important and interesting since nothing comparable has been described in the European literature. Nigerian psychiatrists themselves are in fact not in agreement about the existence of this syndrome. A paper presented at an annual conference of a psychiatric association concerning the existence of this syndrome attracted a lively debate and a great deal of controversy as to whether the patients so diagnosed were in fact not cases of hypomania or mania, or—alternatively—catatonic schizophrenia; other psychiatrists have suggested that there is a hysterical component in this syndrome. It is clear that this kind of condition ought to be the subject of intensive research" (Binitie 1988).

The following case report illustrates the syndrome of acute transient psychosis.

*Case Report.* The author was called to see a 35-year-old black African male university graduate. He was single and had never been married. His presenting symptoms were acute excitement state and sleeplessness of sudden onset. He was reported to have been sitting at his desk writing and drawing architectural diagrams for about 72 hours without sleep. He refused to eat his food or wash himself, but he got up occasionally to drink water or pass urine. He denied any history of substance abuse (for example, alcohol, tobacco, or illicit drugs). There was no past history of head injury, epilepsy, or mental illness. There was also no known family history of mental illness. Physical examination showed no abnormality. Mental state examination revealed an athletic-looking African male. He was uncooperative and initially resisted medical–psychiatric examination. He was excitable but not aggressive or violent. He showed evidence of psychomotor acceleration by either writing or doing his architectural drawing continuously, and was almost completely occupied with these activities. He answered most questions with a statement: "Leave me alone, I am not sick." He also claimed that he was on "the threshold of becoming a great spiritual and world leader". After several hours of unsuccessful attempts to persuade him to take some prescribed tranquillizer tablets and go to bed, force had to be used with the written consent of his next of kin. He was first restrained by assistants, and given an intramuscular injection of 100 mg chlorpromazine. About 30 minutes after the injection, he slept deeply for about 12 hours, interrupted by two visits to the toilet to urinate. When the patient got out of bed the following day, he was quite friendly but resentful of the compulsory treatment that had been given the previous night. He has remained in good mental health and continued to carry out his usual duties about 5 years after this single episode of what was diagnosed as acute transient psychosis.

## *Brain Fag Syndrome*

Controversy continues among African psychiatrists working in West, East, and Central Africa, about the classification of brain fag syndrome as a separate diagnostic category. Prince (1960), working in Nigeria, described the brain fag syndrome among Nigerian students as a symptom complex with the following characteristics:

1. It occurs in Nigerian students, teachers, and other intellectual workers.
2. It is associated with studying.
3. Patients complain of intellectual impairment, plus sensory (chiefly visual) and somatic complaints, most commonly pain or burning in head and neck.
4. These and a variety of other complaints often militate against the student's ability to study.
5. Alteration in affect. An unhappy, tense facial expression is often evident.
6. A characteristic gesture of passing the hands over the scalp and rubbing the vertex of the skull especially when concentration is needed.

"The name 'brain fag' was given to the disturbance by students themselves at the time they consulted Prince" (Anumonye 1983). Another interesting point is the observation of several workers in other African countries, showing that brain fag syndrome was not specific to Nigerian students (German et al 1970, Swift et al 1973, Thebaud et al 1972, Leham 1972, Rahim 1972). Most African psychiatrists recognize some cases of brain fag syndrome as a mixture of anxiety and depressive symptoms and signs. Prince (1960) observed that characteristic complaints associated with study were unpleasant headache, sensation of pain, visual difficulties, and inability to grasp. These symptoms have been called somatization in classical descriptions in the West. The brain fag syndrome may, therefore, be seen as a somatization reaction to study (Prince 1960). On the whole, there is no doubt that the majority of cases have turned out to defeat classification into the standard nosologies. Nevertheless, the theme remains the same—signs and symptoms associated with studying (Swift et al 1973, Morakinyo 1980, Anumonye 1983).

### *Conduct, Behavior, and Emotional Disorders Specific to or Associated with Childhood and Adolescence*

Child psychiatric services are rare in sub-Saharan Africa, in spite of the fact that substantial childhood psychiatric disorders have been highlighted (Odejide et al 1989). Statistical analysis of a sample of 296 children and adolescents seen for consultation at the Accra Psychiatric Hospital, Accra (Ghana), over a 5-year-period (1974 to 1979) showed that the sample contained examples of most of the diagnostic categories of the ICD-9 (Codes 312 to 315). This finding supports Rutter's statement (1965) that his suggested outline of classification is purely phenomenological and operational definitions could be provided for each of the groups. Accordingly, it would be relatively simple to apply it to the individual case in clinical practice (Johnson 1983).

## Conclusion

The majority of African psychiatrists support the view that culture is pathoplastic rather than pathogenic in discussing the influence of culture on the diagnosis and classification of psychiatric disorders. Recent cross-cultural research has demonstrated that there is a substantial prevalence of psychiatric disorders in Africa. A review of the literature shows that there is a need to clarify the nature and prognosis of schizoaffective psychosis; manic-depressive psychosis, depressed type; acute transient psychosis; and somatization in comparison with their nature and prevalence in Western countries. The challenge for contemporary African psychiatrists is to conduct further detailed cross-cultural research using standardized methodologies on these diagnostic categories as well as suicidal behavior and alcohol-related problems.

African psychiatrists and Oceanic psychiatrists with appropriate training and experience have used ICD-9 successfully since it came into effect in 1979. They now look forward to the introduction of ICD-10 with its multiaxial classification system and simplified versions for use in primary health care and general medical care.

*Acknowledgment.* Gratitude is due to Annelise Tvede Johnson for meticulously typing the manuscript.

## *References*

Ampofo O, Johnson-Ramauld FD (1978). Traditional medicine in the African sociocultural context. In *Traditional Medicine and its Role in the Development of Health Services in Africa.* Regional Office for Africa (AFRO), World Health Organization, Brazzaville.

Anumonye A (1983). *Brain Fag Syndrome.* International Council on Alcohol and Addictions (ICAA), Case Postale 140, 1001 Lausanne, Switzerland.

Asuni T (1972). Diagnostic Aspects of Depression from a trans-cultural point of view. In M Lader, R Garcia (eds), *Aspects of Depression: Papers read at World Psychiatric Association Symposium on Aspects of Depression, Madrid, May 1972.*

Binitie A (1975a). A factor-analytic study of depression across cultures (African and European). *British Journal of Psychiatry* 127:559–563.

Binitie A (1975b). The differentiation of masked depression from psychoneurotic disorders. In *Recognition of depression in the African*, pp 31–33. Proceedings of a round-table discussion held July 30, 1975 in conjunction with the IVth Pan-African Congress on Psychiatry, Abidjan, Ivory Coast. CIBA-GEIGY Ltd, Switzerland.

Binitie A (1988). Diagnosis and classification of mental disorders and alcohol- and drug-related problems in Nigeria, pp 65–72. In JE Mezzich, M von Cranach (eds), *International Classification in Psychiatry, Unity and Diversity.* Cambridge University Press, Cambridge.

Cooper JE (1988). The structure and presentation of contemporary psychiatric classifications with special reference to ICD-9 and 10. In N Sartorius, A Jablensky, JE Cooper, JD Burke (eds), Psychiatric Classification in an International Perspective. *British Journal of Psychiatry* 152:21–28 (suppl 1).

Ebie JC (1972). Some observations on depressive illness in Nigerians attending a psychiatric outpatient clinic. *African Journal of Medical Science* 7:207–210.

Field MG (1958). Mental disorders in rural Ghana. *Journal of Mental Science* 104:1043–1051.

Forster EFB (1971). Personal communication.

German GA (1987). Mental Health in Africa: II. The nature of mental disorder in Africa today—Some clinical observations. *British Journal of Psychiatry* 151:440–446.

German GA, Assael MI, Muhanji J (1970). Psychiatric disorders associated with study in mid-adolescent years. In *Proceedings of 2nd Pan-African Psychiatric Workshop, Mauritius, 22–26 June 1970.*

Johnson FYA (1982/83). Depression in Africa: A review of the literature. *Proceedings of Jos Medical Society* 2:36–52.

Johnson FYA (1983). Accra Psychiatric Hospital: Analysis of child and adolescent psychiatric disorders, August 1974–July 1979. *Association for Child Psychology and Psychiatry News* 14:2–7.

Johnson FYA (1987). Depressive Illness in Nigeria: A Review of Research. *The Journal of Jos University Medical Students Association* 2:43–49.

Kasanin J (1933). The acute schizophrenic psychoses. *American Journal of Psychiatry* 13:97–123.

Lambo TA (1960). Further neuropsychiatric observations in Nigera. *British Medical Journal* ii:1696–1704.

Lambo TA (1974). Psychotherapy in Africa. *Psychotherapy and Psychosomatics* 24:311–326.

Leham JP (1972). Psychopathology of Adolescent Students in Abidjan, Ivory Coast. In *Proceedings of the Third Pan-African Psychiatric Conference in Khartoum, Sudan, 1972.*

Majodina MZ, Johnson FYA (1983). Standardized Assessment of Depressive Disorders (SADD) in Ghana. *British Journal of Psychiatry* 143:442–446.

Morakinyo O (1980). A psychophysiological theory of a psychiatric illness (The Brain Fag Syndrome) associated with study among Africans. *Journal of Nervous Mental Disorders* 168, 84.

Odejide AO, Oyewunmi LK, Ohaeri JU (1989). Psychiatry in Africa: An overview. *American Journal of Psychiatry* 146:708–716.

Olatawura MO (1973). The problems of diagnosing depression in Nigeria. *Psychopathologie Africaine* IX:389–403.

Prince R (1960). The Brain Fag syndrome in Nigerian students. *Journal of Mental Science* 106:559–570.

Rahim ETA (1972). Epidemiology of neurosis in Sudan. In *Proceedings of the Third Pan-African Psychiatric Conference in Khartoum, Sudan, 1972.*

Rutter M (1965). Classification and Categorization in Child Psychiatry. *Journal of Child Psychology and Psychiatry* 6:71–83.

Sartorius N, Jablensky A, Gulbinat W (1980). Application of WHO scales for the assessment of depressive states in different cultures. In Epidemiological Research as Basis for the Organization of Extramural Psychiatry. *Acta Psychiatrica Scandinavica.* 62:205–211 (suppl 285).

Spock J (1988). Classification of schizoaffective disorder. *Comprehensive Psychiatry* 29:55–71.

Swift CR, Gosling R (1973). Psychiatric patterns of Tanzanian students. *African Journal of Medical Science* 4:447–452.

Thebaud E, Rigamer EF (1972). Some considerations on Student Mental Health in Liberia. In *Proceedings of the Third Pan-African Psychiatric Conference in Khartoum, Sudan, 1972.*

World Health Organization (1967). Section V: Mental Disorders. In *International Classification of Diseases* (8th rev). World Health Organization, Geneva.

World Health Organization (1978). Section V: Mental Disorders including Glossary. In *International Classification of Diseases* (9th rev). World Health Organization, Geneva.

# 8
# On the Second Edition of the Chinese Classification of Mental Disorders (CCMD-II)

YUCUN SHEN

Illness classification has a long tradition in China. In line with this, the classification of mental disorders in this country is based on a rich cultural heritage. The first edition of the modern Chinese Classification of Mental Disorders (CCMD) was prepared by a specialized committee of the Chinese Medical Association (1985). Its fundamental features were described by Shen et al (1988).

## Preparation of the Second Edition of the Chinese Classification (CCMD-II)

A Task Force on Classification and Diagnostic Criteria of Mental Disorders was organized in 1986 by the Neuropsychiatric Branch of the Chinese Medical Association. Twenty-four leading psychiatrists of China were appointed as members or consultants of this Task Force. The main program of this Task Force were to revise the Chinese Classification of Mental Disorders and update the knowledge derived from related scientific investigations, and to work out operational diagnostic criteria for major mental disorders (see Table 8.1).

The urgent need to revise CCMD-I (1984 version) came from the requirements of psychiatric clinics and research activities within China because the disease patterns of mental disorders had undergone great changes in the past 10 years since urbanization in China. Stimulus for revision also came from abroad, as remarkable achievements had been made in the classification of mental disorders at the international level, such as DSM-III-R (American Psychiatric Association 1987) and ICD-10 (World Health Organization 1989).

Through three years of intensive effort, the Task Force in collaboration with a wide range of psychiatric professionals drafted a new classification

TABLE 8.1. Chinese Classification of Mental Disorder, 2nd Edition (CCMD-II) authorized by the Chinese Medical Association, Neuropsychiatric Branch.

| | |
|---|---|
| 00 | Organic mental disorders and mental disorders caused by physical diseases (F0) |
| 01 | Alzheimer's disease and mental disorders caused by other cerebral degenerative diseases (F00, F02) |
| 01.0 | Alzheimer's disease (F00) |
| 01.00 | Alzheimer's disease, senile type (F00.1) |
| 01.01 | Alzheimer's disease, presenile type (F00.0) |
| 01.02 | Alzheimer's disease, atypical or mixed type (F00.2) |
| 01.1 | Pick's disease (F02.0) |
| 01.2 | Creuzfeldt–Jakob's disease (F02.1) |
| 01.3 | Huntington's disease (F02.2) |
| 01.4 | Parkinson's disease (F02.3) |
| 01.9 | Other cerebral degenerative diseases |
| 02 | Mental disorders caused by cerebral vascular diseases (F01) |
| 02.0 | Mental disorders after brain stroke (F01.0) |
| 02.1 | Multi-infarct dementia (F01.1) |
| 02.2 | Mental disorders caused by subcortical vascular diseases (F01.2) |
| 02.9 | Mental disorders caused by other cerebrovascular diseases (F01.8) |
| 03 | Mental disorders caused by intracranial and physical infections (F06) |
| 04 | Mental disorders caused by brain injury (F05) |
| 05 | Mental disorders caused by intracranial tumor (F06) |
| 07 | Mental disorders caused by epilepsy (F06) |
| 08 | Mental disorders caused by visceral organ diseases (F06) |
| 09 | Mental disorders caused by other brain or physical diseases (F09) |
| (The three digit code) | |
| 0 | Disturbance of consciousness |
| 1 | Psychotic syndrome |
| 2 | Amnestic syndrome |
| 3 | Personality change |
| 4 | Dementia |
| 5 | Neurotic syndrome |
| 9 | Other mental disorder syndrome |
| 10 | Mental disorders caused by psychoactive substance use (F1) |
| 11 | Mental disorders caused by alcohol (F10) |
| 12 | Mental disorders caused by opium and related substances (F11, F14) |
| 13 | Mental disorders caused by sedatives and hypnotics (F13) |
| 14 | Mental disorders caused by analgesics and aenesthetics (other than opioids) |
| 15 | Mental disorders caused by stimulants intoxication (F15) |
| 16 | Mental disorders caused by multipsychoactive substances intoxication (F19) |
| 19 | Mental disorders caused by other psychoactive substance use (specify in the four digit code) (F16, F18, F19) |
| (The three digit code) | |
| 0 | Acute intoxication |
| 1 | Psychotic state |
| 2 | Amnestic syndrome |
| 3 | Personality change |
| 4 | Dementia |
| 5 | Neurotic syndrome |

TABLE 8.1. *Continued.*

| | |
|---|---|
| 6 | Subacute intoxication |
| 7 | Dependence |
| 8 | Withdrawal syndrome |
| 9 | Other syndrome |
| 20 | Schizophrenia (F20) |
| 21 | Schizophrenia, hebephrenic type (F20.1) |
| 22 | Schizophrenia, catatonic type (F20.2) |
| 23 | Schizophrenia, paranoid type (F20.0) |
| 24 | Schizophrenia, undifferentiated type (20.3) |
| 25 | Schizophrenia, simple type (20.6) |
| 26 | Atypical schizophrenia |
| 26.0 | Schizophreniform psychosis (F23.2) |
| 26.1 | Postschizophrenic depression (F20.4) |
| 27 | Schizophrenia, residual type (F20.5) |
| 28 | Schizophrenia, deteriorated type |
| 29 | Other types of schizophrenia (F20.8) |
| 30 | Affective (mood) disorders (F3) |
| 31 | Manic episode (single episode) (F30) |
| 32 | Depression |
| 32.0 | Depression, single episode (F32) |
| 32.1 | Depression, recurrent (F33) |
| 33 | Bipolar affective disorder (F31) |
| 33.0 | Bipolar affective disorder, manic phase (F31.0–F31.5) |
| 33.1 | Bipolar affective disorder, depressive phase (F31.3–F31.5) |
| 33.2 | Bipolar affective disorder, mixed phase (F31.6) |
| 33.9 | Other bipolar affective disorders (F31.8) |
| 40 | Paranoid disorders (F22) |
| 41 | Paranoia (F22.0) |
| 42 | Acute delusional disorders (F23) |
| 43 | Paranoid psychosis (F22.8) |
| 50 | Psychophysiological disorders,† neuroses,* and psychogenic mental disorders |
| (51–53) | Psychophysiological disorders |
| 51 | Eating disorders (F50) |
| 51.0 | Anorexia nervosa (F50.0) |
| 51.1 | Bulimia nervosa (F50.1) |
| 51.2 | Nervous vomiting |
| 52 | Sleep and wakening disorders (F51) |
| 52.0 | Insomnia (F51.0) |
| 52.1 | Hypersomnia (F51.1) |
| 52.2 | Sleep walking (F51.3) |
| 53 | Sexual dysfunctions (F52) |
| 53.0 | Sexual hypoactivity or loss of sexual desire (F52.0) |
| 53.1 | Erective disorder (impotence) (F52.2) |

*Continued*

TABLE 8.1. *Continued.*

| | |
|---|---|
| 53.2 | Premature ejaculation (F52.4) |
| 53.3 | Orgasmic dysfunction (F52.3) |
| 53.4 | Vaginismus (F52.5) |
| 53.5 | Dyspareunia (F52.6) |
| 53.9 | Other sexual dysfunctions (F52.9) |
| (54–56) | Neuroses |
| 54 | Hysteria (F44) |
| 54.0 | Hysterical mental diorder (dissociative hysteria) |
| 54.1 | Hysterical somatic dysfunction (conversion hysteria) |
| 55 | Neuroses with anxiety |
| 55.0 | Anxiety neurosis (F41) |
| 55.00 | Generalized anxiety disorder (F41.1) |
| 55.01 | Panic disorders (F41.0) |
| 55.1 | Obsessive–compulsive disorder (F42) |
| 55.2 | Phobia (F40) |
| 56 | Other types of neurosis (F48.0) |
| 56.0 | Depressive neurosis |
| 56.1 | Hypochondriac neurosis (F45.2) |
| 56.2 | Neurasthenia (F48.8) |
| 56.3 | Other neuroses (F48.8) |
| (57–59) | Psychogenic disorders |
| 57 | Reactive mental disorders (F43.0) |
| 57.0 | Acute psychogenic reaction (F43.0) |
| 57.1 | Delayed psychogenic reaction |
| 57.2 | Persistent psychogenic reaction (F43.1) |
| 57.3 | Neurotic reaction |
| 57.4 | Adjustment reaction (F43.2) |
| 57.9 | Other reactive mental disorders (F48.3) |
| 58 | Induced psychosis (F24) |
| 59 | Mental disorders closely related to the culture |
| 59.0 | *Koro* |
| 59.1 | Eastern-gymnastic-exercise-induced mental disorders |
| 59.2 | Mental disorders closely related to superstitions or witchcraft |
| 59.9 | Other mental disorders closely related to cultural background |
| 60 | Personality disorders and psychosexual disorders (F6) |
| 61 | Personality disorders (F60) |
| 61.0 | Antisocial personality disorder (F60.2) |
| 61.1 | Impulsive personality disorder (F60.3) |
| 61.2 | Paranoid personality disorder (F60.0) |
| 61.3 | Schizoid personality disorder (F60.1) |
| 61.4 | Anankastic personality disorder (F60.5) |
| 61.5 | Histrionic personality disorder (F60.4) |
| 61.9 | Other personality disorders (F60.8) |
| 62 | Psychosexual disorders |
| 62.0 | Homosexuality (F66.x1) |
| 62.1 | Transvestic fetishism (F65.1) |
| 62.2 | Transsexualism (F64.0) |
| 62.3 | Exhibitionism (F65.2) |
| 62.4 | Voyeurism (F65.3) |
| 62.5 | Fetishism (F65.0) |
| 62.9 | Other psychosexual disorders (F65.8) |

TABLE 8.1. *Continued.*

| | |
|---|---|
| 70 | Mental retardation (F7) |
| 71 | Mild mental retardation (F70) |
| 72 | Moderate mental retardation (F71) |
| 73 | Severe mental retardation (F72) |
| 74 | Profound mental retardation (F73) |
| 79 | Other unspecified mental retardation (F78, F79) |
| 80 | Mental disorders in childhood and adolescence‡ (F8, F9) |
| 81 | Child psychosis (F84) |
| 82 | Emotional disorders in childhood (F93) |
| 82.0 | Separation anxiety (F93.0) |
| 83 | Hyperactive syndrome (attention defects disorder) (F80) |
| 84 | Conduct disorder (F91) |
| 85 | Specific developmental disorders (F8) |
| 85.0 | Language and speech developmental disorder (F80) |
| 85.1 | Academic skill developmental disorder (F81) |
| 85.2 | Motor skill developmental disorder (F82) |
| 85.3 | Mixed developmental disorder (F83) |
| 85.9 | Other specific developmental disorders (F88) |
| 86 | Other conduct disorders of childhood or adolescence (F98) |
| 86.0 | Excretion disorders (F98.0, F98.1) |
| 86.00 | Functional enuresis (F98.0) |
| 86.01 | Functional encopresis (F98.1) |
| 86.1 | Eating disorders (F98.2) |
| 86.10 | Pica of childhood (F98.3) |
| 86.2 | Sleep disorders |
| 86.20 | Night terror |
| 86.3 | Stuttering (F98.5) |
| 86.4 | Tic disorders (F98.5) |
| 86.9 | Other unspecified conduct disorders (F98.8) |
| 90 | Other mental disorders and metal health related problems |
| 91 | Schizoaffective psychosis (F25) |
| 91.0 | Schizo-manic psychosis (F25.0) |
| 91.1 | Schizo-depressive psychosis (F25.1) |
| 92 | Periodic psychosis (F29) |
| 99.0 | Other unspecified psychotic disorders (F28) |
| 99.1 | Other unspecified nonpsychotic disorders |
| 99.9 | Mental health related problems |
| 99.90 | No mental disorder |
| 99.91 | Malingering |
| 99.92 | Borderline psychosis (F29) |
| 99.93 | Borderline intellectual functioning |
| 99.94 | Suicide |

Note. Numbers within parentheses after diagnostic term correspond to ICD-10 code.
* The term Neuroses was kept instead of Neurotic Disorders (F4 of ICD-10).
† The term Psychophysiological Disorders was used in CCMD-II instead of Behaviour Syndromes And Mental Disorders Associated with Physiological Dysfunction (F5 ICD-10).
‡ F8, F9 of ICD-10 were combined into one category under the heading, Mental Disorders in Childhood and Adolescence.

system. The feasibility of the draft was clinically tested in 77 mental health institutions with 22,285 patients in outpatient clinics and 8061 cases in inpatient wards.

This revised version, CCMD-II, was then adopted by the steering committee of the Psychiatric Branch, Chinese Medical Association (1989). A listing of its categories is presented in Table 8.1.

## Organization and Content of CCMD-II

The revised version consists of nine categories similar to those in ICD-10, yet the structure of each category was not always the same as in ICD-10. The main principles adopted during the formulation of the CCMD-II were to keep as close as possible to the ICD-10 classification system to facilitate international communication, while trying to maintain the traditional nosological approach as much as possible. Sometimes this effort proved very difficult.

The similarities and differences between ICD-10 and CCMD-II are as follows:

The following five categories of ICD-10 are categorized very similarly in CCMD-II: F0, Organic, Including Symptomatic, Mental Disorders; F1, Mental and Behavior Disorder Due to Psychoactive and Other Substance Use; F3, Mood (Affective) Disorders; F6, Disorders of Adult Personality and Behavior, and F7, Mental Retardation.

Schizophrenia, delusional disorders and induced delusional disorders are considered by Chinese psychiatrists to be heterogeneous in nature. In CCMD-II, Paranoid Disorders are separated from Schizophrenia and categorized as an independent unit as it was in ICD-9 and CCMD-I. Induced delusional disorder as a subgroup was arranged under the category entitled Psychogenic Mental Disorders.

Reactive psychoses have been recognized as a disease entity of psychogenic origin since the 1950s by Chinese psychiatrists. In CCMD-II terminology, Reactive Mental Disorders, were maintained and categorized under the title, Psychogenic Mental Disorders. Under reactive mental disorders the following subgroups were listed: acute psychogenic reaction, delayed psychogenic reaction, persistent psychogenic reaction, neurotic reaction, adjustment reaction, and other reactive mental disorders.

*Koro* is a special mental syndrome, closely related to Chinese culture. Its occurrence was closely related to the idea or doctrine, stated in ancient Chinese traditional medicine, that "shrinking of the penis into the abdomen is a fatal sign." The statement of this mental syndrome had been discovered in the historical literature of Hainan, south of Canton province, written in 1862 to 1864 (Mao et al 1990). In Chinese mental health literature, epidemics of *Koro* were reported in 1962 and 1968 in

Hainan. In one recent epidemic of *Koro* in Hainan and Leizhou of Canton (1984) 3000 to 4000 local inhabitants were attacked. The core symptoms of *Koro* syndrome were acute anxiety and fear of sudden death together with the sensation of the penis shrinking into the abdomen in men or of nipples turning into bread in women (Chen et al 1990). Epidemics of *Koro* were also reported in Singapore (1967), Thailand (1976) and India (1982). Cases were reported in Taiwan and Hong Kong. Chinese ethnic groups were much more affected than other ethnic groups in these regions. This synrome was also listed in CCMD-II as a syndrome of Mental Disorders Closely Related to Culture under the category, Psychogenic Mental Disorder.

Some comments are offered next on the classification of depressive episode, Mood (Affective) Disorders in ICD-10. The principle of classification of depressive episode in ICD-10 is based on severity and characteristics of course (single or recurrent). This was adopted in CCMD-II. Clinical tests of this new system were conducted on 88 cases of functional depression, as compared with the classification system in CCMD-I (corresponding to ICD-9) (Shen et al 1990). It was found that under depressive episodes, different kinds of depression were coded as: reactive, neurotic, and unspecified. That classification is judged insufficient for clinical practice without additional etiological considerations (biological, psychosocial). Therefore, classification systems are recommended to overcome this problem.

## Conclusion

Comments and discussion on the revised classification, CCMD-II, has already begun among Chinese psychiatrists in mental health professional journals. Comments to CCMD-II from professionals abroad would be sincerely appreciated for further improvement of the classification system in China.

## *References*

American Psychiatric Association (1987). *Diagnostic and Statistical Manual of Mental Disorders* (3rd ed, rev). American Psychiatric Association, Washington, DC.

Chen G-Q, et al (1990). Social psychiatry and epidemic Koro: Questionnaire survey in Hainan and Leizhou. *Chinese Mental Health Journal* 4:148.

Chinese Medical Association (1985). Chinese Classification of Mental Disorders (CCMD). *Chinese Neuropsychiatric Journal* 18:317–318.

Chinese Medical Association (1989). Chinese Classification of Mental Disorders, 2nd ed (CCMD-II). Hunan Medical University Press, Hunan, China.

Mao G-M, et al (1990). Social psychiatry and epidemic Koro: Literature review of epidemic Koro. *Chinese Mental Health Journal* 4:145.

Shen Y-C, et al (1988). Principles of the Chinese Classification of Mental Disorders (CCMD). In JE Mezzich, et al (eds), *International Classification in Psychiatry: Unity and Diversity*. Cambridge University Press, Cambridge.
Shen Y-C, Liang S, Dai Z (1990). Common types of depressive disorders in the elderly seen in an outpatient psychiatric clinic. Presented at the International Conference on Psychiatric Diagnosis, *World Psychiatric Association Section in Classification*. September 6 (ICPD'90 Abstract p 36) Tokyo.
World Health Organization, Division of Mental Health (1989). *ICD-10 1989 Draft of Chapter V. Clinical Description and Guidelines*. World Health Organization, Geneva.

# 9
# Perspectives on Psychiatric Diagnosis from Southeast Asia

R. SRINIVASA MURTHY

The mental health professionals of the countries of Southeast Asia have been part of the international efforts to develop national and international classificatory systems. Wig and Sing (1966) proposed a classification of psychiatric disorder for use in India at the time of the *International Classification of Diseases*, 8th revision (ICD-8), World Health Organization (WHO). Wig et al (1985) have summarized the problems of psychiatric diagnosis and classification in the region. In addition, the applicability of the *Diagnostic and Statistical Manual of Mental Disorders*, 3rd edition (DSM-III) (with its strengths and weaknesses) has been considered (Wig 1983, 1990). Another major development in psychiatric diagnosis is the study of phenomenology, course, and outcome of mental disorders in the region (Kapur and Pandurangi 1980, Wig et al 1982, Saxena 1987, 1989a, ICMR 1989b). A further important point is the existence of ancient classification systems in India in the Ayurveda system of health (Dube 1978).

The development of international classification of mental disorders during the last three decades represents systematic efforts to understand the nature of mental disorders and develop a system of professional information sharing. As we enter the last decade of the century, we pass two important milestones. These are (1) a crystallization of international thinking in classification in the form of ICD-10 and (2) a rapid growth in mental health awareness in the developing world. The second development in mental health has major implications, because the developing world represents 80% of the population and their needs are likely to be different from those of the Western world. This aspect forms an important background to this chapter.

International classification has gone through a number of developments from the time of the historic review by Stengel in 1959. His efforts led to a common nomenclature in the form of ICD-8 (WHO 1965) and the development of structured interview schedules like the Present State Examination (PSE), which was followed by the development of a glossary

(1972) with a greater scope for a common "language" for professional communication. The next major effort was international consultations, followed by the field trials of the draft classificators' system (Kramer 1979). These international developments were also reflected in the simultaneous development of the DSM system in the United States. The systematic step-by-step process of the last 30 years of work in the classification system both emphasizes the need for continuous effort and portends the need for systematic efforts in the future. This time point is only a stop point and not the end point. In spite of all the positive developments, there are major hurdles, as Kendell (1988) has pointed out: "Perhaps I should apologise for raising so intently the unresolved issue [of what mental disorder is]. I am convinced, though, that we must start to think more deeply than we have in the past about what we really mean by the term 'mental disorder' which we use so frequently and so readily, and why it is that we have such difficulty defining it adequately or perhaps are so reluctant to try."

These general developments are important for mental health professionals in developing countries. The clarity in classification that is emerging in Western countries (eg, the DSM system in the United States) against a background of well-established systems of care, can be confusing for mental health professionals in developing countries when the reality of work in a developing country is different. Working in a developing country we often identify with the experience noted in DSM-I (1952): "Only about 10% of the total cases seen fell into any of the categories ordinarily seen in public mental hospitals." I discuss here this problem based on my experience of work in the following areas: (1) epidemiology in the general population, (2) primary health care (PHC) work, (3) training of PHC personnel, (4) newer research on schizophrenia/acute psychosis, (5) clinical experience, and (6) review of literature.

## Epidemiological Studies

The prevalence of mental disorders has been studied in more than a dozen centers in India. We have recently completed a major total population survey covering 32,000 people in about 100 villages. The earlier studies categorized the patients seen in the surveys by percentage using the following classification terms: alcohol dependence (70%), schizophrenia (71%), depression (64%), anxiety neurosis (57%), depressive neurosis, hysteria (43%), organic psychosis (36%); in lesser frequency, other ICD categories were used. What is striking is the near paucity of patients diagnosed as belonging to the large number of known categories of ICD system.

In our study, we found the prevalence rates and pattern of mental disorders, as summarized in Table 9.1.

TABLE 9.1. Rural population epidemiology (1990) based on a population of 32,402.

| ICD category | Disorder | Rate/ 1000 | % |
|---|---|---|---|
| 290 | Senile psychosis | 4 | 0.12 |
| 291 | Alcoholic psychosis | 5 | 0.15 |
| 295 | Schizophrenia | 63 | 1.94 |
| 296 | Affective psychoses | 42 | 1.20 |
| 297 | Paranoid states | 4 | 0.12 |
| 300 | Neuroses | 149 | 4.59 |
| 302 | Sexual deviation | 1 | 0.03 |
| 303 | Alcohol dependence | 275 | 8.48 |
| 305 | Nondependent use of drugs | 109 | 3.36 |
| 307 | Special symptoms | 512 | 15.80 |
| 312–315 | Childhood disorders | 61 | 1.87 |
| 317–318 | Mental retardation | 121 | 3.67 |
| 345 | Epilepsy | 404 | 12.46 |
| | Other | 5 | 0.15 |
| | Total | 1,757 | 54.22 |

It is salient to note the near absence of sexual disorders and personality disorders, and the high proportion of those with special symptoms under ICD-9 category 307. The question is: Is this a reflection of a true difference in the pattern of mental disorders? Against the background of data available from India, it is necessary to take note of this possibility in future investigations.

## Mental Disorders in Primary Health Care

Currently, most of the developing countries have extremely limited mental health care facilities. Consequently, those who have mental disorders either live in the community or seek help from general health facilities. A series of studies has been carried out using accepted methodology to find out the nature and the extent of mental disorders at PHCs. The rates vary from 14% (Harding et al 1980) to 10% (Sriram et al 1987), and has been considered in detail elsewhere in this volume (Srinivasa Murthy).

An observation made by the investigators of these studies was that the patients present clinically diagnostic problems. Most of them do not fit into a known category and present wide and varying symptoms. This has led to the consideration of their problems as psychosocial distress syndrome, emotional distress syndrome, and functional complaints, descriptive terms like psychalgia, myalgia, sexual neurosis, and so forth have been used. The classificatory system for this group has to be different from that for the mental health specialists (Srinivasa Murthy in this volume). This need is all the more urgent in developing countries where the beginnings of mental health care are occurring primarily at the primary health care level of the health care system. In other words, fulfilling this need is urgent for countries of Southeast Asia more than for those in the West. The acceptance of the mental health concepts by PHC personnel could largely depend on the classificatory system developed and its ease of application.

## Training of the PHC Personnel

As a part of the community-based mental health care in developing countries, the PHC personnel form the main care providers. Experience has shown that they would not be able to use a classificatory system of more than half a dozen categories. Our own experience and that of others involved in training, as reflected in the manuals for PHC personnel, emphasize this point (Table 9.2). A required classificatory system should be one small in number of categories, simple to use, and related to care provision at the PHC level.

## Newer Research into Psychiatric Syndromes

The WHO contributed to the international awareness of the universality of schizophrenia as well as to the differences in the pattern of symptoms and course of the disorder throughout countries (IPSS 1978). A recently completed study in India has reported varied presentation of schizophrenia in three centers in India and confirmed the good prognosis over the 5-year follow-up period. If these two observations are accepted, the need for differential diagnostic criteria will follow. Let me illustrate this point. In the ICMR study (ICMR 1989a) the inclusion criteria were modified to use 3 months as duration of illness and to drop marital status as a variable to suit the study needs. As part of the WHO field trial of ICD-10, the nine Indian centers have emphasized the need for (1) inclusion of catatonic symptoms and (2) decreased emphasis on first-rank symptoms and greater importance of Bleulerian symptoms. There is an emerging con-

TABLE 9.2. Commonly used diagnostic categories in the manuals of mental health for PHC personnel.

| Category |
|---|
| Psychoses, acute and chronic |
| Neuroses |
| Mental retardation |
| Childhood disorders |
| Alcoholism |
| Epilepsy |
| Emergencies |

sensus to consider schizophrenia in India in this light. Studies from other developing countries could throw light on other aspects of schizophrenia, such as the frequency of first rank symptoms and so forth.

Another example is the studies of acute psychosis (Kapur and Pandurangi 1979, Singh and Sachdev 1980, ICMR 1989b). Of these studies, the ICMR study is the most recent and has played a role toward inclusion of this category under F.23 in ICD-10. The findings of this study led to the recognition of a category other than schizophrenia and affective psychoses. The presentation of acute psychosis, with its early recognition, regular treatment, and good outcome has significant public health implications for the mental health professionals in developing countries. This development can contribute to the larger goal of integrating mental health with primary health care.

The trance states, as part of religious experiences, have been traditionally viewed as a hysterical phenomenon with psychodynamic explanations. Recent studies of Simons et al (1988) and Ervin et al (1988) from Malayasia support the possibility of an organic state in the form of an altered state of mind at the limbic system level with associated biochemical changes. Similar is the *latah* paradox (Simons and Hughes 1985) which appears now to arise from a heightened reaction patern to sudden stimulus and the social response and to it. These limited experiences and newer attempts to understand them emphasize the need to avoid "transferring" in this region passively the diagnostic systems across countries and cultures.

## Conclusion

Collated experience in Southeast Asia emphasizes the following points: (1) a more practical classification is needed in this region and in other developing countries to meet the differing presentation of mental disorders, and (2) mental health activities need to be integrated with primary health care. A better classification is needed for mental health professionals, and for primary health personnel to understand the magnitude and the nature of disorders. All of these points are important and should be seen as complementary. This is not to say that international classification is not relevant, but to emphasize the need for both international consensus and opportunities forr national classifications.

## *References*

Dube KC (1978). Nosology and therapy of mental illness in Ayurveda. *Comparative Medicine East and West* VI:250–259.

Ervin FR, Palmour RM, Pearson BE, Prince RA, Simons RC (1988). The psychobiology of Trance-II. *Transcultural Psychiatric Research Review* 25: 267–284.

Harding TW, de Arango MV, Baltazar J, Climent CE, Ibrahim AHA, Ignacio LL, Srinivasa Murthy R, Wig N (1980). Mental disorders in primary health care: A study of their frequency and diagnosis in four developing countries. *Psychological Medicine* 10:231–241.

Indian Council of Medical Research (1989a). Study of course and outcome of schizophrenia—a five year follow-up study. *ICMR*, New Delhi, India.

Indian Council of Medical Research (1989b). The phenomenology and natural history of acute psychosis: Report of a collaborative study at Bikaner, Goa, Patiala, Vellore. *ICMR*, New Delhi, India.

Kapur RL, Pandurangi AK (1979). A comparative study of reactive psychosis and acute psychosis without precipitating stress. *British Journal of Psychiatry* 133:544–560.

Kendell RE (1988). Priorities for the next decade. In JE Mezzich, M von Cranach (eds), *International Classification in Psychiatry: Unity and Diversity*. Cambridge University Press, Cambridge.

Kramer M (1979). The ICD-9 classification of mental disorders: A review of its development and contents. *Acta Psychiatrica Scandinavica* 59:241–262.

Mezzich J, Von Kranach M (eds) (1988). *International Classification in Psychiatry: Unity and Diversity*. Cambridge University Press, Cambridge.

Saxena S (1987). Simple dissociative disorder. A subcategory in DSM-III-R (Letter to Editor). *American Journal of Psychiatry* 144:524–525.

Simons RC, Ervin FR, Prince RH (1988). The psychobiology of trance-I. *Transcultural Psychiatric Research Review* 25:249–266.

Simons RC, Hughes CC (1985). *Culture-Bound Syndromes*. Reidel, Boston.

Singh G, Sachdev JS (1980). A clinical and follow up study of atypical psychosis. *Indian Journal of Psychiatry* 22:167–172.

Sriram TG, Kumar K, Moily S, Chandrasekhar CR, Isaac MK, Srinivasa Murthy R (1987). Minor psychiatric disturbances in primary health care: A study of their prevalence and characteristics using a simple case detection technique. *Indian Journal of Social Psychiatry* 3:212–226.

Stengel R (1959). Classification of mental disorders. *Bulletin of the World Health Organization* 21:601–663.

Wig NN (1983). DSM-III—Its strengths and weaknesses: A perspective from the third world. In RL Spitzer, IBW Williams, AE Skodol (eds), *International perspectives on DSM-III*. American Psychiatric Press, Washington, DC.

Wig NN (1990). Third world perspective on diagnosis and classification. In N Sartorius, A Jablensky, DA Regier, JD Burke, RMA Hirshfield (eds), *Sources and Traditions of Classification in Psychiatry*. Hogrefe & Huber, Toronto.

Wig NN, Mangalwedhe K, Bedi H, Srinivasa Murthy R (1982). A follow-up study of hysteria. *Indian Journal of Psychiatry* 24:120–125.

Wig NN, Setyonegoro K, Shen Yu Cun, Sell H (1985). Problems of psychiatric diagnosis and classification in the third world. In *Mental Disorders, Alcohol and Drug-Related Problems: International Perspective on Their Diagnosis and Classification*. Excerpta Medica International Congress 669:50–60.

Wig NN, Singh GA (1966). A proposed classification of psychiatric disorders for use in India. *Indian Journal of Psychiatry* 9:158–171.

World Health Organization (1978). Report of the International pilot study of schizophrenia, vol 2. WHO, World Health Organization, Geneva.

# 10
# Japanese Experiences in Psychiatric Diagnosis

## A. Overview of Japanese Experience in Diagnostic Classification: Past and Present Classification of Mental Disorders in Japan

Akira Fujinawa

The development of modern Japanese psychiatry began after the Meiji Reformation in 1868. A new classification of mental disorders was developed that did not follow not the traditional diagnostic procedures from the preceding Edo Era, from 1603 to 1867. This was because modern Japanese psychiatry, as was the case with other medical specialities, was based on modern European medicine, which was introduced in translated forms.

This movement was initiated by the translation of the textbook of Maudslay, a British psychiatrist. The Meiji government subsequently decided that the Japanese legal, military, and medical systems should follow those of Germany. In the late period of the Edo Era, some Japanese physicians studied the medicine of Netherlands, the only European country whose people were permitted to enter Japan. Some Japanese physicians already realized, before the Meiji Reformation, that the origins of Dutch medicine resided in Germany. The government invited German professors to Japan so that they could teach German medicine directly to Japanese students.

In 1886, a Psychiatric Section was founded in the Medical Depart-ment of the Tokyo Imperial University, which was later renamed Tokyo University. The first professor of medicine was Hajime Sakaki; he lived from 1857 to 1897, and was a contemporary of Emil Kraepelin. Sakaki studied in Germany from 1882 to 1886, under Westfal and Mendel. After returning to Japan, he became the director of psychiatry at Tokyo University. He created a classification and diagnostic system of mental diseases and started statistical research based on it.

His work was carried on by Shuhzoh Kure, his successor. We could say that it was Kure who really established Japanese psychiatry, in clinical practice as well as research. He studied in Heidelberg, Vienna, and Paris from 1897 to 1901. Kure immediately grasped the value of Kraepelin's research, which had just become systematized, and through his efforts ensured that it had a long-standing influence in Japan. Kraepelin was a professor at Heidelberg when Kure was studying there. During that period, Kraepelin prepared the fifth edition of his famous textbook of psychiatry and constructed the dichotomous theory of dementia praecox and manic-depressive psychosis.

It should be noted that the starting point of Japanese psychiatry corresponded to the period when European psychiatry was just developing and was based on modern scientific principles. After Kure, a number of Japanese psychiatrists studied in Germany and France and witnessed the contemporary evolution of European psychiatry. Thus the history of the nosological development of Japanese psychiatry is in line with the history of modern European psychiatry.

Kraepelin's theory was sometimes a target of criticism even in Germany, although the majority of opinion always supported him. Similarly, in Japan there were several schools that held different views from those held at Tokyo University. One example is the Kyoto University school, which originated with Shin'ichi Imamura. He graduated from Tokyo University and studied in Germany and Austria from 1899 to 1903 under Obersteiner. After returning to Japan he was appointed first professor of psychiatry at Kyoto University and remained in that position for nearly 40 years. In 1916 he went to Paris for further study.

Although Imamura accepted Kraepelin's theory, he was also interested in the theories of Wernicke, Kleist, and several French psychiatrists. He tried to integrate them to create his own concept of mental disease entities, which differed from the theories of Tokyo University.

One of the chief characteristics of the Kyoto group was their refusal of the dichotomous view of endogenous psychosis. Instead, they introduced the notion of atypical psychosis and created a trichotomous view. The concept of atypical psychosis, similar to the theory of periodic psychosis by Leonhard, was developed from the empirical data of their genetic research.

Another school that proposed nosological concepts was that directed by Chitani. He adopted the theory of mono-psychosis of Neuman and Griesinger. The school of Masatake Morita created its own theory concerning a certain type of neurosis particular to Japan, namely Taijin-Kyofoshu, a kind of social phobia.

These different concepts never replaced Kraepelin's theory as the major basis of Japanese psychiatry. However, it is obvious that they made a great contribution by providing a sophisticated and flexible way of thinking that supplemented the major classification system.

It was only after World War II that the influence of American psychiatry reached Japan. The psychodynamic school of psychiatry was widely accepted in the United States from 1940 to 1960. Although this model was introduced into Japan soon after the war, it did not result in a change in the diagnostic system. Essential classification categories remained within the framework proposed by Kraepelin.

It should be noted that Kurt Schneider's concept of clinical psychopathology has had a strong influence on a considerable number of Japanese psychiatrists. The first-rank symptoms were widely accepted just after their first publication.

In the process of developing ICD-8 and 9, Masaki Kato, a former director of the National Institute of Mental Health of Japan participated as Japan's representative. The ICD-8 and the ICD-9 were adopted by the Ministry of Health and Welfare of Japan as a tool for compiling statistics on mental disorders.

During the 1960s when most young psychiatrists lost interest in descriptive classification, efforts to improve diagnostic procedures were maintained among biologically oriented psychiatrists. They sought a standard classification system that could be shared and used internationally. It was this group of psychiatrists that responded immediately when the *Diagnostic and Statistical Manual of Mental Disorders*, 3rd edition (DSM-III) was published by the American Psychiatric Association.

They formed a discussion group, The Clinical Use of DSM-III in Japan, and a working group, The Adaptation and the Clinical Examination of DSM-III. The latter developed in 1981 into the Japenese Society for International Diagnostic Criteria in Psychiatry (JSIDCP).

After the revision of the Mental Health Act in 1988, the Ministry of Health and Welfare of Japan asked the author to chair a committee on the Development of Diagnostic Criteria for Mental Disorders in Japan. After 3 years of cooperative work by the committee and 20 psychiatric specialists, we completed the translation of the Japanese version of the *International Classification of Diseases*, 10th revision (ICD-10), a nationwide field trial of it, and the preparation of the Japanese Clinical Modification of the draft of ICD-10.

During these procedures it was found that the ICD-10 has a fairly high clinical reliability. Nevertheless, several problems emerged that may be specific to Japan. Some of these are discussed in other contributions in this section.

# B. Mental Disorders Related to Substance Use in Japan

NOBUKATSU KATOH AND KATSUMASA MIYASATO

In the *International Classification of Diseases*, 10th revision (ICD-10) draft (1989), mental and behavioral disorders caused by psychoactive and other substances are specified by 3-digit codes. These disorders are classified into the following 10 categories (F10–19) by substance: alcohol, opioids, cannabinoids, sedatives or hypnotics, cocaine, other stimulants (including caffeine), hallucinogens, volatile solvents, multiple drugs, and other. The clinical symptoms are further specified by 4- and 5-digit codes, and are classified into 10 categories, from acute intoxication to mental or behavioral disorders induced by alcohol or drugs, unspecified (Fix. 0–9).

Controversy still remains about how this draft conforms to DSM-III-R, and the differences between this draft and conventional classification.

## Terminology

It is necessary to arrange many kinds of technical terms—general–objective, habitual, and pharmacological terms. There is still controversy concerning the use of such terms as drugs, substance, psychoactive substance, and alcohol. No clear reason is given why in this draft such a conventional term as "abuse" is excluded.

## Disorders Resulting from the Use of Alcohol

These are included within two categories: (1) a syndrome induced by other drugs, and (2) an independent syndrome often symptomatologically dealt with from the historical standpoint of alcohol, where alcohol is regarded as not a drug but as a luxury good, reflecting the variety of psychiatric studies. The subclassifications considering this point and *delirium tremens* are appreciable. Because the symptomatological characteristics of other drugs are not sufficiently shown, it is necessary to consider this point.

Although few more modifications seemed possible, we wish to refer to our comments about ICD-10, and show our fundamental concept and the outline of our classification in the process of formulating the *Japanese Clinical Modification* (JCM).

## Disorders Resulting from the Use of Psychoactive Substances

The following major modifications were made in JCM (Table 10B.1): (1) the title was simplified; (2) for clinical convenience, the system conforming to *Diagnostic and Statistical Manual of Mental Disorders*, 3rd edition, revised (DSM-III-R) was used; (3) description only of the diagnostic criteria was given; (4) anxiolytics were included in the sedative and hypnotic subcategories; (5) psychotic conditions closely related to the psychoactive substance use were mentioned in each substance item.

Following are the most distinct differences between JCM and ICD-10. The classification was made according to the types of pathogenetic substances. The disorder resulting from the use of amphetamine was adopted based on the special social situation in Japan. Disorders resulting from the use of caffeine and the multipsychoactive substances were classified as independent categories. The classification according to type of psychoactive substance and the clinical condition are included under disorders resulting from the use of alcohol.

Disorders resulting from the use of alcohol (Table 10B.2) are:

1. Acute alcoholic intoxication: Diagnostic criteria are (a) recent ingestion of alcohol (without evidence suggesting that the amount is insufficient to cause intoxication in most people); (b) maladaptive behavioral changes (eg, lack of inhibition of sexual or aggressive impulses, mood lability, impaired judgment, impaired social or occupational functioning; (c) at least one of the following signs: slurred speech, lack of coordination, unsteady gait, nystagmus, flushed face; (d) not a result of any physical or other mental disorders.

TABLE 10B.1. Japanese Clinical Modification draft (1989), psychoactive substance use disorders.

| Disorder resulting from use of |
|---|
| 1. Alcohol |
| 2. Opioids |
| 3. Cannabinoids |
| 4. Sedatives or hypnotics |
| 5. Cocaine |
| △6. Amphetamines |
| △7. Caffeine |
| 8. Hallucinogens |
| 9. Tobacco |
| 10. Volatile solvents |
| 11. Other and unidentified substances |
| △12. Multiple psychoactive substances |

Note. △, central nervous system stimulant.

TABLE 10B.2. Subclassification of disorders resulting from use of alcohol (Japanese Clinical Modification).

| Subclassification |
|---|
| 1. Alcohol acute intoxication |
| 2. Alcohol idiosyncratic intoxication |
| 3. Alcohol abuse |
| 4. Alcohol dependence syndrome |
| 5. Alcohol withdrawal state |
| 6. Alcohol withdrawal delirium |
| 7. Alcohol hallucinosis |
| 8. Alcohol amnestic disorder |
| 9. Alcohol dementia |
| 10. Other disorders induced by alcohol |

2. Other disorders resulting from the use of alcohol are alcoholic idiosyncratic intoxication, alcohol abuse, alcoholic dependence syndrome, alcoholic withdrawal state, alcoholic withdrawal delirium, alcoholic hallucinosis, alcoholic amnestic disorder, alcoholic dementia, and other or unspecified alcoholic disorder.

Disorders resulting from the use of other substances were similarly classified according to the types of pathogenetic substances, such as opioids, cannabinoids, sedatives or hypnotics; disorders resulting from the use of cocaine, amphetamines, caffeine, hallucinogens, tobacco, and volatile solvents; and disorders resulting from multiple drug use and use of other and unidentified substances.

In Japan, there are many cases of mental disorders that result from the abuse of methamphetamines after the Second World War. We classified these as acute intoxication, abuse, dependence, withdrawal state, delirium, hallucinatory–delusional disorder and other mental disorders. We classified disorders resulting from the use of caffeine into the two items of caffeine intoxication and other mental disorders. On the other hand, disorders resulting from the use of tobacco were classified into nicotine dependence, nicotine withdrawal state, and other mental disorders.

## Tasks for Further Clarification

As mentioned earlier, several unsettled problems in the ICD-10 still remain, and we drew up our Japanese diagnostic criteria with this fact in mind.

We continue to coordinate the differences between ICD-10, DSM-III-R, and JCM, and to discriminate between common worldwide subjects and specific situations in each country. The cases particular to a given country are most correctly and distinctly diagnosed by the diagnostic criteria of each country. Compatibility with ICD-10 should always be maintained.

## *References*

American Psychiatric Association (1987). *Diagnostic and Statistical Manual of Mental Disorders* (3rd ed, rev). American Psychiatric Association, Washington, DC.

World Health Organization (1989). *ICD-10 1989 Draft of Chapter V Categories F00–F99*. World Health Organization, Geneva.

# C. Diagnostic Classification of Psychotic Disorders in Japan

SABURO TAKAHASHI

Two outstanding features in Japanese psychiatry that have occurred since the introduction of *Diagnostic and Statistical Manual of Mental Disorders*, 3rd edition (DSM-III) will be discussed here. One is the impact of DSM-III, the other is the issue of definition of atypical psychosis.

## Impact of DSM-III in Japan

Until the publication of DSM-III in 1980, Japanese psychiatry did not appear to have much interest in the international classification and standardization of nomenclature of mental disorders. After DSM-III was introduced by our group (Takahashi et al 1982), it was somewhat enthusiastically accepted by many younger Japanese psychiatrists, and the trend changed toward positive use of international diagnostic systems, such as the forthcoming *International Classification of Diseases*, 10th revision (ICD-10).

Based on my own clinical experience in psychiatry for more than 30 years, diagnostic disagreement has been observed on many different occasions. However, Japanese psychiatrists seemed to have neglected this issue until we conducted a multi-institutional study of DSM-III diagnoses as compared with Japanese conventional diagnoses.

A project team, supported by a grant-in-aid from the Japanese Ministry of Education, was organized by the members of Japanese Society for the International Diagnostic Criteria in Psychiatry (JSIDCP), of which the author served as the head. We conducted research into basic issues of psychiatric diagnosis, such as agreement in diagnosis between ICD-9 and DSM-III, and reliability of use with videotaped materials, involving more than 100 clinicians from 7 institutions (Hanada and Takahashi 1982, Hanada et al 1982, Hanada and Takahashi 1983a, Takahashi et al 1982).

As shown in Table 10C.1, DSM-III diagnosis had a good reliability index, with an overall K of 0.80, which was better than 0.75, the value when using conventional diagnosis. Of several categories, K for schizophrenia and affective disorders were higher than K for other categories. A much lower K was obtained for ICD-9 other nonorganic psychosis (0.43) than the value for DSM-III psychotic disorders NOS (0.82) (Hanada and Takahashi 1983a, 1983b).

Another interesting fact was obtained through video study: diagnostic reliability vs clinical experiences in years. Difference between the K for DSM-III diagnosis and the one for conventional diagnosis was large when clinicians have little clinical experience (K = 0.79), and diagnostic skills appeared to reach a plateau (K = 0.84) after 4 years of training (Hanada and Takahashi 1982, Hanada and Takahashi 1983a) (Table 10C.2).

Our results indicate that a diagnostic system such as DSM-III, with clear descriptions of operational criteria, is very useful. Even clinicians trained many years before publication of DSM-III, improved their diagnostic skills.

After the presentation of our data, Japanese psychiatrists started to use DSM-III in everyday practice. Terms such as operational criteria, interrater reliability, reliability index, and so on began to be referred to in

TABLE 10C.1. A multicenter study of diagnostic reliability using videotaped materials.

| DSM-III diagnosis | Base rate | K | Conventional diagnosis (ICD-9) | K |
|---|---|---|---|---|
| Axis I | | 0.80 | Overall | 0.75 |
| Organic mental disorders | 0.061 | 0.59 | Organic psychotic conditions | 0.70 |
| Substance use disorders | 0.092 | 0.73 | Drug dependence and abuse | 0.76 |
| Schizophrenic disorders | 0.208 | 0.95 | Schizophrenic psychoses | 0.83 |
| Paranoid disorders | 0.065 | 0.88 | Paranoid states | 0.56 |
| Psychotic disorders NEC | 0.075 | 0.82 | Other nonorganic psychoses | 0.43 |
| Affective disorders | 0.221 | 0.93 | Affective psychoses | 0.83 |
| Anxiety disorders | 0.158 | 0.68 | Neurotic disorders | 0.75 |
| Somatoform disorders | 0.126 | 0.54 | Physical conditions arising from mental factors | 0.57 |
| Other | 0.047 | 0.08 | | |
| Axis II | | | | |
| Personality disorders | 0.159 | 0.33 | | |

Note. A total of 103 clinicians from seven institutions participated in this study; videotaped materials of 14 cases were evaluated.

TABLE 10C.2. Improvement of diagnostic reliability in the course of training and experience.

| | K | |
|---|---|---|
| Years of clinical experience | DSM-III diagnosis | Conventional diagnosis |
| Less than 1 | 0.77 | 0.64 |
| 1–2 | 0.75 | 0.69 |
| 3–4 | 0.73 | 0.71 |
| 5–6 | 0.84 | 0.79 |
| 7–10 | 0.89 | 0.72 |
| 11–20 | 0.84 | 0.81 |
| More than 20 | 0.87 | 0.79 |

psychiatric conferences in Japan. This trend, which continued for several years, increased awareness of the importance of diagnostic criteria among Japanese clinicians (Takahashi et al 1988, Takahashi 1988).

We conducted another study of diagnostic stability on 300 patients who were hospitalized when DSM-III was first used to diagnose all inpatients at Shiga University of Medical Science Hospital (1980 to 1983). When the diagnoses on discharge were regarded as representing the true diagnoses, it was found that diagnoses made at the initial evaluation at the outpatient department agreed with the former in 81 of 100 occasions, or 0.81, for schizophrenia, and 0.83 for affective disorders, while both agreement and K were low for psychotic disorders not elsewhere classified (Takahashi and Hanada 1985) (Table 10C.3).

The field trial for ICD-10 Draft recently conducted by the National Institute of Mental Health in Japan, may exert a great influence on conservative Japanese diagnostic method. Some 600 psychiatrists, rep-

TABLE 10C.3. Stability of psychiatric diagnosis at the outpatient department.

| DSM-III diagnosis at the outpatient department | Base rate | Agreement with final diagnosis on discharge | K |
|---|---|---|---|
| Axis I overall | | 0.73 | 0.60 |
| Organic mental disorders | 0.114 | 0.76 | 0.70 |
| Substance use disorders | 0.028 | 0.88 | 0.75 |
| Schizophrenic disorders | 0.166 | 0.81 | 0.64 |
| Paranoid disorders | 0.028 | 0.25 | – |
| Psychotic disorders NEC | 0.062 | 0.67 | 0.59 |
| Affective disorders | 0.304 | 0.83 | 0.70 |
| Anxiety disorders | 0.028 | 0.63 | 0.43 |
| Somatoform disorders | 0.031 | 0.78 | 0.58 |
| Adjustment disorders | 0.044 | 0.38 | 0.45 |
| Other | 0.107 | 0.53 | – |
| Axis II | | | |
| Personality disorders | 0.035 | 0.80 | 0.35 |

resenting one-tenth of the clinicians practicing psychiatry in Japan, took part in a multicenter field trial from 1989 to 1990. They had to confront the inferiority of their conventional diagnoses to ICD-10, which has clearly defined and well designed categories. Diagnostic discrepancy was often clear when two experienced interviewers were requested to make an independent judgment using the conventional diagnosis and ICD-10 Draft diagnosis. Data in detail will be presented by Kitamura elsewhere (Kitamura 1990). In general, it can be said that clinicians in Japan have developed good diagnostic skills for psychotic disorders, particularly for schizophrenia.

## Definition of Atypical Psychosis in Japan

A working group for the diagnostic classification of functional psychoses was organized by seven members of JSIDCP, and meetings were held to discuss the criteria for psychotic disorders and mood disorders (Takahashi et al 1985). They agreed that the most controversial area in Japan was that of acute transient psychotic disorders, or what we conventionally called atypical psychosis.

Agreement was satisfactory with high inter-rater K for schizophrenia using conventional procedures in the recent field trial conducted by NIMH (Kitamura 1990). The K results were as high as 0.90 for schizophrenia, and 0.75 for depression and 0.75 for mania, respectively. On the contrary, the concept of atypical psychosis was rather confusing, although the diagnosis of atypical psychosis was very frequently given in some schools, and several excellent papers were reported on the concept of atypical psychosis from the school of psychiatrists from Kyoto University. In the trial mentioned above, K for atypical psychosis was 0.67 (Kitamura 1990).

The concept of atypical psychosis proposed by the Kyoto school is essentially an expanded and modified version of the unsystematized and cycloid psychoses described by Leonhard, and includes all of the conditions with intermediate signs and symptoms different from typical schizophrenic and from manic-depressive symptomatology. A hierarchical structure was also proposed, composed of six stages (ie, manic-depressive mood disturbance, depersonalization state, acute delusional–hallucinatory state, catatonia-like syndrome, oneiroid state, and confusional state) according to severity.

Clinicians at the Kyoto school explain that a good number of nonorganic psychotic patients have features of atypical psychosis, thus the clinicians diagnose patients with atypical psychosis probably as frequently as with the two major psychoses.

On the other hand, because of the influence of DSM-III and the ICD-10, some Japanese psychiatrists began to use this term as a synonym for acute transient psychotic state, and others used it to describe the schizoaffective state and mixture of three components of schizophrenic, mood, and confusional or delirious states. According to our survey of professors of psychiatry in 80 medical schools in Japan, the majority of respondents considered the concept of atypical psychosis to include the following five subcategories: acute delusional episode, cycloid psychosis, acute confusional episode, acute schizophrenia-like episode, and acute delusional–hallucinatory state (Table 10C.4) (Takahashi et al 1988). Apparently these five categories are all distinct in their acute and transient characteristics.

The accumulated answers of subcategories were illustrated using Quantification Method Type 3, which is a kind of cluster analysis, the scores of two main factors were shown on the two-dimensional plane. Categories of Numbers 1, 4, 6, 9, 10 and 11 (see Table 10C.4) formed the largest group, which indicated that most of the respondents preferred the combination of these six categories for the classification of atypical psychosis.

Half of the respondents preferred the term atypical psychosis when asked what name was most suitable for a group of so-called atypical psychosis. They considered that there was a rather large group that was distinct from two typical major groups (Table 10C.5). The ad hoc NIMH, NCNP, Committee for Diagnostic Criteria to modify ICD-10 (ICD-10 JCM Committee) also preferred the term atypical psychosis to that of acute and transient psychotic disorders. This may reflect the strong influence of Kyoto school on Japanese psychiatry, particularly on the concept of functional psychoses. In the course of revising ICD-10 into a draft of Japanese Clinical Modification (JCM), there was strong resistance to the naming of acute and transient psychotic disorders proposed in ICD-10. The JCM committee also proposed different terminology (eg,

TABLE 10C.4. Cumulative number of subtypes of so-called atypical psychosis.

| Subcategory | No. |
|---|---|
| 1. Acute delusional episode | 60 |
| 2. Cycloid psychosis | 53 |
| 3. Psychogenic delusional disorder | 29 |
| 4. Acute confusional state | 50 |
| 5. Acute schizophrenia-like episode | 43 |
| 6. Acute delusional–hallucinatory episode | 39 |
| 7. Oneiroid, confusional, or catatonic episode | 29 |
| 8. Acute dissociative–confusional psychosis | 24 |
| 9. Acute schizophrenia-form psychosis | 23 |
| 10. Acute affective disorder-form psychosis | 24 |
| 11. Other acute transient episode | 48 |
| 12. Schizoaffective disorder | 29 |

Note. Takahashi et al 1988.

TABLE 10C.5. A survey of diagnostic criteria and classification for a group of so-called atypical psychoses (1987).

| Term | No. |
|---|---|
| Atypical psychosis | 47 |
| Acute psychotic disorders | 3 |
| Acute affective psychosis | 1 |
| Other nonorganic psychosis (ICD-9) | 2 |
| Acute or transient psychotic disorders (ICD-10 Draft, 1987) | 28 |
| Acute and transient psychotic disorders (ICD-10 Draft, 1986) | 19 |
| Psychotic disorders not elsewhere classified (DSM-III) | 3 |
| Total | 103 |

acute confusion, acute delusional disorder, and other acute and transient psychotic disorders) for subcategories of this class instead of ICD-10 terminology. The committee believes that the category called atypical psychosis in Japan covers a relatively wide but clearly demarcated phenomenology (Kitamura 1990).

## *References*

Hanada K, Takahashi S (1982). A DSM-III field trial in Japan. *Japanese Journal of Clinical Psychiatry* 11:171–181 (in Japanese).

Hanada K, Takahashi S (1983a). A Multi-institutional collaborative study on diagnostic reliability using videotaped materials, pp 77–108. In T Doi, A Fujinawa (eds), *Significance of Diagnosis in Psychiatry*. Tokyo University Press, Tokyo (in Japanese).

Hanada K, Takahashi S (1983b). Multi-institutional collaborative studies of diagnostic reliability of DSM-III and ICD-9 in Japan, pp 273–290. In RL Spitzer, JBW Williams, AE Skodol (eds), *International Perspectives on DSM-III*. American Psychiatric Press, Washington DC.

Hanada K, Takahashi S, Honda Y, Anzai N, Yamaguchi N, Kato N, Maeshiro H, Noguchi T, Takahashi R, Takemura M, Kazamatsuri H (1982). A Multi-institutional study using DSM-III diagnostic criteria and diagnosis of so-called endogenous psychoses in Japan. *Psychiatria et Neurologia Japonica* 84:794–799 (in Japanese).

Kitamura T (1990). A field trial of ICO-10 and results, pp 3–83. In A Fujinawa, *Studies on Formulation of Diagnostic Criteria for Mental Disorders, Annual Report 1989*. NCNP, Ministry of Health and Welfare (in Japanese).

Takahashi S, Hanada K (1985). Stability of psychiatric diagnosis in outpatient clinic. *Clinical Psychiatry* 27:879–887 (in Japanese).

Takahashi S, Hanada K, Fujinawa A (1982). Japanese translation of *Quick Reference to the Diagnostic Criteria from DSM-III by The American Psychiatric Association*. Igaku Shoin, Tokyo (in Japanese).

Takahashi S, Hanada K, Fujinawa A (trans) (1988). *Quick Reference to the Diagnostic Criteria from DSM-III-R by The American Psychiatric Association*. Igaku Shoin, Tokyo (in Japanese).

Takahashi S, Takahashi R, Kasahara Y, Kimura B, Nomura J, Fujinawa A, Nakane N (1985). Classification and diagnostic criteria of so-called endogenous psychoses prepared by the JCIDCP Committee. *Clinical Psychiatry* 27:761–770 (in Japanese).

Takahashi S (trans) (1988). *Diagnostic and Statistical Manual of Mental Disorders*, 3rd Edition Revised by The American Psychiatric Association. Igaku Shoin, Tokyo (in Japanese).

Takahashi S, Iida H, Fujinawa A (1988). A survey of diagnostic criteria and classification for a group of so-called atypical psychoses. *Clinical Psychiatry* 30:1107–1113 (in Japanese).

# D. The New Classification of Mood Disorders in Japan

Koichi Hanada

The traditional classification of psychiatric disorders in Japan placed manic-depressive illness under the rubric of endogenous psychoses, together with schizophrenia and atypical psychosis. The diagnosis of manic-depressive illness was thought to be rather simple and clear. However, the classification of mood disorders was not systematic: Many different subtypes based on different concepts were used without clear differentiating criteria by different clinicians.

The *International Classification of Diseases*, 9th revision (ICD-9), which has been the official classification system for statistics in Japan since 1979, was not widely used in Japanese clinical settings.

## The Impact of DSM-III

The introduction of the *Diagnostic and Statistical Manual*, 3rd edition (DSM-III) in the early 1980s had a strong impact on psychiatric diagnosis and classification in Japan. Many Japanese psychiatrists who were frustrated by the low reliability of the traditional psychiatric diagnosis were attracted by the operational diagnostic criteria provided by DSM-III for almost all mental disorders. Thus, many Japanese psychiatrists became interested in diagnostic issues.

In 1981, a multi-institutional collaborative study on the psychiatric diagnosis was conducted by 103 psychiatrists from 7 university psychiatric departments (Hanada and Takahashi 1983). In this study, two clinicians interviewed the same patient and independently made diagnoses according to both the traditional system and DSM-III criteria. The results showed that the use of operational diagnostic criteria such as DSM-III improved the diagnostic reliability of affective disorders, as well as that of most of other mental disorders. Many psychiatrists, especially those in the younger generation, accepted DSM-III and used it as a diagnostic tool in their clinical practices and research.

## Proposal of Diagnostic Criteria

The Japanese Society for the International Diagnostic Criteria in Psychiatry (JSIDCP), established in 1981, nominated working groups to prepare diagnostic criteria for major mental disorders, and the working group on the functional psychoses proposed a classification and diagnostic criteria for the so-called endogenous psychoses in 1985. The proposed classification and diagnostic criteria for affective disorders was based mainly on ICD-9, not including neurotic depression and persistent mood changes (Table 10D.1). It consisted of only bipolar and unipolar subtypes with subclassifications based on three severity levels: mild, severe, and with psychotic features. However, this classification has not been used widely.

TABLE 10D.1. Proposed diagnostic criteria for depression by JSIDCP (1985).

A. Decreased vitality, depressed mood, and diminished psychomotor activity are observed and sustained every day for at least 2 weeks

B. Following symptoms are helpful but not essential for the diagnosis:
   1. Decrease in appetite and weight loss
   2. Sleep disturbance
   3. Deranged circadian rhythm or diurnal variation of mood, vital signs, or sleep
   4. Easy fatigability or various somatic complaints
   5. Agitation or inhibition
   6. Low self-esteem, feeling of self-reproach or guilt
   7. Loss of interest in daily life, including loss of libido
   8. Diminished ability to think or concentrate, or indecisiveness
   9. Thinking of death or suicide
   10. Syntonic or adhesive character

C. Although there is no disturbance in basic interpersonal relationship and no disturbance in adjustment to daily life in the period between episodes, the disability to perform social functioning to the full is sustained

D. If schizophrenic symptoms are present and mood-incongruent, depressive syndrome is predominant in clinical picture

E. Not due to any of the following:
   1. Substance use
   2. Organic mental disorders
   3. Apparently transient reactive depressive state (eg, bereavement)
   4. Schizophrenic disorder
   5. Borderline personality disorder

TABLE 10D.2. Mood disorder results of ICD-10 draft field trial in Japan: Reliability of the conventional and ICD-10 diagnoses for 696 patients in 59 university hospitals.

| Diagnosis | | K | Base rate |
|---|---|---|---|
| Conventional diagnosis | | | |
| Depression | | 0.68 | 23.9% |
| Mania | | 0.70 | 5.5% |
| Depressive neurosis | | 0.52 | 10.1% |
| ICD-10 diagnosis | | | |
| F3 | Mood (affective) disorders | 0.80 | 40.5% |
| F30 | Manic episode | 0.70 | 1.9% |
| F31 | Bipolar affective disorder | 0.86 | 9.2% |
| F32 | Depressive episode | 0.73 | 21.6% |
| F33 | Recurrent depressive disorder | 0.65 | 7.5% |
| F34 | Persistent affective disorders | 0.57 | 4.2% |
| F38 | Other mood (affective) disorders | 0.67 | 0.6% |

## Field Trial and Clinical Modification of ICD-10 in Japan

The ICD-10, the forthcoming revision, will be the official classification system in Japan. To facilitate the use of ICD-10 in daily practice, provision needs to be made for classification and diagnostic criteria in Japanese that is compatible with the original ICD classification and is appealing to Japanese users. A working group, with Akira Fujinawa as chair, was organized in 1987, under the sponsorship of the Ministry of Health and Welfare to create the official diagnostic criteria for mental disorders in Japan by modifying ICD-10. The group conducted a nationwide field trial and reliability study of ICD-10 draft in autumn 1989.

In all, 292 clinicians in 59 university psychiatric departments formed diagnostic pairs, and interviewed 696 patients, and made both ICD-10 and conventional diagnoses independently. The results for mood disorders are shown in Table 10D.2. This result showed generally better diagnostic reliability of ICD-10 than conventional diagnosis. The Japanese clinical modification (ICD-10-JCM) was prepared based on these experiences. Major modification of ICD-10-JCM for mood disorder consisted of reorganization of the severity subclassification in episodic mood disorders. The remaining problems include the differentiation of mood disorders with psychotic symptoms from schizoaffective disorder.

## *Reference*

Hanada K, Takahashi S (1983). Multi-institutional collaborative studies of diagnostic reliability of DSM-III and ICD-9 in Japan, pp 273–290. In R Spitzer, JBW Williams, AE Skodol (eds), *International Perspectives on DSM-III*. American Psychiatric Press, Washington, DC.

# E. Neurosis Spectrum Disorders in Japan

Itaru Yamashita and Tsukasa Koyama

The Japanese Society for International Diagnostic Criteria in Psychiatry (JSIDCP) decided to organize a subcommittee in 1984 to evaluate the diagnostic criteria for neuroses and related conditions in the *Diagnostic and Statistical Manual of Mental Disorders*, 3rd edition (DSM-III) and the *International Classification of Diseases*, 10th revision (ICD-10) draft, and to formulate criteria readily usable for clinicians in Japan.

The subcommittee was composed of six members; I. Yamashita (chairperson), T. Iwasaki (vice-chairperson), T. Kasahara, M. Nakamura, T. Oguchi and T. Takahashi. One member was a psychoanalyst and another had worked long on the clinical application of DSM-III in Japan.

## A Few Basic Problems

The subcommittee had to deal with a few basic questions at the very beginning of its activity:

1. There is no diagnostic category of Neurotic Disorders in either DSM-III (American Psychiatric Association 1980) or ICD-10-Draft (World Health Organization 1988). To quote from the Introduction of the DSM-III Manual: "In DSM-III, the Neurotic Disorders are included in Affective, Anxiety, Somatoform, Dissociative and Psychosexual Disorders." Should the subcommittee proceed along the lines of DSM-III and modifiy some parts of it so that the DSM-III classification could be more easily used in clinical practice?
2. The ICD-10 is expected to be officially published in the near future and used as the common diagnostic criteria worldwide. What then is the purpose of formulating another set of criteria only for Japanese psychiatrists?
3. There are conventional classifications of neurotic disorders in Japan, which mostly conform to ICD-9 (World Health Organization 1975) and were almost uniform in their descriptions in many textbooks and widely used clinically. Is it necessary at present to make itemized, operational criteria for neurotic disorders and risk confusing clinicians accustomed to the conventional classifications?

The subcommittee members discussed the above matters and agreed (1) to obtain as many opinions as possible from prominent members of JSIDCP and to develop a classification on the basis of their opinions, and (2) to describe symptoms in the itemized form as concisely as possible so that the classification may serve as an intermediary step that can bridge the gap between the conventional and the forthcoming ICD-10 classifications.

## The Formulation of Criteria

According to the previously mentioned agreements, the subcommittee had sent questionnaires four times, one by one, at various stages of the preparation of criteria, to chairpersons of psychiatric departments of medical schools and directors of mental hospitals, 70 in number, all of whom were JSIDCP members. They were very cooperative and contributed greatly to the formation of the criteria.

The first questionnaire in 1985 asked several overall questions on neuroses. To the question about the omission of the diagnostic class of neuroses in DSM-III, 2 members wholly favored the omission, 8 agreed in principle, 12 answered that the term of neuroses is necessary, and 38 were of the opinion that the category of neuroses is necessary.

Also, to the question on the actual use of DSM-III criteria for neurotic disorders, 8 members reported that they had been using them in practice, 19 only for research purposes, 3 were considering using them, and 24 had no plan to use them.

The second questionnaire, which soon followed the first one, asked mainly about the DSM-III criteria. The majority of responses indicated reluctance to the partitioning of neurotic disorders into anxiety, somatoform, and dissociative disorders in DSM-III, and preferred the ICD-9 classification of neurotic disorders including various subtypes without subcategorization, although all the members showed appreciation of clear descriptions of symptoms in DSM-III.

Accordingly, the subcommittee started to prepare the first draft of criteria, maintaining the framework of ICD-9 and conventional classifications and taking into consideration the descriptions of DSM-III and ICD-10-Draft (1986) (World Health Organization 1988) and the members' own experiences with neurotic patients.

The third and fourth questionnaires were sent to the JSIDCP members with the subcommittee's drafts, asking for their opinions and corrections. The manuscripts were revised repeatedly, and the criteria were finally developed in the autumn of 1986.

During 1986–87, the final version was tested for clinical use in 29 universities and hospitals by 132 psychiatrists (Yamashita et al 1988). The DSM-III, conventional, and subcommittee's criteria were applied at the same time to classify 386 patients. The concordance rate between the conventional and sucommittee's classifications was 81.3%. A total of 94.2% of patients with concordant diagnoses by the two classifications could be classified into the corresponding categories of DSM-III. No alteration of the categories and items of the subcommittee's criteria was made by this field study because the trial was not aimed particularly at testing the sensitivity and specificity of the criteria.

## The Classification of The JSIDCP Subcommittee

The headlines of the classification of neurosis spectrum disorders by the subcommittee (Yamashita et al 1989) is shown in Table 10E.1, the criteria for milieu reactions and neurotic disorders in Table 10E.2, and, as an example of eight subtypes of neurotic disorders, the criteria for depressive neurosis are presented in Table 10E.3.

As seen in the tables, there are several points in the classification that differ from DSM-III categories: (1) it retains the framework of conventional and ICD-9 classifications and has no categories corresponding to anxiety, somatoform, and dissociative disorders in DSM-III. (2) It has two main categories: milieu reactions and neurotic disorders. The former roughly corresponds to F43, reaction to severe stress, and adjustment disorders in ICD-10-Draft, and the latter to categories other than F43, namely F40–42 and 44–48, in the same Draft. (3) As to subtypes of

TABLE 10E.1. Neurosis spectrum disorders.

- I. Milieu reaction (308, 309)
  - 1. Acute milieu reaction (308)
  - 2. Adjustment disorder (309)
- II. Neurotic disorders (300)
  - 1. Anxiety neurosis (300.0)
    - a. Panic type
    - b. Generalized anxiety type
    - c. Mixed type
  - 2. Phobic neurosis (300.2)
    - a. Agoraphobia
    - b. Social phobia
    - c. Nosophobia
    - d. Simple phobia
  - 3. Obsessive-compulsive neurosis (300.3)
  - 4. Hysterical neurosis (300.1)
    - a. Conversion type
    - b. Dissociative type
    - c. Regressed type
    - d. Mixed type
  - 5. Hypochondriacal neurosis (300.7)
    - a. Nosophobic type
    - b. Multiple complaints type
    - c. Autonomic dysfunction type
    - d. Pain type
  - 6. Depressive neurosis (300.4)
  - 7. Depersonalization neurosis (300.6)
  - 8. Other neurotic disorders (300.8)

TABLE 10E.2. Criteria for milieu reaction and neurotic disorders.

I. Milieu reaction
   A. There is a serious life event that is extremely distressing to most individuals (eg, natural disaster, sudden separation from intimate persons, migration, serious interpersonal conflict, certain religious experiences)
   B. There must be a clear temporal and psychological connection between the impact of an event and the onset of symptoms (if the connection is not clear enough, diagnosis of neurotic or personality disorders should be considered according to their criteria)
   C. At least one symptom in the following categories is present
      1. Psychic symptoms such as anxiety, depression, irritability, daze, syncope or transient hallucination
      2. Somatic symptoms such as headache, vomiting, diarrhea or general fatigue
      3. Conduct disorders such as aggressive behavior, fugue or refusal to work (school)
   D. The symptoms are severe enough to cause
      1. Serious subjective distress and/or
      2. Marked restriction of social or occupational activities
   E. The symptoms subside rapidly when life situation improves
   F. The symptoms are not due to schizophrenia, mood disorder, or any physical disorder
II. Neurotic disorders
   A. At least one of these symptoms is present: anxiety, phobia, obsession-compulsion, hysteria, hypochondriasis, depression, depersonalization
   B. The symptoms are severe enough to cause for a considerable period of time (usually longer than 1 month)
      1. Serious subjective distress and/or
      2. Marked restriction of social or occupational activities
   C. In principle, patients have considerable insight and unimpaired reality testing (ie, they do not confuse their morbid subjective experiences and fantasies with external reality)
   D. A psychological connection between the symptoms and the personality traits should be recognized
   E. The symptoms are not due to schizophrenia, mood disorder, organic disorder, drug abuse, epilepsy, or milieu reaction

neurotic disorders, neurasthenia is omitted and depressive neurosis is retained. (4) As a result, the subcommittee's classification closely resembles F4 categorization of ICD-10-Draft. Actually, they fit each other quite well if the term "neurosis spectrum disorders" of the former is replaced by "neurotic, stress-related, and somatoform disorders" of the latter, the term "hysterical neurosis" by "dissociative (conversion) disorders," "hypochondriacal neurosis" by "somatoform disorders," and "nosophobic type" of hypochondriacal neurosis by "hypochondriacal disorder," etc. (5) The process of sorting out patients in the subcommittee's classification is different from those in DSM-III and ICD-10. Patients are diagnosed at first as milieu reactions or neurotic disorders according to their criteria, and then classified into their subtypes.

The most common responses of clinical psychiatrists to this classification are that it looks like a compromise between conventional and ICD-10 classifications and it is easily used in everyday practice. It can be used

Table 10E.3. Criteria for depressive neurosis.

A. Depressive mood, decreased energy and interest in everyday activities are clearly present
B. The following symptoms are not present
   1. complete loss of pleasure in all activities
   2. manifest delusion of guilt
   3. marked diurnal variation of mood (worse in the morning)
   4. any manic episode in the past
C. There is a clear temporal and psychological connection between the impact of life event(s) and the onset and course of symptoms; the symptoms subside when life situation improves
D. It is clearly understandable that the depressive state has been brought about by the interaction between personality trait (eg, immature, dependent, perfectionistic or excessively enthusiastic) and a life situation not severe enough to cause milieu reaction

References
1. Psychomotor retardation is often relatively slight
2. Guilt feeling and self-reproach are often slight, while aggressive attitude toward others is sometimes manifest
3. Depressed mood can often be relieved temporarily by comfort or compliments from others
4. The symptoms may often follow other neurotic disorders (anxiety, hypochondriacal, obsessive–compulsive, etc)
5. Mood disorder should be considered when the symptoms continue even if life situation improves
6. Depressed type of milieu reaction should be differentiated from depressive neurosis by item A of milieu reaction and by item D stated above

jointly with DSM-III, particularly when DSM-III is requested for research purposes.

## Conclusion

The subcommittee of the JSIDCP formulated a classification for neurotic disorders and related conditions, taking into acount the conventional, DSM-III, and ICD-10 classifications and the opinions of prominent JSIDCP members on these classifications. The classification retains the framework of ICD-9 and includes itemized criteria for each disorder. Its overall style and contents are similar to those of the ICD-10 and are regarded as easily usable in psychiatric practice.

## *References*

American Psychiatric Association (1980). *Diagnostic and Statistical Manual of Mental Disorders* (3rd ed). American Psychiatric Association, Washington, DC.

World Health Organization (1975). *International Classification of Diseases* (9th rev). World Health Organization, Geneva.

World Health Organization (1988). *International Classification of Diseases* (10th rev) (Draft). World Health Organization, Geneva.
Yamashita I, Iwasaki T, Oguchi T, Takahashi T, Nakamura M, Kasahara T (1988). Japanese survey of diagnostic criteria for neurotic disorders. *Japanese Journal Psychiatry Neurology* 42:407–408.
Yamashita I, Iwasaki T, Oguchi T, Kasahara T, Takahashi T, Nakamura M (1989). Tentative diagnostic criteria for neurosis spectrum disorders. *Clinical Psychiatry* (Japan) 31:345–352.

# F. Classification of Sleep Disorders in Japanese Psychiatry

YUTAKA HONDA

Six different international diagnostic classifications of sleep disorders are available, as shown in Table 10F.1. The classification by the Association of Sleep Disorders Centers (ASDC) and the Association for the Psychophysiological Study of Sleep (APSS) in 1979 had great significance and clinical impact in situations where there was no systematic classification of sleep disorders in the world (Association of Sleep Disorders Centers 1979). It substantially facilitated international exchange of research activities concerning sleep disorders. However, it lacked operational diagnostic criteria, multiaxial structure, compatibility with ICD-9, and reliability study through field trials. Another problem was the adoption of classification based on the chief complaint of either insomnia or hypersomnia. An essentially single sleep apnea syndrome can be classified into both DIMS (insomnia) and DOES (hypersomnia).

The *Diagnostic and Statistical Manual of Mental Disorders*, 3rd edition, Revised (DSM-III-R) (American Psychiatric Association 1987), is clear

TABLE 10F.1. International classifications of sleep disorders.

| Classification | No. of disorders |
|---|---|
| 1. 1979 ASDC-APSS classification of sleep and arousal disorders | 67 |
| 2. DSM-III-R category of sleep disorders (1987) | 13 |
| 3. JSIDCP classification of sleep disorders | 21 |
| 4. ICD-10 Chapter V | 6 nonorganic |
| Chapter VI | 10 organic |
| 5. 1990 International classification of sleep disorders, by American Sleep Disorders Association (ASDA) | 87 |
| 6. Japanese Clinical Modification of ICD-10 diagnostic criteria for sleep disorders | 19 |

and practical and uses atheoretical descriptions, operational diagnostic criteria, and a multiaxial approach. However, it is too simple, and important sleep disorders such as narcolepsy and periodic hypersomnia are listed only as "hypersomnia related to a known organic factor." Furthermore, the differential diagnoses given for various hypersomnias are not satisfactory for sleep specialists.

In Japan, the Japanese Society for International Diagnostic Criteria in Psychiatry (JSIDCP) was organized in 1981, and the Subcommittee for the Classification of Sleep Disorders was organized as one of nine disorder-focused subcommittees that were created to establish convenient and practical diagnostic classifications and criteria for Japanese psychiatrists. The draft classification of sleep disorders for Japanese psychiatrists contained 21 diagnostic entities. The basic precepts of our JSIDCP classification were as follows: (1) The classification should be made on the basis of clear descriptions of clinical syndromes and clinical course without using any theoretical principle. (2) It should be useful in clinical settings in the Japanese psychiatric climate. (3) Operational diagnostic criteria should be adopted. (4) A multiaxial system should be used to describe biological test results on another axis. (5) Concurrent psychiatric and somatic disorders should be noted as additional diagnoses. (6) The classification should maintain compatibility with other international diagnostic classifications such as the *International Classification of Diseases*, 10th revision (ICD-10) and DSM-III-R. (7) Important sleep disorders such as narcolepsy, periodic somnolence (recurrent hypersomnia), and sleep–apnea syndrome should be adopted as independent diagnostic categories.

The ICD-10 (World Health Organization [1992]) has divided the classification of sleep disorders into two parts. The nonorganic sleep disorders are classified in Chapter V (mental, behavioral, and developmental disorders that are coded as F), and the organic sleep disorders are classified in Chapter VI (neurological disorders that are coded as G). The explanatory descriptions and diagnostic guidelines are provided for nonorganic sleep disorders in Chapter V, but no such descriptions are available for any of the disorders of Chapter VI. One of the serious problems in the ICD-10 classification of sleep disorders is its dichotomous principle of classification according to the etiology of organicity. In clinical practice, however, there are many patients in whom specific causes of sleep disorders are unclear. In addition, there are also many patients whose onset of sleep disorders are associated with both psychosocial and organic factors. Furthermore, it is not clear what should be considered as organic causes. When extrinsic factors are mild, or temporally only remotely associated, their significance as the cause of a sleep disorder is often not clear. Furthermore, judgment of whether a disordered state of sleep in a certain patient is caused by organic factors or not requires extensive clinical testing prior to a final clinical judgment. Ruling in and out differential diagnoses requires time, facilities, and expense, and even when a pathological somatic finding is obtained, the judgment of its causative significance is often difficult. For example, when mild objective findings of cerebral cortical atrophy on CT are obtained, it is not easy to exclude the concurrent presence of nonorganic hypersomnia or insomnia.

Narcolepsy is currently classified as an organic sleep disorder in ICD-10, but exogenous organic causal factors have not been demonstrated. Sometimes the onset of narcolepsy even appears to be preceded by psychosocial events. There have been no positive findings suggestive of any specific neuropathological abnormalities in the brain of the autopsied cases of narcolepsy. It is well known that sleep-onset REM periods and positive HLA-DR2 are characteristic biological findings in narcolepsy, but these findings are also present in healthy subjects and are not considered as pathological findings indicating brain organic damage. Thus, it can be said that sufficient evidence is absent to classify narcolepsy as an organic disorder.

On the other hand, there are many cases of excessive daytime sleepiness in the family members of narcolepsy patients. These cases may be etiologically similar to narcolepsy, but they must be diagnosed as nonorganic hypersomnia according to ICD-10 guidelines. However, if these same cases were accidentally complicated with hypnagogic hallucinations or sleep paralysis, they would be rediagnosed as narcolepsy and reclassified under organic sleep disorder. Hypnagogic hallucinations and sleep paralysis are commonly found in 10 to 20% of the normal population, and are not by themselves pathological. Therefore, it is unreasonable to regard the presence of these symptoms as the evidence of organic pathology. Therefore narcolepsy should justly be classified into Chapter V as a member of psychiatric disorders rather than in Chapter VI neurological disorders.

The Kleine-Levin syndrome was initially adopted as an independent category of mental disorder in the ICD-10 draft, but it was moved into the neurological disorders section without any explanation. In Japan, the Kleine-Levin syndrome has been considered as a subtype of periodic somnolence, or recurrent hypersomnia, with disinhibition of appetite during the somnolent period. Patients with periodic somnolence sometimes exhibit various psychiatric pictures, including hypomanic mood changes, hallucinations and delusions, atypical psychoses and dysthymic mood disorders. Therefore, periodic somnolence has been treated primarily by psychiatrists in Japan. Similar situations may be present in other countries, and patients with periodic somnolence may be treated by psychiatrists with various psychiatric diagnoses, such as atypical psychosis or periodic mental disorder, and only the Kleine-Levin syndrome with classical bulimia appeared in the foreground.

In Japan, the administrative section of the government for the medical care of both narcolepsy and periodic somnolence is the Section of Mental

Health of the Ministry of Health and Welfare. Thus, it is practically and essentially very difficult to classify individual patients with sleep disorders into either nonorganic mental disorders or organic neurological disorders.

Adoption of a single category of sleep disorders as a class of disorders of neuroscience is most appropriate. In view of the absence of clinical descriptions and diagnostic guidelines for Chapter VI organic sleep disorders, all sleep disorders would be most beneficially classified under Chapter V with precise clinical descriptions and diagnostic guidelines.

The recent publication of International Classification of Sleep Disorders (ICSD) by the American Sleep Disorders Association (ASDA) (1990) contains 87 sleep disorders. Its structure solved many problems of the preceding classifications. This ICSD classification does not adopt the dichotomy of organic and nonorganic etiologies. On the other hand, it is complicated and contains many disorders that are unfamiliar to most medical practitioners who are not sleep specialists. Field trials are needed to validate the diagnostic criteria for these extensive categories. Since the ICSD doesn't observe the organic/nonorganic dichotomy, it is not compatibile with ICD-10 code numbers. For example, parasomnias are distributed into five different areas of medicine, such as F, G, I, P and R, and some have dual codes of both F and G according to the present ICD coding system. This indicates that reconsideration on the part of ICD-10 is necessary.

The research group on Establishment and Clinical Application of Integrated Diagnostic Criteria for Mental Disorders in Japan was organized in 1987 with Akira Fujinawa, director of the National Institute of Mental Health in Japan, as chairperson. The group translated the ICD-10 Draft and performed a large-scale field trial. They then prepared a Japanese clinical modification (JCM) of the diagnostic criteria for ICD-10. This JCM largely used the concepts and results of the diagnostic criteria prepared by the subcommittees of JSIDCP (Honda 1985, Honda and Sasaki 1988, 1990). The outline of JCM of sleep disorders is shown in Table 10F.2 and consists of 19 disorders. Dyssomnia, circadian rhythm sleep disorders and parasomnias were adopted as the three major categories of sleep disorders. Disorders related to other medical disorders or known organic factors were included in each category in order to be compatible with ICD-10 Chapter VI codes. The causative organic disorders can be noted in another axis. Associated mental disorders can be noted as additional diagnoses. The compatible code numbers are randomized and duplex over F51 and G47 codes. This is due to the structure of ICD-10. Clinical knowledge for the diagnosis and treatment of sleep disorders is increasing rapidly. The framing of sleep disorders of ICD-10 appears as not large enough to house various new advances. On the other hand, biological findings obtained by polysomnography, molecular biology, and brain imaging will provide more clues for the classification by using biological markers. New diagnostic criteria and

TABLE 10F.2. Japanese Clinical Modification of the ICD-10 classification of sleep disorders.

| | ICD-10 codes |
|---|---|
| A. Dyssomnias | |
| 1. Primary insomnia | F51.0 |
| 2. Psychophysiological insomnia (neurotic insomnia) | F51.0 |
| 3. Primary hypersomnia | F51.1 |
| 4. Narcolepsy | G47.4 |
| 5. Sleep–apnea syndrome | G47.3 |
| 6. Recurrent hypersomnia (periodic somnolence) | |
| 7. Idiopathic hypersomnia | G47.1 |
| 8. Dyssomnia related to other medical disorders or known organic factors | G47.0 |
| 9. Dyssomnia, NOS | G47.9 |
| B. Circadian rhythm sleep disorders | |
| 1. Delayed sleep phase disorder | F51.2, G47.20 |
| 2. Non-24 hour circadian rhythm sleep disorder | F51.22, G47.22 |
| 3. Disorganized circadian rhythm sleep disorder | F51.23, G47.23 |
| 4. Circadian rhythm sleep disorder, related to other medical disorders or known organic factors | F51.2, G47.2 |
| 5. Circadian rhythm sleep disorder, NOS | F51.29, G47.29 |
| C. Parasomnias | |
| 1. Sleep-walking disorder | F51.3, G47.81 |
| 2. Sleep-terror disorder | F51.4, G47.82 |
| 3. Nightmare disorder | F51.5 |
| 4. Parasomnia, NOS | |
| D. Sleep disorder, NOS | F51.9, G47.9 |

Abbreviation. NOS not otherwise specified.

classification by using both these biological findings and more specific clinical symptomatology will be an important step forward for the future classification of sleep disorders.

## *References*


American Psychiatric Association (1987). *Diagnostic and Statistical Manual of Mental Disorders*, Third Edition, Revised (DSM-III-R), pp 297–313. American Psychiatric Association, Washington, DC.

American Sleep Disorders Association (1990). *International Classification of Sleep Disorders: Diagnostic and Coding Manual*. American Sleep Disorders Association, Rochester, MN.

Association of Sleep Disorders Centers (1979). Diagnostic classification of sleep and arousal disorders. *Sleep* 2:1–137.

Honda Y (1985). Activities of the Subcommittee for Sleep Disorders. *Folia Psychiatrica et Neurologica Japonica* 39:460–461.

Honda Y, Sasaki T (1988) Classification of sleep and arousal disorders. *Psychiatric Mook* 21:102–126 (in Japanese).

Honda Y, Sasaki T (1990). Draft of ICD-10 and sleep disorders. *Japanese Journal of Clinical Psychiatry* 19:1075–1082 (in Japanese).
World Health Organization (1992) *Tenth Revision of the International Classification of Diseases ICD-10*. World Health Organization, Geneva.

# G. Childhood Psychiatric Disorders in Japan

KOSUKE YAMAZAKI

The following three issues are important for discussing diagnostic classification for child psychiatric disorders:

First, at what stage should impairment or disorder be assessed? When dealing with the wide stages of development from infancy to adolescence, the stage at which we are to sort through and extract for symptoms or characteristic behaviors should be determined. Then there is the problem of how to evaluate the effect of parent–child relationships on the child's behavior, whether we are to confine our observations to second- or third-party behavior interaction, and whether to restrict ourselves to cross-section evaluations or to include longitudinal section evaluations as well.

Second, there is the question of how to define the boundaries in the concepts of various disorders. Children, who are in the midst of psychological development, are still in an undifferentiated state. For this reason, the various factors coming into play in formulating the symptoms and behavior are intricately interwoven, making clinical differentiation no simple task. In particular, what criteria could there be for the differentiation and diagnosis of infants whose behavior is as yet undifferentiated? Furthermore, to what degree can we expect to separate the symptoms appearing in the adolescent or adult with developmental disorders?

Third, there is the problem of how to extract those basic symptoms and behavior disorders that override such factors as age, stage of development, gender, living environment, education and therapeutic history. Multiaxial approaches have been incorporated to elucidate these issues. But to what extent can we expect to collect reliable data in the daily clinical setting?

## Surveys on Child Psychiatric Disorders by Multifacility Joint Studies

The Committee on Child and Adolescents of the Japanese Society for International Diagnostic Criteria in Psychiatry (JSIDCP) conducted a survey on *Diagnostic and Statistical Manual of Mental Disorders*, 3rd edition (DSM-III) diagnoses in 725 subjects under age 20 who visited clinics of the 12 member institutions of the committee between March and September 1986. The survey showed the diagnosis of pervasive developmental disorders as the most common at 23.5%, followed by mental retardation at 12.3%. When specific developmental disorders (1.3%) were added to these figures, the rate of developmental disorders became 37.1%. Symptomatologically, when attention deficit disorder, appearing at 6.3%, with its close resemblance to developmental disorders was added to this score, the total became 43.4%, portraying developmental disorders as a central issue in child and adolescent mental health care in Japan. This is followed by adjustment disorder (10.3%), schizophrenic disorders (6.5%), somatoform disorders (5.4%) and anxiety disorders (4.6%).

In this survey, the question of how to classify school refusal and violence in the family, which are serious social issues in our country, became a big problem. Many respondents included them under adjustment disorders or anxiety disorders, but it is highly probable that this judgment was largely affected by the mention of 309.23, Adjustment Disorder with Work or Academic Inhibition, with many respondents feeling that there was no truly appropriate classification for the behavior.

## Evaluation of School Refusal

Hence, an evaluation on the classification of school refusal, which has been a phenomenon receiving much attention as a social issue in Japan (Yamazaki et al 1987, Yamazaki et al 1990) but without specific designation in the international diagnostic classifications was performed. First, we conducted a questionnaire survey of 154 general psychiatrists, child psychiatrists, and psychiatry professors, asking how they perceived school refusal. As a result, 47.1% answered that school refusal should be treated as a clinical diagnostic entity. Among them, 73.5% believed that it should be left as a state diagnosis, 22.4% opted for syndrome diagnosis, whereas only 4.1% believed that it ought to be taken as an independent clinical diagnosis.

Next, we evaluated the degree of conformity we could expect in diagnosis if school refusal was used as a state diagnosis. The committee discussed several cases, and selected Case 1, a 13-year-old boy who was unanimously diagnosed as school refusal, and Case 2, a 16-year-old girl presenting with school refusal as the primary complaint, but in whom aggressiveness towards the mother, state of mental agitation, auditory hallucinations, and suicidal ideation were seen, who was not diagnosed as school refusal. Detailed records of these two cases were sent to 213 psychiatrists, asking them for diagnoses by the traditional classifications, *International Classification of Diseases*, 9th revision (ICD-9) and DSM-III.

The results of analysis showed that conformities of diagnosis by ICD-9 and DSM-III were both quite low, even though diagnostic conformity was high with regard to the usual clinical diagnosis of school refusal. And in Case 1, without any pronounced clinical characteristics apart from school refusal, a large variation was seen in the response using DSM-III, with its clear-cut clinical standards, whereas diagnostic conformity was higher in using ICD-9, with its inscription, including school refusal. And in Case 2, a case that suggests schizophrenia, but in whom a definitive diagnosis is difficult, conformity of response was found to be higher by DSM-III than by ICD-9. It should be kept in mind that there is a tendency to emphasize the obsessive mentality behind this phenomenon in Japan, due to the concept of school phobia being first introduced into the country.

## Developmental Disorders

The fact that the position of "developmental disorders" was placed within the systematic diagnostic classification of psychiatric disorders holds great significance.

In ICD-10, the specific developmental disorders and pervasive developmental disorders were included under F80–89, developmental disorders, alongside F70–F79, mental retardation. On the other hand, in DSM-III-R, developmental disorders were classified in Axis II, combining mental retardation, pervasive developmental disorders, and specific developmental disorders. If we use this diagnostic classification, it is possible to arrive at an overlapping diagnosis of both autism and mental retardation. However, these two are different, according to definition as well as in concept. In other words, in DSM-III and DSM-III-R, it is stated, "In mental retardation, there are generalized delays in development, but the person behaves as if he or she were passing through an earlier normal developmental stage," whereas autism is characterized as being "distortion in development over a pervasive area." There is similar mention regarding autism in ICD-10: "There are disorders primarily defined in terms of deviance rather than delay in developmental functions; this applies especially to autism." We must be cautious of the way of thinking that places delay and distortion next to each other, allowing for simple overlapping diagnoses (Yamazaki 1992).

The JSIDCP Committee on Child and Adolescents conducted clinical surveys and research on a serial basis, and proposed the inclusion of attention-deficit hyperactivity disorder (ADHD) under developmental disorders, as a result of accumulated clinical experience and prognostic pictures. The reasons for this proposal are:

1. The clinical symptoms are closely similar, with many cases being difficult to label one or the other.

2. In contrast to the diagnostic model of physical disabilities, the lower the level of development, the greater the overlap of symptoms and the higher the development, the greater the differentiation of symptoms.
3. The prognostic picture of many cases of high functioning autism, specific developmental disorders are ADHD show closely similar symptoms.

## *References*

Yamazaki K (1992). Early signs of infantile autism, pp. 169–175. In H Naruse, EM Ornitz (eds), *Neurobiology of Infantile Autism*. Elsevier Science Publishers, Amsterdam.

Yamazaki K, Inomata J, MacKenzie JA (1987). Self-expression, interpersonal relations, and juvenile delinquency in Japan, pp 180–204. In CM Super (ed), *The Role of Culture in Developmental Disorder*. Academic Press, Boston.

Yamazaki K, Inomata J, Makita K, MacKenzie JA (1990). Culture japonaise et caractéristiques des manifestations névrotiques dans l'enfance et l'adolescence, pp 493–503. In C Chiland, JG Young (eds), *Nouvelles approches de la santé mentale de la naissance à l'adolescence pour l'enfant et sa famille*. Presses Universitaires de France, Paris.

# H. Present and Future of Psychiatric Diagnosis in Japan

YUJI OKAZAKI

A major change in psychiatric diagnosis over the last 20 years has been the adoption of operational diagnostic criteria that have improved diagnostic reliability through a reduction of criterion variance (Feighner et al 1972, Spitzer et al 1981). Also, the introduction of a multiaxial system has contributed greatly to the systematic description of complicated clinical information. During the last 2 decades, psychiatrists have faced the challenge of having to be familiar with new systems and concepts. The mutual influence of different diagnostic systems developed in different nations produced similar diagnostic criteria for psychiatric disorders. Despite this development, some conflicts between the new systems and conventional diagnostic systems appeared. In addition, some dissociation between new diagnostic categories and conventional treatments has arisen.

One important task for the future will be to validate both diagnostic criteria and diagnostic categories. However, without appropriate education and training, no diagnostic system can be internationally useful and acceptable. Even when the same diagnostic criteria are applied, differences in diagnosis across countries may still occur because of the influence of underlying concepts that are deeply rooted in the culture and the nature of psychiatric practice of each country.

Accordingly, training in evaluation is very important for researchers and clinicians who use common criteria. Only after this has been accomplished can a common diagnostic system be properly adopted internationally. Establishment of such validity can also help to resolve the discrepancy between diagnosis and treatment.

In the near future, it may be possible to map all human genes. With advances in computer technology and the ability to analyze individual gene codes, it may be possible to describe the genotypes of individual physical constitutions, psychiatric disorders, and even personality traits. However, all neuron networks in the brain are not thought to be controlled solely by gene codes. Furthermore, there is evidence to support the influence of nongenetic factors in the development of psychiatric disorders. These two factors are necessary in establishing the clinical validity of each category. Such validity can be established through syndrome identification, demarcation of syndrome boundaries, outcome studies, family studies, therapeutic trials, and identification of biological correlates (Robins and Guze 1970, Kendell 1989).

For the development of valid diagnostic criteria, we need to examine the possible roles of polythetic and monothetic approaches. In this case, a study on the relationship between narcoleptic symptoms and HLA types by Honda (1990) (Table 10H.1) presents a good example. If it is established that HLA-DR2 antigen correlates specifically to both cataplexy and excessive daytime sleep episodes of narcolepsy, it will then be enough to make a specific symptom-based diagnosis by confirming the existence of cataplexy. In other words, the presence of cataplexy should be indispensable in the symptomatological diagnostic criteria for narcolepsy (monothetic approach). A polythetic approach for the diagnosis of narcolepsy involves the presence of excessive daytime sleepiness (EDS) and one out of the four following symptoms cataplexy, hypnagogic hallucinations, sleep paralysis, and sleep-onset REM. Using this approach, however, HLA–DR2-negative patients can also be diagnosed as having "narcolepsy." In Table 10H.1 this would mean that 13 HLA–DR2-negative EDS patients can be diagnosed as having "narcolepsy." As long as there is no difference in the effectiveness of the treatment of EDS with psychostimulants such as methylphenidate between narcolepsy with cataplexy and essential hypersomnia (EHS) without cataplexy, a polythetic diagnostic approach is fairly useful. However, the psychostimulant is not effective in cataplexy, which responds to clomipramine. Thus, in the case of narcolepsy, polythetic diagnosis shows poorer predictive validity than monothetic diagnosis. Cataplexy appears to be an attacklike symptom different from other narcoleptic symptoms associated with sleep

TABLE 10H.1. Combinations of major narcoleptic symptoms and HLA-DR2 frequencies among 246 patients with narcolepsy and EHS.

| C | HH | SP | SOREM | HLA-DR2 (+) | HLA-DR2 (−) | Frequency of DR2(+) (%) | Diagnostic criteria: Honda | ASDC-APSS | Roth |
|---|---|---|---|---|---|---|---|---|---|
| + | + | + | + | 125 | 0 | 100.0 | N | N | N |
| + | + | + | − | 32 | 0 | 100.0 | N | N | N |
| + | + | − | + | 10 | 0 | 100.0 | N | N | N |
| + | + | − | − | 3 | 0 | 100.0 | N | N | N |
| + | − | + | + | 4 | 0 | 100.0 | N | N | N |
| + | − | + | − | 1 | 0 | 100.0 | N | N | N |
| + | − | − | + | 7 | 0 | 100.0 | N | N | N |
| + | − | − | − | 10 | 0 | 100.0 | N | N | N |
| − | + | + | + | 4 | 1 | 80.0 | E | N | N |
| − | + | + | − | 8 | 8 | 50.0 | E | N | N |
| − | + | − | + | 0 | 0 | − | E | N | N |
| − | + | − | − | 0 | 0 | − | E | N | N |
| − | − | + | + | 2 | 0 | 100.0 | E | N | N |
| − | − | + | − | 2 | 1 | 66.7 | E | N | N |
| − | − | − | + | 2 | 3 | 40.0 | E | N | N |
| − | − | − | − | 13 | 10 | 56.5 | E | | N |

Note. From Honda 1990, with permission.
Abbreviations. C, cataplexy; E, essential hypersomnia (EHS); HH, hypnagogic hallucinations; N, narcolepsy; SOREM, sleep-onset REM; SP, sleep paralysis.

phenomena. Such kind of identification of a symptom specific to a disease is an essential process in the symptomatological validation of a psychiatric disorder.

Both hierarchical stratification of clinical symptoms and correlation of symptoms with biological parameters are important steps in validating psychiatric diagnosis. There are various possible hierarchical dimensions such as attacklike vs non-attacklike, regular vs irregular, persistent vs transient, and so on. Most psychiatric symptoms that are the expression of brain dysfunction must show some order in their nature and presentation. Furthermore, it is also important to standardize the assessment procedures of biological studies. It is only through the refinement of both symptomatology and biological investigation that a translation between phenomenotype and biotype (Andreasen 1987) can be achieved.

It is necessary to develop a psychiatric diagnostic system that can satisfy different purposes and demands such as treatment, research, and primary care. It is for this reason that ICD-10 was developed as a set of diagnostic measures (Sartorius 1988). The introduction of a multiaxial system that describes many aspects of clinical data is very useful not only for treatment and research, but also for communication among psychiatrists (Mezzich 1988). Finally, the evaluation of coping ability needs to be introduced as a new axis because of its usefulness in deciding treatment planning and the possibility of predicting clinical course and prognosis.

## Conclusion

During the next few decades, as a result of improvement in methodology and statistical analysis, the field of psychiatric diagnosis should approach maturity and become truly international and valid. It is expected that the time will soon come when advances in psychiatric diagnostics will change the basic structure of ICD-10 from its present form to a more biological and scientific orientation.

## *References*

Andreasen NC (1987). The diagnosis of schizophrenia. *Schizophrenia Bulletin* 13:9–22.

Feighner JP, Robins E, Guze SB, Woodruff RA, Winokur G, Munouz R (1972). Diagnostic criteria for use in psychiatric research. *Archives of General Psychiatry* 26:57–63.

Honda Y (1990). Genetic aspects of narcolepsy, pp 217–234. In M Thorpy (ed), *Handbook of Sleep Disorders*. Marcel Dekker, Inc, New York.

Kendell RE (1989). Clinical validity, pp 305–321. In LN Robins, JE Barrett (eds), *The Validity of Psychiatric Diagnosis*. Raven Press, New York.

Mezzich JE (1988). On developing a psychiatric multiaxial schema for ICD-10. *British Journal of Psychiatry* 1:38–43 (suppl 1).

Robins E, Guze SB (1970). Establishment of diagnostic validity in psychiatric illness: Its application to schizophrenia. *American Journal of Psychiatry* 126: 983–987.

Sartorius N (1988). International perspectives of psychiatric classification. *British Journal of Psychiatry* 152:9–14 (suppl 1).

Spitzer RL, Endicott J, Robins E (1981). *Research diagnostic Criteria (RDC) for a Selected Group of Functional Disorders* (3rd ed). New York State Psychiatric Institute, Biometrics Research Department, New York.

# Part II
# ICD-10 Field Studies

# 11
# Progress in the Development of the Classification of Mental Disorders in the ICD-10

NORMAN SARTORIUS

On the 17th of May 1990 the World Health Assembly, the supreme decision making body of the World Health Organization (WHO), resolved that it will formally adopt the proposals for the 10th revision of the *International Classification of Diseases* (ICD-10) that the Director-General of WHO presented to it. The new revision thus came into force and all member states began introducing it as their official classification from the 1st of January 1993 onwards. Preparations for this change started in May 1990. These included the translation of the text of the 10th revision by WHO into the official languages of the Organization and by numerous ministries of health into the languages of the member states; training in the use of the revision at country level for different staff using the ICD; the development of computer software; and the preparation of national guidelines for the use of the classification.

## Organization of the Mental Health Components of ICD-10

The ICD-10 contains a significantly revised chapter on mental and behavioral disorders. Each category in the chapter is accompanied by a brief glossary definition—a feature that makes this chapter unique in the ICD-10. The definitions have been introduced because it was felt that the categories included in the mental disease chapter may be particularly at risk of being differently interpreted in various countries. They were produced through extensive consultation with many experts and nongovernmental organizations. Among the latter was also the World Psychiatric Association, which has made a particularly useful contribution to the development of the ICD-10. An example of a glossary definition is given below:

F32 *Depressive episodes*

In typical mild, moderate, or severe depressive episodes, the patient suffers from lowering of mood, reduction of energy, and decrease in activity. Capacity for enjoyment, interest, and concentration is reduced, and marked tiredness after even minimum effort is common. Sleep is usually disturbed and appetite diminished. Self-esteem and self-confidence are almost always reduced and, even in the mild form, some ideas of guilt or worthlessness are often present. The lowered mood varies little from day to day, is unresponsive to circumstances and may be accompanied by so-called "somatic" symptoms, such as loss of interest and pleasurable feelings, waking in the morning several hours before the usual time, depression worst in the morning, marked psychomotor retardation, agitation, loss of appetite, weight loss, and loss of libido. Depending upon the number and severity of the symptoms, a depressive episode may be specified as mild, moderate, or severe.

The glossary is not the only document that has been developed to accompany the classification of mental and behavioral disorders in the ICD-10: Numerous other materials have also been produced and compose jointly the family of texts linked to the ICD-10 and prepared for mental health service research, training, and statistical reporting. These texts include:

1. The Clinical Guidelines accompanying the ICD-10 chapter dealing with mental disorder.
2. The ICD-10 Diagnostic Criteria for Research on mental disorders.
3. The primary health care adaptation of the classification of mental disorders included in the ICD-10.
4. Crosswalks and reference materials allowing comparisons with classifications produced by national psychiatric associations (eg, *Diagnostic and Statistical Manual*, 3rd edition (DSM-III) of the American Psychiatric Association) or by nongovernmental associations with a special interest (eg, the classification of epilepsy, the classifications of pain, sleep disorders, etc). The "crosswalk" between the ICD revisions (8th, 9th, 10th) has been recently produced by WHO.
5. A multiaxial presentation of the ICD-10. The ICD categories will be used to compose contents of three axes: An axis for clinical syndromes (on which more than one diagnosis, from Chapter F or from another ICD disease chapter may be noted); an axis classifying environmental circumstances of importance for the disease; an axis indicating the level of disability that the disease or syndrome has caused: and another multiaxial version for use in child psychiatry—possibly using six axes—to record the psychiatric syndrome, specific developmental delays, overall intelligence, possible somatic comorbidity, psychosocial factors of importance in the development of the disease, and level of functioning.
6. Computer software allowing the analysis of data obtained by the use of standardized instruments produced by WHO and their summation in a diagnostic category.

7. A series of related classifications (eg, the classification of impairment, disability and handicap, the classification of reasons for contact with health services, and a classification of services for the mentally ill).

8. Standardized assessment instruments for use in clinical work (eg, the Schedules for the Clinical Assessment in Neuropsychiatry [SCAN] (Wing et al 1990) and the International Personality Disorder Examination [IPDE] (Loranger et al 1991) and in epidemiological investigations (eg, The Composite International Diagnostic Interview [CIDI]) (Robins et al 1988).

9. Standard case histories and videotaped material that can be used for training (for example, in the framework of a research project or in postgraduate training) and for the assessment of reliability between interviewers who are making their diagnosis using ICD-10 categories.

All of these texts are being developed simultaneously in several languages. This is a novelty in the development of ICD materials: For previous revisions, the English-language version was prepared first then tested and after finalization offered for translation into other languages. This is a more efficient way of proceeding, but it carries two dangers: First, that the experience and diagnostic usage of the many experts in different parts of the world will not be considered early enough and sufficiently in producing the classification; and second, that, once produced, the classification will not be acceptable because it will not contain provisions for the classification of diagnostic statements made in countries that do not use English as their first foreign language.

## The Core Classification of Mental Disorders

The classification of mental disorders proposed to the World Health Assembly for approval in 1990 was a product of joint work by many people and the result of many years of work. This work started as an international program on the standardization of psychiatric diagnosis, classification, and statistics launched by WHO in the late 1960s (Sartorius 1976, Kramer et al 1979). Among the results of this program, two were of particular importance for the development of the ICD-10: The first was the development of methods for research into psychiatric diagnosis (Shepherd et al 1968) and the second was the establishment of a worldwide network of individuals and institutions participating in this work. This background work facilitated the initiation of a major new program of research and development started by WHO in collaboration with the US Alcohol, Drug Abuse and Mental Health Administration in the late 1970s (Jablensky et al 1983) and later supported by numerous other agencies, institutions, and associations. A first step was a comprehensive review of knowledge about mental disorders, carried out by individual experts in different parts of the world. The reviews were then presented to small groups of experts, each dealing with a set of problems—such as, for example, affective disorders. The findings and recommendations of these groups served as background documents for a major conference on psychiatric classification held in Copenhagen in 1982 (World Health Organization Drug Abuse and Mental Health Administration 1985).

The Copenhagen conference was followed by a period of several months devoted to the drafting of definitions for each of the categories of the classification. These were drafted by specialists in a variety of countries and circulated for comment and review to numerous experts in different parts of the world. Once their views had been received, drafts of the definitions were amended and then released for yet wider circulation.

## Field Trials of the Diagnostic Guidelines

At the same time, WHO launched a series of trials of the diagnostic guidelines that were to accompany the new classification. These tests were conducted with the aim of establishing whether the definitions and the arrangement of categories were comprehensible, easy to use, and translatable into other languages. The classification was used in reliability exercises to establish whether psychiatrists and others likely to deal with psychiatric patients could reach the same diagnosis when faced by the same information and whether they found it possible to accommodate the universe of syndromes and diagnoses that they saw in their practice into the categories that were proposed in a reliable way.

These trials grew into the largest collaborative program on classification and diagnosis that has ever been undertaken. More than 100 centers in some 40 countries participated in the trials, using the classification that by then had been translated into some 15 languages. A list of countries and numbers of centers in each is given in Table 11.1.

The results of the tests of the diagnostic guidelines were most encouraging (Sartorius et al 1993). The classification was found to be easy to use. The definitions were found to be clear and easy to understand; the variety of clinical syndromes in different countries could be covered by the system proposed; the reliability of ratings made by psychiatrists was at acceptable levels (generally with a kappa of 0.70 or more) and the translations could be rendered equivalent and acceptable to the different psychiatric schools, worldwide.

In the conduct of this work, the World Health Organization relied on the help of Field Trial Coordinating Centers (FTCC) located in Campinas, Brazil; Shanghai, China; Risskov, Denmark; Alexandria, Egypt; Lübeck, Germany; Bangalore, India; Naples, Italy; Nagasaki, Japan; Luxembourg; Wellington, New Zealand; Madrid, Spain; Nottingham, United Kingdom; Rockville, Maryland, United States of America. Each of these centers

TABLE 11.1. Countries in which the field trials of the classification of mental disorders contained in the ICD-10 were conducted.

| Country | Centers | Clinicians | Assessments |
|---|---|---|---|
| Australia | 3 | 8 | 257 |
| Austria | 1 | 2 | 24 |
| Bahrain | 1 | 3 | 132 |
| Belgium | 1 | 2 | 10 |
| Brazil | 3 | 11 | 269 |
| Canada | 6 | 39 | 1,051 |
| China | 2 | 6 | 184 |
| Colombia | 1 | 3 | 50 |
| Czechoslovakia | 1 | 4 | 120 |
| Denmark | 5 | 75 | 1,383 |
| Egypt | 1 | 4 | 192 |
| France | 5 | 16 | 581 |
| Germany | 7 | 122 | 1,626 |
| Greece | 1 | 2 | 58 |
| India | 8 | 30 | 675 |
| Indonesia | 1 | 7 | 60 |
| Italy | 1 | 9 | 225 |
| Japan | 5 | 61 | 2,192 |
| Korea | 1 | 7 | 282 |
| Luxembourg | 1 | 2 | 40 |
| Mexico | 2 | 5 | 90 |
| Netherlands | 1 | 2 | 70 |
| New Zealand | 2 | 8 | 291 |
| Nigeria | 1 | 3 | 72 |
| Pakistan | 3 | 20 | 422 |
| Peru | 1 | 3 | 49 |
| Poland | 2 | 10 | 248 |
| Spain | 7 | 55 | 539 |
| Sudan | 1 | 2 | 44 |
| Sweden | 1 | 3 | 70 |
| Switzerland | 4 | 19 | 282 |
| Thailand | 1 | 2 | 20 |
| Turkey | 1 | 7 | 245 |
| United Kingdom | 12 | 70 | 1,257 |
| Uruguay | 1 | 8 | 193 |
| USA | 14 | 67 | 1,705 |
| Yugoslavia | 1 | 3 | 30 |
| Total | 110 | 700 | 15,038 |

coordinated the work of 15 to 20 other centers, usually grouped by geographical proximity, by being able to use the same language, or by previous collaborative relationships. The tremendous amount of work that has been necessary to complete these trials has been carried out by the centers using their own resources or resources that their countries provided for this work.

The results of the field trials facilitated the finalization of the clinical guidelines that accompany the ICD-10 chapter on mental disorders. The road was thus opened for work on the research diagnostic guidelines, for assessment of the multiaxial presentations of the ICD-10, and for preparation of the classification for primary health care.

## Diagnostic Criteria for Research

The first of these tasks—a year-long program to test the diagnostic criteria for research—began in October 1990. The trials were carried out in numerous centers around the world. In addition to the centers that participated in the first series of studies, a number of new centers joined the work. The centers were offered a standard, core protocol involving reliability tests and detailed annotations of the criteria as well as a series of options for other studies. On this occasion, the trials in a number of centers also include comparisons with national classifications. Some of the centers decided to concentrate on only one or two diagnostic groups: Others examined the whole range of diagnostic categories. As the trials were completed, the formulation of the criteria was amended and the material was circulated to obtain further comments before finalization. During the course of these trials, consultations with groups working on national classifications (eg, the DSM-IV of the American Psychiatric Association) continued to take place. These consultations were most helpful to both the ICD-10 and national classification groups and are an expression of the commitment by WHO and researchers worldwide to seek full translatability and compatibility between the ICD-10 and the national classifications, and there is every likelihood that this goal will be achieved.

## Multiaxial Presentations

The tests of the multiaxial presentation of the ICD-10 for use in psychiatric practice with adults have also begun in Austria, Denmark, Spain, and the United States, and were then expanded to many other centers. Close collaboration with the Section on Classification of the World Psychiatric Association has been maintained in this work throughout and it is hoped that it will continue. It is expected that the multiaxial presentation will be published shortly after publication of the ICD-10 Diagnostic Criteria for Research. The multiaxial classification of mental disorders in children has also been developed and will be published in 1994. The multiaxial presentation of the ICD-10 for adults has three axes. The first includes all diagnoses present in a particular patient. This arrangement has been made because it was felt that such a presentation would—better than anything else—demonstrate that the division of morbid states in a mental and a physical group was neither useful nor justifiable in light of the current state of our knowledge. The second axis, of disability, is to classify degrees of inability to perform in social roles—an inability to a large extent dependent on factors other than impairment and the disease itself. Environmental circumstances relevant to the diagnosis and management were placed on the third axis to exemplify the importance of their proper assessment and to facilitate international and, in particular, cross-cultural comparisons.

## Primary Health Care Version (ICD-10 PHC)

The development of the version of the ICD-10 classification of mental disorders for primary care is of particular importance. This is the version most likely to affect the care that is provided to people with mental disorders. If an attractive and easy-to-use classification can be produced, it is very likely that it will find wide application: This may break the vicious circle currently hampering the improvement of services for those with mental disorders. The vicious circle is particularly present in third world countries where training in psychiatry for the general practitioner and staff working in general and primary contact care has been insufficient in quality and quantity for a long time. As a consequence, mental disorder is not recognized in primary health care and not reported. The fact that statistics from primary care facilities (because of nonrecognition) show very low numbers of people requesting care for mental illness is then often taken as evidence that mental disorder is rare in the developing countries, and that training of staff in recognizing it or treating it is a luxury.

The introduction of a simplified classification taught in undergraduate training would help improve patient care and allow more accurate estimations of frequency of mental health problems seen in general health care. This, in turn, would help to change attitudes to such problems and might influence the ordering of priorities in the health systems of the third world.

## ICD-10 Timetable

The timetable for WHO's work in the development of materials linked to the ICD-10 is given in Table 11.2.

The Primary Care Version of the *International Classification of Diseases* (10th Revision) Chapter V, Mental and Behavioural Disorders (ICD-10 PHC) focuses on 24 conditions which are frequently seen in primary care and which can be managed effectively by general practitioners. The classification is accompanied by one flipcard for each of the categories. The cards contain diagnostic guidelines on one side and management guidelines on the other. The draft ICD-10 PHC was tested in the field for its

TABLE 11.2. Timetable for the development of materials supporting the use of the classification of mental and behavioral disorders in ICD-10.

| Materials | 1990 | 1991 | 1992 | 1993 | 1994–1997 | 1998 |
|---|---|---|---|---|---|---|
| ICD-10 short definitions | Adopted by assembly | Publish | Coder's training in use of ICD | Entry into use worldwide | Monitor use | Begin 11th revision process |
| Clinical guidelines | Finalized and submitted for publication | Publish | Monitor use | | Monitor use | Revision of text (if needed) |
| Diagnostic criteria for research | First draft | Complete field tests | | Publish | Monitor use | Revision of text (if needed) |
| Multiaxial classification (children) | Second draft | Complete field tests | Publish | Monitor use | Monitor use | |
| Multiaxial classification (adults) | First draft prepared | Begin field tests | | | Publish | Revision of text (if needed) |
| PHC version of ICD-10 | | Prepare first draft | Field tests | Publish | | Monitor use |
| Classification of disabilities | | | First draft | Field tests | Publish | Monitor use |
| Crosswalks | | Produced as document | | Update | Update and publish | |
| Training materials | | Produce drafts | | Update | Update and publish | |

Note. The various materials will be released for use as they become ready, and the experience in their use monitored by the Field Centers collaborating with WHO in this area. The comments and reports on experiences in different countries will be systematically reviewed by groups of experts and used in the revision of texts, tentatively scheduled for 1998.

applicability and acceptance of its style and content in 154 centers from 58 countries. The trials help to obtain data in three different parts: (i) the applicability and usefulness, (ii) reliability and validity, (iii) appropriateness of the ICD-10 PHC for primary care practice. Initial results suggests that the ICD-10 PHC version is applicable and useful.

## Conclusion

The WHO's long-term goal in the field of mental health is to produce a common language for the field of mental health so that those who work in it can communicate their experience and learn from each other. The "family" of ICD publications is an important contribution to this effort. Other components aim to develop tools for the assessment of patients and for the assessment of quality of care provided to the mentally ill. Several multicenter studies are under way to develop these instruments and are likely to produce them in the foreseeable future so that a comprehensive and coherent system of assessment and reporting about mental disorders can be offered for international use.

Much progress has been made in the development of this "family": None of it would have been possible without the selfless, generous, and highly expert contributions of many people and institutions worldwide. The continuing existence of this network will continue to be of vital importance for further development of this work, which has such direct relevance to the improvement of mental health services, better training in mental health matters, and collaboration in research nationally and across borders, worldwide.

## *References*


Jablensky A, Sartorius N, Hirschfeld R, Pardes H (1983). Diagnosis and classification of mental disorders and alcohol and drug-related problems: A research agenda for the 1980's. *Psychological Medicine* 13:907–921.

Kramer M, Sartorius N, Jablensky A, Gulbinat W (1979). The ICD-9 classification of mental disorders: A review of its development and contents. *Acta Psychiatrica Scandinavica* 59:241–262.

Loranger A, Hirschfield R, Sartorius N, Regier D (1991). The WHO/ADAMHA international pilot study of personality disorders: Background and purpose. *Journal of Personality Disorders* 5:296–306.

Robins LE, Wing JE, Wittchen H-U, Kelzer JE, Babor TF, Burke JD, Farmer A, Jablensky A, Pickens R, Regier DA, Sartorius N, Towle LH (1988). The composite international diagnostic interview: An epidemiologic instrument suitable for use in conjunction with different diagnostic systems and in different cultures. *Archives of General Psychiatry* 45:1069–1077.

Sartorius N (1976). Classification: An international perspective. *Psychiatric Annals* 6:22–35.

Sartorius N, Kaelber CT, Cooper JE, Roper MT (1993). Progress toward achieving a common language in psychiatry: Results from the field trial of the clinical guidelines accompanying the WHO classification of mental and behavioral disorders in ICD-10. *Archives of General Psychiatry* 50:115–124.

Shephard M, Brooke EM, Cooper JE, Lin T (1968). An experimental approach to psychiatric diagnosis: An international study. *Acta Psychiatrica Scandinavica* (suppl 20).

Wing JE, Babor TF, Jablensky A, Regier DA, Sartorius N (1990). SCAN: Schedule for clinical assessment in neuropsychiatry. *Archives of General Psychiatry* 47:589–593.

World Heath Organization (1985). *WHO/Alcohol, Drug Abuse and Mental Health Administration (ADAMHA). Mental disorders: International perspectives on their diagnosis and classification* (International Congress Series, 669). Excerpta Medica, Amsterdam.

# 12
# Field Trials of the ICD-10 Chapter on Mental Disorders in Japan

Yoshibumi Nakane, Yoshiro Ohkubo, Ryo Takahashi,
Itaru Yamashita, Masahisa Nishizono, and Tooru Takahashi

The *International Classification of Diseases* (ICD), developed by the World Health Organization (WHO) to diagnose and to classify both physical and mental diseases, has been adopted by many countries worldwide. Every 10 years the system has been revised. In 1950 in Japan, ICD-6 was introduced through the direct supervision of the Statistical Data Division of the Ministry of Health and Welfare. In 1979, ICD-9 was officially adopted for use in medical statistics. Since then, ICD-9 has been widely used in both clinical and research settings in the psychiatric as well as other medical fields.

With the publication of both the *Diagnostic and Statistical Manual of Mental Disorders*, 3rd edition (DSM-III) and the revised edition (DSM-III-R) by the American Psychiatric Association (APA) (1980, 1987), diagnostic classification of mental disorders in Japan has received considerable interest, especially in terms of aiding the selection of a homogeneous group of subjects in biological studies of psychiatric illness. Because of the absence of an original classification system in Japan, the idea of establishing specific operational diagnostic criteria and the development of multiaxial diagnosis by the APA had a significant impact. This interest in diagnostic systems was not restricted to only DSM-III, but extended to other diagnostic classification systems as well, especially the ICD (Nakane et al 1984, Nakane and Takahashi 1984, Takahashi et al 1985).

In 1984, the first draft of the latest revised edition of ICD-9, namely ICD-10, was prepared by WHO. Since then several other drafts have followed. In Japan, the Ministry of Health and Welfare introduced the second draft of ICD-10 in 1986. Interest in the revised system has gradually increased, and since 1987, many papers in the field of psychiatry relating to Chapter V of the Classification have been published (Hanada 1990, Honda and Sasaki 1990, Iwasige and Nakamura 1990, Kitamura et al 1990, Okazaki 1990, Okubo et al 1990, Takahashi 1990,

Takahashi and Ishida 1990, Tanaka and Nakamura 1990). As originally scheduled, ICD-10 was officially adopted at the general meeting of the World Health assembly in May 1990. In Japan, the classification will be officially adopted around 1994.

As described in Chapter 11 of this volume, various versions of ICD-10 are being prepared to serve different purposes. The materials included in the ICD–10(F) "family" are: (1) Clinical Descriptions and Diagnostic Guidelines (WHO 1992), (2) Diagnostic Criteria for Research, (3) Multiaxial Classification, (4) Simple Classification for Primary Health Care, (5) Glossary, and (6) Lists of Crosswalks between the Classifications of ICD-8, ICD-9 and ICD-10. At this stage, and since the core classification was officially accepted in May 1990, several revisions have been made to the Clinical Descriptions and Diagnostic Guidelines, Chapter V (Table 12.1).

As drafts of ICD-10, Chapter V were prepared, the Division of Mental Health of WHO planned and organized corresponding international field trials. The main purposes of these trials were: (1) to evaluate the usefulness of the Clinical Descriptions and Diagnostic Guidelines of ICD-10, Chapter V; (2) to evaluate how appropriately the diagnostic classification system describes various psychiatric disorders, and how applicable they are to patients; and (3) to provide information about the extent of agreement between evaluators using the diagnostic classification system. In Japan, WHO Collaborating Centers were requested to conduct these field trials. In 1986 and 1987, the field trials were conducted with the collaboration of five institutions: Tokyo Medical and Dental University (Field Trial Coordinating Center), Nagasaki University, Fukuoka University, Hokkaido University, and the National Institute of Mental Health. In this chapter, the summary of the results obtained in the

TABLE 12.1. Revision stages of ICD-10 (F) Clinical Descriptions and Diagnostic Guidelines.

| Revision | Description |
|---|---|
| MNH/MEP/87.1 | 1986 Draft of Chapter V, categories F00–F99, mental, behavioral and developmental disorders; 1986 draft for Field Trials |
| MNH/MEP/87.1 rev.1 | 1987 Draft of Chapter V, categories F00–F99, mental, behavioral and developmental disorders; June 1987 draft for Field Trials |
| MNH/MEP/87.1 rev.2 | 1988 Draft of Chapter V, categories F00–F99, mental, behavioral and developmental disorders; September 1988 draft |
| MNH/MEP/87.1 rev.3 | 1989 Draft of Chapter V, categories F00–F99, mental and behavioral disorders (including disorders of psychological development); April 1989 draft |
| MNH/MEP/87.1 rev.4 | 1990 Draft of Chapter V, categories F00–F99, mental and behavioral disorders (including disorders of psychological development); May 1990 draft |

Japanese field trials previously reported in Japanese (Okubo et al 1990) is discussed.

## Method

The Japanese translated version of the 1986 *Draft of ICD-10, Clinical Descriptions and Diagnostic Guidelines* (WHO 1987) was used in the Japanese field trials: It is the core unit of the ICD-10 family and is designed for both clinical work and education. Each diagnostic category consists of concept description, diagnostic guidelines, and differential diagnosis. Each category is described in either a four- or five-digit code. The first three digits show the main category of diagnosis. The fourth digit shows the subclassification, and the fifth digit (optional) shows any special features of the category. For example, F20.00 describes Paranoid Schizophrenia, Continuous Course. The second digit F20.00 indicates Schizophrenic Disorders; Schizotypal States, and Behavioral Disorders; the third character F20.00, Schizophrenia; the fourth character F20.00, Paranoid (subtype of schizophrenia); and the fifth character F20.00, Continuous Course (type of course of disorder).

The field trials were conducted according to the protocol devised by WHO. The time frame for each stage of the study—translation, familiarization, preparation of case summaries, joint assessment of patients, assessment of case summaries and further comments and discussion—was arranged for between 1 to 20 weeks (Table 12.2). Familiarization was a preliminary step in which diagnostic training with 5 to 10 patients was conducted for researchers to become familiar with the use of the ICD-10 draft. Actual assessment of patients was based on either joint clinical interviews or case summaries. The field trials based on case summaries alone consisted of two stages: preparation and assessment. Each of the five participating institutions prepared four case summaries, and sent each of the four cases to the other four collaborating centers for assessment. All in all, each center assessed 16 cases.

As shown in Table 12.3, 60 psychiatrists and 1 clinical psychologist participated in the trials, and a total of 129 patients were assessed. Each

TABLE 12.2. Time schedule for ICD-10 field trial in Japan.

| Task | Schedule | Date |
|---|---|---|
| Translation and printing | Preliminary | 1 June 1986 |
| Familiarization | Weeks 1–2 | 15 June 1986 |
| Preparation of case summaries | Weeks 3–6 | 30 June 1986 |
| Joint assessment of patients | Weeks 7–16 | 31 July 1986 |
| Assessment of case summaries | Weeks 17–18 | 31 August 1986 |
| Further comments and discussion | Weeks 19–20 | 30 September 1986 |
| Conclusion of the field trials | | 31 October 1986 |

TABLE 12.3. Participating clinicians and evaluated patients.

| Institution | Clinicians | Patients |
|---|---|---|
| Tokyo Med. Dent. University | 18 | 36 |
| Nagasaki University | 6 | 36 |
| Hokkaido University | 18 | 36 |
| Fukuoka University | 11 | 39 |
| National Institute of Mental Health | 8* | 42 |
| Total | 61* | 129 |

*Includes one psychologist.

case was diagnosed according to the individual judgment of the clinician without consultation with other clinicians. Clinicians gave both a main diagnosis and a subdiagnosis for each patient. Furthermore, clinicians' evaluations of the diagnosis itself were obtained: (1) goodness-of-fit of main diagnosis chosen was evaluated using a five-level scale, (2) degree of confidence of diagnosis was evaluated using a three-level scale, (3) degree of difficulty in making a diagnosis according to the guidelines provided by ICD-10 was evaluated using a three-level scale, and (4) adequacy of clinical description and of diagnostic guidelines was also evaluated.

## Results and Discussion

### *Agreement Rate*

Although the ICD-10 draft allows for categories to be coded by either four or five digits, in this chapter we only report on the basis of the four-digit code. The diagnosis (four-digit code) given by the largest number of evaluators was defined as the major diagnosis of the patient being evaluated. For 12 of the 129 cases, several different diagnoses were given by equal numbers of evaluators so that a major diagnosis could not be identified. For these cases, a smaller code number of the chosen categories was selected as the major diagnosis. In summary, this field trial using 129 subjects yielded 52 categories (four-digit code) that were selected as major diagnoses.

Table 12.4 shows the number of cases of two-digit classification of major diagnoses and the inter-rater agreement for three- and four-digit categories. In this trial, there were no cases included in the F7 (Mental Retardation) and F8 (Developmental Disorders) categories. In relation to two-digit categories selected as the major diagnosis, 50 cases were given the diagnosis of F2, Schizophrenia, Schizotypal States, and Delusional Disorders, 38 cases were given the diagnosis of F3, Mood Disorders, 22 cases were given the diagnosis of F4, Neurotic, Stress-Related, and Somatoform Disorders.

TABLE 12.4. Inter-rater agreement (%) by major classes of mental disorders.

| Class | Description | Cases | 3-Digit | 4-Digit |
|---|---|---|---|---|
| F0 | Organic, including symptomatic, mental disorders | 3 | 73.6 | 69.7 |
| F1 | Mental and behavioral disorders due to psychoactive substance use | 5 | 97.8 | 80.8 |
| F2 | Schizophrenia, schizotypal states, and delusional disorders | 50 | 78.6 | 69.3 |
| F3 | Mood (affective) disorders | 38 | 73.3 | 64.0 |
| F4 | Neurotic, stress-related, and somatoform disorders | 22 | 65.7 | 52.8 |
| F5 | Physiological dysfunction associated with mental and behavioral factors | 2 | 100.0 | 97.2 |
| F6 | Abnormalities of adult personality and behavior | 7 | 73.0 | 45.8 |
| F9 | Behavioral and emotional disorders with onset usually occurring in childhood or adolescence | 2 | 57.6 | 57.6 |
| | Total | 129 | 74.6 | 63.8 |

The mean agreement rates for F2, F3 and F4 (four-digit codes) were 69.3%, 64.0% and 52.8% respectively. The mean agreement rate for all cases on the four-digit code was 63.8% and for the three-digit code, 74.6%.

As shown in Table 12.5, the major three-digit categories were F20, Schizophrenia with 30 cases, F31, Depressive Episode with 17 cases, F22, Persistent Delusional Disorders with nine cases, F33, Recurrent Depressive Disorders with eight cases and F45, Somatoform Disorder with seven cases. Agreement rates for the categories were 81.6%, 74.6%, 80.1%, 85.3% and 72.3%, respectively.

TABLE 12.5. Inter-rater agreement (%) on 3-digit diagnostic categories.

| Category | Description | Cases | 3-Digit |
|---|---|---|---|
| F06 | Other mental disorders due to brain disease, damage or dysfunction, or to physical disease | 2 | 60.4 |
| F10 | Disorders resulting from use of alcohol | 5 | 97.8 |
| F20 | Schizophrenia | 30 | 81.6 |
| F21 | Schizotypal states | 5 | 58.4 |
| F22 | Persistent delusional disorders | 9 | 80.1 |
| F23 | Acute or transient psychotic disorders | 5 | 86.8 |
| F31 | Depressive episode | 17 | 74.6 |
| F32 | Bipolar affective disorder | 4 | 90.0 |
| F33 | Recurrent depressive disorders | 8 | 85.3 |
| F40 | Phobic disorder | 4 | 72.2 |
| F41 | Other anxiety disorder | 2 | 45.6 |
| F44 | Dissociative disorder | 3 | 74.1 |
| F45 | Somatoform disorder | 7 | 72.3 |
| F50 | Eating disorders | 2 | 100.0 |
| F60 | Personality disorders | 6 | 71.4 |

TABLE 12.6. Inter-rater agreement (%) on 4-digit diagnostic categories.

| Category | Description | Cases | 4-Digit |
|---|---|---|---|
| F10.3 | Disorders resulting from use of alcohol, harmful use | 3 | 84.7 |
| F10.4 | Disorders resulting from use of alcohol, withdrawal state | 2 | 75.0 |
| F20.0 | Paranoid schizophrenia | 23 | 75.4 |
| F20.1 | Hebephrenic schizophrenia | 4 | 82.6 |
| F21.0 | Schizotypal disorder | 4 | 48.5 |
| F23.8 | Other acute psychotic disorder | 2 | 54.5 |
| F31.0 | Severe depressive episode | 16 | 77.2 |
| F32.1 | Bipolar affective disorder, currently depressive | 2 | 97.2 |
| F33.0 | Recurrent severe depressive disorder | 6 | 60.4 |
| F33.2 | Recurrent depressive disorder, variable | 2 | 60.4 |
| F34.1 | Dysthymia | 4 | 26.7 |
| F36.1 | Schizo-depressive disorder | 3 | 44.6 |
| F40.0 | Agoraphobia | 2 | 46.2 |
| F43.2 | Adjustment disorder | 4 | 50.1 |
| F44.5 | Psychogenic disorders of voluntary movement | 2 | 86.1 |
| F45.0 | Multiple somatoform disorder | 2 | 69.6 |
| F45.2 | Hypochondriacal syndrome | 2 | 41.0 |
| F45.4 | Pain syndrome without specific organic cause | 3 | 48.4 |
| F60.6 | Anxious personality disorder | 2 | 59.1 |

Table 12.6 shows the four-digit diagnostic categories used as major diagnoses in more than two cases. The most frequent categories given were F20.0, Paranoid Schizophrenia in 23 cases, F31.0 Severe Depressive Episode in 16 cases, and F33.0, Recurrent Severe Depressive Disorder in six cases. Table 12.6 also shows the inter-rater agreement rates for each of these diagnoses. Table 12.7 shows the diagnostic categories for the F2 group alone, and the inter-rater agreement rates for both the three- and four-digit codes.

## *Goodness-of-Fit Rating, Confidence of Rating, and Ease and Difficulty of Diagnosis*

As shown in Table 12.8, the mean percentage of people who indicated a good goodness-of-fit rating was 86.9% (very good fit, 41.2%; good fit, 45.7%). This means that most of the evaluators who made a diagnosis that reflected the major diagnosis considered that their diagnosis represented a good fit. For some individual categories, however, the goodness-of-fit rating was low. Poor fit or less was given to F34.1, Dysthymia (52.5%); F21, Schizotypal States (50.7%); F21.0, Schizotypal Disorder (46.7%); and F23.8, Other Acute Psychotic Disorder (46.7%).

Table 12.8 also shows the evaluation of confidence of rating. Generally, the confidence of rating was high—93.0% (very confident, 41.3%; moderately confident, 51.7%). In other words, most evaluators were

TABLE 12.7. Inter-rater agreement (%) for F2 categories.

| Category | Disorder | Cases | 3-Digit | 4-Digit |
|---|---|---|---|---|
| F20 | Schizophrenia | 30 | 81.6 | 73.1 |
| F20.0 | Paranoid schizophrenia | 23 | 81.9 | 75.4 |
| F20.1 | Hebephrenic schizophrenia | 4 | 95.8 | 82.6 |
| F20.2 | Catatonic schizophrenia | 1 | 16.7 | 16.7 |
| F20.3 | Undifferentiated schizophrenia | 1 | 62.5 | 62.5 |
| F20.4 | Postschizophrenic depression | 1 | 100.0 | 50.0 |
| F21 | Schizotypal states | 5 | 58.4 | 50.8 |
| F21.0 | Schizotypal disorder | 4 | 55.5 | 48.5 |
| F21.1 | Simple schizophrenia | 1 | 70.0 | 60.0 |
| F22 | Persistent delusional disorders | 9 | 80.1 | 75.1 |
| F23 | Acute or transient psychotic disorders | 5 | 86.8 | 61.3 |
| F23.0 | Acute delusional disorder | 1 | 100.0 | 50.0 |
| F23.1 | Psychogenic delusional disorder | 1 | 100.0 | 60.0 |
| F23.2 | Schizophrenia-like episode | 1 | 100.0 | 87.5 |
| F23.8 | Other acute psychotic disorder | 2 | 67.0 | 54.5 |
| F28 | Other nonorganic psychotic disorders | 1 | 33.3 | 33.3 |
| | Total | 50 | 78.6 | 69.3 |

confident about their diagnosis. Those diagnostic categories that had the lowest confidence rating (ie, low level of confidence in diagnosis) were F45.2, Hypochondriacal Syndrome (39.6%); F34.1, Dysthymia (29.2%); and F60, Personality Disorder, (20.1%).

In relation to the ease or difficulty of rating (see Table 12.8), 35.4% of the evaluators found making diagnoses very easy, 49.7% found them moderately easy, and 14.9% found them difficult to make. In general, 85.1% of the evaluators did not have any difficulty in making a diagnosis.

TABLE 12.8. Goodness-of-fit rating, confidence of rating, and ease or difficulty of diagnosis (%).

| | % |
|---|---|
| Goodness-of-fit rating | |
| Very good fit | 41.2 |
| Good fit | 45.7 |
| Poor fit | 10.1 |
| Difficult differential diagnosis | 2.5 |
| Not covered by any disorder | 0.5 |
| Confidence of rating | |
| Very confident | 41.3 |
| Moderately confident | 51.7 |
| Low level of confidence | 7.0 |
| Ease or difficulty of diagnosis | |
| Very easy | 35.4 |
| Moderately easy | 49.7 |
| Difficult | 14.9 |

When we look at individual categories, we find that evaluators had the most difficulty with the following categories: F23.8, Other Acute Psychotic Disorder (54.5%); F34.1, Dysthymia (37.6%); F41, Other Anxiety Disorder (36.5%); and F45.2, Hypochondriacal Syndrome (34.0%).

## *Adequacy of Descriptions*

Clinicians were asked to evaluate the adequacy of the Clinical Descriptions and Diagnostic Guidelines. In those cases in which clinicians rated the same diagnostic categories several times, their lowest evaluations were used. Results showed the following evaluation of the adequacy of description of the categories in general: good, 26.5%; adequate, 65.4%; and inadequate, 9.1%. In general, 90.9% of the clinicians felt that the descriptions were adequate or better. Those categories for which the descriptions were felt not to be adequate included: F23.8, Other Acute Psychotic Disorder (25.0%); F60, Personality Disorder (21.2%); F36.1, Schizo-Depressive Disorder (17.2%); F22.0, Delusional Disorders (16.4%); and F34.1, Dysthymia (15.6%).

## *Correlation Among Ratings*

Table 12.9 shows the correlation coefficients between the five evaluation variables—inter-rater agreement, goodness-of-fit, confidence of diagnosis, ease of making a diagnosis, and adequacy of description of categories. Correlation coefficients were calculated for 34 diagnostic categories, all of which had been made by at least two clinicians. Significant intercorrelations were found for all five factors ($P < 0.05$). In other words, a category that was high on one rating tended to be high on the other ratings.

The relationship between inter-rater agreement and adequacy of diagnostic category description was examined by looking at the dispersion of each of the categories (for three- or four-digit codes) in which two or more clinicians had given the same diagnosis. The results are shown in Figure 12.1. Those categories with both a good description rating

TABLE 12.9. Correlations between evaluations.

| | Agreement | | | | |
|---|---|---|---|---|---|
| Goodness | 0.61 | Goodness | | | |
| Confidence | 0.61 | 0.80 | Confidence | | |
| Ease | 0.70 | 0.81 | 0.70 | Ease | |
| Adequacy | 0.60 | 0.66 | 0.60 | 0.78 | Adequacy |

Note. (N = 34, Pearson $P < 0.05$).

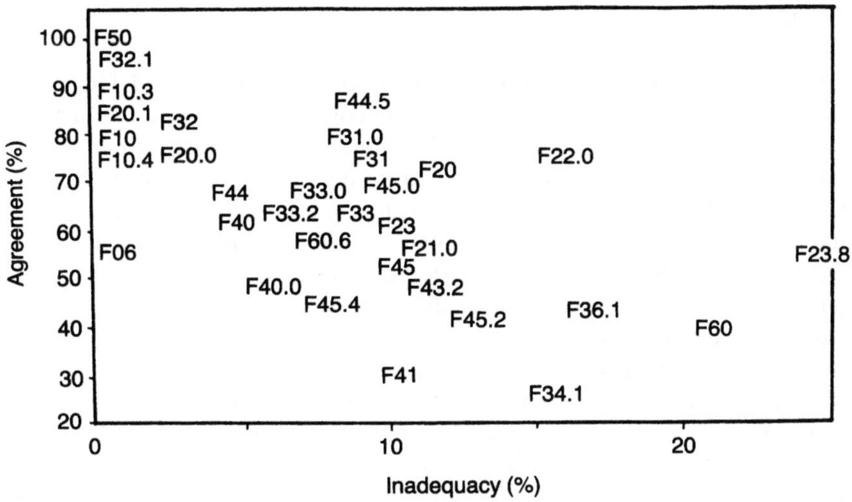


FIGURE 12.1. Adequacy of clinical descriptions and inter-rater agreement in the ICD-10 field trials in Japan.

(horizontal axis) and higher inter-rater agreement (vertical axis) can be found in the upper left region, and include F10, Disorders Resulting From Use of Alcohol; F10.3, Disorders Resulting From Use of Alcohol, Harmful Use; F10.4, Disorders Resulting From Use of Alcohol, Withdrawal Use; F20.0, Paranoid Schizophrenia; F20.1, Hebephrenic Schizophrenia; F32, Bipolar Affective Disorder; F32.1, Bipolar Affective Disorder, Currently Depressive; and F50, Eating Disorders. These categories were also high on the other evaluations of goodness-of-fit, confidence of diagnosis, and ease of diagnosis.

Most of those categories that were low on inter-rater agreement were also low in the evaluation of the adequacy of their description. In the lower right region one can see that these categories include F23.8, Other Acute Psychotic Disorder; F34.1, Dysthymia; F36.1, Schizo-Depressive Disorder; F41, Other Anxiety Disorder; F45.2, Hypochondriacal Syndrome; and F60, Personality Disorder. These categories also had low evaluations on each of the other factors of goodness-of-fit, confidence of diagnosis, and ease of diagnosis. In these field trials, there appears to be a problem in using these categories.

As one can see, there was generally a good correlation between adequacy of description and inter-rater agreement. The major exceptions were F22.0, Delusional Disorders, which had high inter-rater agreement but whose description was found to be inadequate; and F06, Other Mental Disorders Due to Brain Disease, Damage or Dysfunction, or to Physical Disease, which had low inter-rater agreement but whose description was rated as being adequate.

## Conclusion

Field trials for ICD-10 Chapter V, Clinical Description and Diagnostic Guidelines (1986 Draft) in Japan were conducted as part of an international WHO project. Sixty-one clinicians from five institutions participated in the field trials and examined a total of 129 patients using ICD-10. The diagnostic evaluations were based on the following measures: general diagnostic agreement between raters; goodness-of-fit, confidence, ease and difficulty of diagnosis; and adequacy of diagnostic description. In general, satisfactory results for each of the five variables were obtained. Inter-rater agreement for the three-digit code diagnostic categories was 74.6% and for the four-digit code categories, 63.8%.

Although general ratings were satisfactory, problems with certain categories were noted. They included F23.8, Other Acute Psychotic Disorder; F34.1, Dysthymia; F36.1, Schizo-Depressive Disorder; F45.2, Hypochondriacal Syndrome; and F60, Personality Disorder. Our experience suggested some problems in the descriptions of these categories. Subsequent revisions to ICD-10, especially to F23, Acute or Transient Psychotic Disorders; F36, Schizoaffective; and F60, Personality Disorders as a result of the findings obtained from the field trials from all around the world, have led to an improvement in the diagnostic categories, and we think to a better diagnostic system.

*Acknowledgment.* The study reported in this chapter was conducted with the cooperation of five institutions: Tokyo Medical and Dental University, Nagasaki University, Fukuoka University, Hokkaido University, and the National Institute of Mental Health. We would like to acknowledge the contribution of all the collaborating researchers from these institutions. We would also like to acknowledge the help of Yasuko Imamura, Mark Radford, and Aki Nakano in the preparation of this chapter.

## *References*

American Psychiatric Association (1980). *Diagnostic and Statistical Manual of Mental Disorders* (3rd ed) (DSM-III). American Psychiatric Association, Washington, DC.

American Psychiatric Association (1987). *Diagnostic and Statistical Manual of Mental Disorders* (3rd ed, rev) (DSM-III-R). American Psychiatric Association, Washington, DC.

Hanada K (1990). Mood disorders in ICD-10 draft. *Japanese Journal of Clinical Psychiatry* 19:1059–1066 (in Japanese).

Honda Y, Sasaki T (1990). Draft of ICD-10 and sleep disorders. *Japanese Journal of Clinical Psychiatry* 19:1075–1082 (in Japanese).

Iwasige T, Nakamura M (1990). Neurotic disorders in ICD-10 (September 1988 draft). *Japanese Journal of Clinical Psychiatry* 19:1067–1074 (in Japanese).

Kitamura T, Kurita H, Fujinawa A (1990). ICD-10 and new trends in diagnostic criteria for psychiatric disorders. *Clinical Psychiatry* 32:686–694 (in Japanese).

Nakane Y, Ohta Y, Araki K (1984). Clinical usability of DSM-III: Diagnosis of schizophrenia—ICD-9 and DSM-III. *Clinical Psychiatry* 26:121–128 (in Japanese).

Nakane Y, Takahashi R (1984). Application of PSE and DSE-III in the same group of mental illness, pp 246–250. *Proceedings of World Psychiatric Association Regional Symposium, Japan 1982*. Japanese Society of Psychiatry and Neurology, Tokyo.

Okazaki Y (1990). Psychotic disorders in ICD-10 draft. *Japanese Journal of Clinical Psychiatry* 19:1049–1058 (in Japanese).

Okubo Y, Komiyama M, Takahashi R, Nakane Y, Yamashita I, Takahashi T, Nishizono M (1990). Collaborative multi-centre field trial of ICD-10, Chapter V (1986 draft), Clinical Descriptions and Diagnostic Guidelines in Japan: A report from the WHO project on field trials of ICD-10, Chapter V. *Clinical Psychiatry* 32:869–880 (in Japanese).

Takahashi S (1990). The structure and the characteristics of ICD-10 draft, 1988. *Japanese Journal of Clinical Psychiatry* 19:1041–1047 (in Japanese).

Takahashi S, Ishida N (1990). Some revised features of DSM-III-R. *Archives of Psychiatric Diagnostics and Clinical Evaluation* 1:5–18 (in Japanese).

Takahashi S, Takahashi R, Kasahara Y, Kimura B, Nomura J, Fujinawa A, Nakane Y (1985). Classification and diagnostic criteria of so-called endogenous psychoses prepared by the JCIDCP Committee. *Clinical Psychiatry* 27:761–770 (in Japanese).

Tanaka Y, Nakamura K (1990). Review of activities in the preparation of the tenth revision and the present status of ICD-10. *Japanese Journal of Clinical Psychiatry* 19:1035–1040 (in Japanese).

World Health Organization (1987). *Tenth Revision of the International Classification of Diseases, Chapter V (F): Mental, Behavioural and Developmental Disorders, Clinical Descriptions and Diagnostic Guidelines—1986 Draft for field trials MNH/MEP/87.1.* WHO, Geneva.

World Health Organization (1992). *The ICD-10 Classification of Mental and Behavioral Disorders: Clinical Descriptions and Diagnostic Guidelines*. World Health Organization, Geneva.

# 13
# The ICD-10 Chapter on Mental Disorders Versus Conventional Diagnosis in Japan

TOSHINORI KITAMURA

Ample evidence has been accumulated to suggest that psychiatrists all too often disagree over the diagnosis of the same subjects (Kendell et al 1971, Kitamura et al 1986, Leff 1977). This has led to close scrutiny of the reasons for such disagreement, and lately, to the development of structured interview guides and operational diagnostic criteria, enabling research psychiatrists to reduce such biases.

Despite these attempts of research workers to operationalize symptom assessment and diagnosis, it is widely recognized that clinical psychiatrists tend to cling to their own conventional diagnostic systems (Kendell 1973, 1981, Saugstad and Odegard 1983). Their insistence on the use of conventional diagnostic systems and nomenclature may partly explain why standard classificatory or diagnostic systems for mental illness are, although desirable, not yet internationally accepted.

Therefore, when research psychiatrists or administrators develop or introduce a new set of diagnostic criteria, they must compromise with conventional or local diagnostic systems and terminologies so as to make the former more acceptable in both research and clinical practice.

In a questionnaire survey, Kitamura et al (1989a, 1989b) reported that, when compared to the Research Diagnostic Criteria (RDC) (Spitzer et al 1981) categories, Japanese psychiatrists used almost the same diagnostic rubrics yet for different, occasionally very different, clinical pictures. Japanese psychiatrists embraced a wider concept of schizophrenia and distinct categories for atypical psychoses, neurosis and character disorder (Table 13.1).

When Akira Fujinawa, Director of the National Institute of Mental Health, was appointed in 1987 as the chairperson of an *ad hoc* committee on diagnostic criteria for psychiatric disorders by the Ministry of Health and Welfare, he thought that the main task of his committee would be to introduce the forthcoming *International Classification of Diseases*, 10th

TABLE 13.1. Comparison of RDC and Japanese conventional diagnoses.

| RDC | Japanese |
|---|---|
| Schizophrenia | |
| Acute | |
| Chronic | |
| DSSRS | Schizophrenia |
| Schizotypal personality disorder | |
| Schizoaffective disorder | |
| Depressed/schizophrenic | |
| Depressed/affective | Paranoid state |
| Manic/schizophrenic | Atypical psychosis |
| Manic/affective | |
| Manic disorder | Mania |
| Major depressive disorder | Depression |
| Minor depressive disorder | |
| Panic disorder | Anxiety neurosis |
| Briquet's disorder | Hysteria |
| Obsessive–compulsive disorder | Obsessive–compulsive disorder |
| Phobic disorder | Phobia |
| Generalized anxiety disorder | Neurosis |
| Intermittent depressive disorder | |
| Cyclothymic personality | Character disorder |
| Antisocial personality | |

Note. From Kitamura et al (1989b).

revision (ICD-10) Chapter V smoothly into Japanese psychiatric practice (Fujinawa 1989). For the committee to execute this task, it seemed most appropriate to conduct a multicenter field trial of the ICD-10 Draft to see how well Japanese psychiatrists could understand the new classifications and diagnoses, and where, if any, clinical modifications should be added to suit conventional diagnostic habits in Japan.

After careful translation of Chapter V, a multicenter field trial was conducted. Some 600 psychiatrists participated in the trial: About one-tenth of the whole group of psychiatrists practicing in Japan (Table 13.2). They represented 95 mental hospitals, 45 psychiatric clinics, and 59 university departments of psychiatry. Trials were conducted for psychotic conditions in mental hospitals; for either psychotic, neurotic, or mood

TABLE 13.2. Multicenter field trial of the ICD-10.

| Sites | No. | Patients (*N*) | Target Conditions |
|---|---|---|---|
| Mental hospitals (Japanese Association of Psychiatric Hospitals) | 95 | 584 | Psychotic |
| Clinics (Japanese Association of Neuro-Psychiatric Clinics) | 45 | 309 | Psychotic/neurotic/mood |
| University Departments of Psychiatry | 59 | 696 | All |

conditions in clinics; while all cases were examined in university departments. The data from the university departments will be described briefly.

In the field trial conducted in university departments, a pair of psychiatrists interviewed psychiatric patients of consecutive admission or new outpatient referrals. These interviews were conducted either jointly or in a test–retest design. The two interviewers were requested to make independent judgments according to conventional diagnoses, and the ICD-10 Draft diagnoses.

The inter-rater reliability of the conventional diagnosis, expressed as kappa coefficient (Cohen 1960), was found to be generally high except for depressive neurosis (Table 13.3). This finding may be spurious because, of nine categories, four showed a marked decrease in the reliability coefficients when examined in a test–retest design. High and stable diagnostic agreement was observed only for schizophrenia, hypochondriasis, and psychogenic reaction.

Because of different rubrics used in the conventional and ICD-10 classifications, it is not easy to compare the results of the reliability study. Nevertheless, the ICD-10 two-digit categories enjoyed high agreement in the inter-rater design (Table 13.4). No marked reduction of reliability was seen when examined in the test–retest design except for Substance Use Disorders and Personality Disorders. The absolute values of the reliability coefficients were generally higher for the ICD-10 categories.

These findings encouraged us to use the forthcoming ICD-10 in diagnosing psychiatric patients in Japan. However, detailed analyses of the field trial data as well as comments made by the trial participants led the committee to discuss further the contents of the criteria in the ICD-10. In so doing, we found that some criteria and terminology used in the ICD-10 were ambiguous or complicated and that there were some categories that were named so differently from the conventions in Japan that they might be rejected. Our efforts in the clinical modification of the ICD-10 aimed

TABLE 13.3. Reliability of conventional diagnosis in Japan.

| Conventional Diagnosis | Inter-rater $\kappa$ | Test–Retest $\kappa$ | Total $\kappa$ |
|---|---|---|---|
| Schizophrenia | 0.90 | 0.82 | 0.86 |
| Atypical psychosis | 0.67 | 0.56 | 0.65 |
| Depression | 0.75 | 0.50 | 0.67 |
| Mania | 0.80 | 0.26 | 0.70 |
| Anxiety neurosis | 0.84 | 0.23 | 0.72 |
| Depressive neurosis | 0.55 | 0.52 | 0.52 |
| Hypochondriasis | 0.72 | 0.66 | 0.69 |
| Psychogenic reaction | 0.81 | 0.70 | 0.78 |
| Organic disorders | 0.69 | 0.82 | 0.68 |

Note. Excluded if the base rate is less than 0.03.

TABLE 13.4. Reliability of ICD-10 diagnosis.

| ICD-10 diagnosis | Description | Inter-rater κ | Test–Retest κ | Total κ |
|---|---|---|---|---|
| F0 | Organic, including symptomatic, mental disorders | 0.86 | 0.93 | 0.80 |
| F1 | Mental and behavioral disorders due to psychoactive substance use | 0.92 | 0.49 | 0.87 |
| F2 | Schizophrenia, schizotypal, and delusional disorders | 0.92 | 0.86 | 0.89 |
| F3 | Mood (affective) disorders | 0.82 | 0.78 | 0.80 |
| F4 | Neurotic, stress-related, and somatoform disorders | 0.83 | 0.73 | 0.79 |
| F5 | Behavioral syndromes and mental disorders associated with physiological dysfunction and hormonal disturbances | 0.89 | – | 0.82 |
| F6 | Disorders of adult personality and behavior | 0.60 | 0.48 | 0.56 |

Note. Excluded if the base rate is less than 0.03.

to overcome these issues. Some topics of the evolving Japanese Clinical Modification (JCM) are to be reported elsewhere.

In the Introduction Section of the ICD-10 1989 Draft, it is stated that the term psychotic has been retained as a convenient descriptive term. It seems to us that the term psychotic or psychosis is all too conveniently used in the ICD-10 as well as in other psychiatric literature. The ICD-10 Draft states in the Introduction that the term psychotic indicates hallucinations, delusions, and a limited number of abnormal behaviors such as gross excitement, severe and prolonged social withdrawal, marked psychomotor retardation, and catatonic symptoms. This definition of the term psychotic, however, is not consistent throughout the text of the ICD-10. For example, F30.2, Mania with Psychotic Symptoms, defined in the ICD-10 Diagnostic Criteria for Research (DCR), includes only delusions and hallucinations. F32.3, Severe Depressive Episode with Psychotic Symptoms includes stupor together with hallucinations and delusions. Thus, abnormal behaviors other than depressive stupor are recognized as psychotic in the Introduction but neglected in the section of Mood Disorders. In the section of Psychoactive Substance Use Disorders, F1x.5, Psychotic Disorder, encompasses even depressive and manic symptoms.

It seems that the authors of the ICD-10 wished to avoid using psychosis as a main category. Thus, F2 was labelled as Schizophrenia, Schizotypal and Delusional Disorders rather than as Psychotic Disorders. Nevertheless, F2's wastebasket categories were given terms F28, Other Nonorganic Psychotic Disorder, and F29, Nonorganic Psychosis, Not Otherwise Specified. Since other main categories simply add Other or Not Otherwise Specified to their main category terms to produce appending categories, it may be extrapolated that F2 should have been labelled Psychotic Disorders. However, if F2 is so named, every condition under this rubric should by definition manifest at least one psychotic feature. Unfortunately, this definition of Psychotic Disorders will lead to the elimination of Simple Schizophrenia, a psychosis without psychotic symptoms, from the F2 categories.

On the other hand, if the term psychotic is not specific to any particular diagnosis but can be used for different categories, the Fujinawa Committee felt that its use could be better expanded from F0, F1, F2, and F3 to some categories of F4, Neurotic Disorders. For we have had the experience that patients with some neurotic disorders, particularly social phobia, hypochondriasis, and a limited number of subcategories of somatoform disorders, occasionally manifest strong but false beliefs undifferentiable from true delusions. The Committee thought it would be more acceptable among Japanese psychiatrists to combine neurotics presenting delusional beliefs with those not presenting such beliefs than to separate the two conditions into F22, Persistent Delusional Disorders and F4, Neurotic Disorders.

The Japanese Clinical Modification (JCM), therefore, involves a moderate revision of the original ICD-10 Draft. First, the Committee labelled F2 as Psychotic Disorders. Here, Psychotic Disorders means nonorganic conditions characterized by either psychotic (ie, positive) symptoms or negative (ie, defect) symptoms (Table 13.5). The distinction between the positive and negative symptoms in the JCM is similar to that used by many other researchers (Andreasen 1985, Crow 1985). In the JCM, however, symptoms such as audible thought, thought insertion, thought withdrawal, thought broadcasting and passivity were separated from delusions to delineate a distinct symptom group, Ego Disturbance. This modification follows the German tradition of psychopathology.

In the JCM, the term psychotic is used for clinical features containing psychotic but not necessarily negative symptoms, and delusional for clinical features that contain delusions but not necessarily other psychotic symptoms. Hence, in the JCM, F0 and F1 have organic psychotic cate-

TABLE 13.5. Definition of psychosis in the Japanese Clinical Modification (JCM) of ICD-10.

| Symptom | |
|---|---|
| Either psychotic (positive) | Or Defect (Negative) |
| Hallucinations | Affective flattening or blunting |
| Delusions | Alogia |
| Ego disturbance | Avolotion–apathy |
| Formal thought disorders | Anhedonia–asociality |
| Catatonia | |

gories, F3 has a subcategory With Psychotic Features and F4, With Delusional Development.

Another issue that required careful examination was the allocation of diagnostic labels frequently used in everyday practice in Japan but not specified in the ICD-10 Draft. For example, these include atypical psychosis, anthropophobia, olfactory reference syndrome, dysmorphophobia, and coenesthopathic disorder (disorder of abnormal bodily sensations).

As already addressed briefly, atypical psychosis in Japan covers a relatively wide but clearly demarcated nonorganic phenomenology, although admittedly its concept may vary between schools (Mitsuda 1962). The Fujinawa Committee agreed that the JCM would adopt this term to correspond to the original ICD-10's Acute and Transient Psychotic Disorders other than Acute Schizophrenia-Like Psychotic Disorder and all categories of Schizoaffective Disorders.

The other four categories are unique in that Japanese psychiatrists consider that these neurotic conditions often manifest delusions of reference or of other kinds, or even hallucinations usually of somatic type. They also think that the transition from the nondelusional to the psychotic among this population is smooth rather than discrete, as is usually maintained in the Western literature. The committee coined the term With Delusional Development to reflect this idea.

In the JCM, Anthropophobia or Phobia, Anthropophobic Type, can be translated as Social Phobia of the Original ICD-10 whereas Olfactory Reference Syndrome, Dysmorphophobia, and Coenesthopathic Disorder (ie, Disorder of Abnormal Bodily Sensation) were all categorized as subtypes of Somatoform Disorders because of their somatic manifestations. However, following the ideas of the ICD-10 very strictly, each of these conditions seems to be best allocated under different categories. If accompanied by delusional development, they should be diagnosed as Delusional Disorder. We feel it more convenient to bring these conditions together under a single heading that reflects their somatoform nature. This decision is, however, tentative, and further research may be warranted to refine the classification.

## Conclusion

The Fujinawa Committee hopes that the JCM will provide an impetus for more research on better classification and diagnostic criteria that will, in turn, lead to further revision of the JCM. And, of course, these forward steps should always be taken in the context of strong international cooperation, and in close collaboration with the headquaters of the World Health Organization.

*Acknowledgment.* The present study was supported by a grant from the Mental Health Services Research Fund, Ministry of Health and Welfare, 1989.

## *References*

Andreasen NC (1985). Positive vs. negative schizophrenia: A critical evaluation. *Schizophrenia Bulletin* 11:380–389.

Cohen J (1960). A coefficient of agreement for nominal scales. *Educational and Psychological Measurement* 20:37–46.

Crow TJ (1985). Two-syndrome concept: Origins and current states. *Schizophrenia Bulletin* 11:471–486.

Fujinawa A (ed) (1989). *Development of Diagnostic Criteria of Mental Illnesses: Annual Report to the Ministry of Health and Welfare.* National Institute of Mental Health, Ichikawa (in Japanese).

Kendell RE (1973). The influence of the 1968 glossary on the diagnosis of English psychiatrists. *British Journal of Psychiatry* 123:527–530.

Kendell RE (1981). The international classification and diagnoses of English psychiatrists 1968–1980. *British Journal of Psychiatry* 139:177–180.

Kendell RE, Cooper JE, Gourlay AJ, Copeland JR (1971). Diagnostic criteria of American and British psychiatrists. *Archives of General Psychiatry* 25:123–130.

Kitamura T, Kato M, Sakio E, Shima S (1986). Application of Research Diagnostic Criteria and International Classification of Diseases to case vignettes. *Journal of Clinical Psychiatry* 47:78–80.

Kitamura T, Shima S, Sakio E, Kato M (1989a). Psychiatric diagnosis in Japan. I. A study on diagnostic labels used by practitioners. *Psychopathology* 22:239–249.

Kitamura T, Shima S, Sakio E, Kato M (1989b). Psychiatric diagnosis in Japan. II. Reliability of conventional diagnosis and discrepancies with RDC diagnosis. *Psychopathology* 22:250–259.

Leff J (1977). International variation in the diagnosis of psychiatric illness. *British Journal of Psychiatry* 131:329–338.

Mitsuda H (1962). The concept of atypical psychoses: From the aspect of clinical genetics. *Folia Psychiatrica et Neurologica Japonica* 16:214–221.

Saugstad LF, Odegard O (1983). Persistent discrepancy in international diagnostic practices since 1970. *Acta Psychiatrica Scandinavica* 68:501–510.

Spitzer RL, Endicott J, Robins E (1981). *Research Diagnostic Criteria (RDC) for a Selected Group of Functional Disorders* (3rd ed). Biometric Research New York State Psychiatric Institute, New York.

# 14
# Affective Disorders in China, Korea, and Japan and the Challenges of ICD-10

He Qin Yan, Yoshibumi Nakane, and H.Y. Lee

According to a series of cohort studies of mental disorders in Asia, the prevalence rates of affective disorders have been found to be generally lower than those of Western countries. Is this difference due to culture and to social influence or to different diagnostic trends? Our study attempts to explore whether reported differences in prevalence rates actually exist; and if not, to reach agreement concerning the resolution of those differences (Nakane et al 1988). With the cooperation of the WHO Regional Office for the Western Pacific, the Department of Neuropsychiatry of Nagasaki University School of Medicine and the Shanghai Mental Health Center conducted a comparative study of affective disorders. Yonsei University of Korea participated in the early stages of the study.

## Methods

After meetings of the researchers from the three centers, we decided to adopt the 9th edition of the Present State Examination (PSE-9), which has often been used in international studies. We also decided to use the Standardized Assessment of Depressive Disorders (SADD), which was developed for use in the WHO collaborative study, and the Hamilton Rating Scale for Depression. Furthermore, to clarify differences in the diagnostic classification of depression among the centers, we examined the agreement rates of symptom evaluation and diagnostic classification through repeated evaluation exercises with members of the various centers. Through these exercises, differences in symptom evaluation of patients with affective disorder were examined and, as a result, reasonably good agreement in patient evaluation was achieved.

After that, each center selected five cases: two cases with typical depression, two cases with atypical depression, and one case having several other psychiatric symptoms as well as depression, and interviewed the five cases according to the revised PSE (including a section containing SADD items). These interviews were conducted and videotaped in the corresponding native language. Each center then sent the videotaped interviews, an English transcript, and a brief case history including description of life-style and family situation for each case to the other two centers.

At each center, five researchers who had attended the evaluation training at the preparatory stage of the study evaluated the clinical symptoms of each 15 patients (five each selected by the three centers) and gave a clinical diagnosis for each case according to *International Classification of Diseases*, 9th revision (ICD-9), *Diagnostic and Statistical Manual of Mental Disorders*, 3rd edition (DSM-III) and its own conventional diagnostic criteria. The Nagasaki center collected 255 diagnoses (15 cases diagnosed by 15 researchers) and conducted statistical analyses.

## Results

Among the 15 cases selected from the three centers, 10 were males (mean age, 35 years) and 5 were females (mean age, 44 years). There was no significant difference in age or sex of subjects between the centers.

Table 14.1 shows the distribution of the general diagnoses for all 15 patients using the ICD-9 3-digit code. Neurotic disorders was the most common diagnosis and affective psychoses was the next most common. About 89% of the diagnoses fell under these two classifications, the agreement rates between these diagnoses show that the kappa values across the 15 cases varied from 0.37 to 1.00, whereas the overall kappa value was 0.48.

Table 14.2 shows the distribution of diagnoses using DSM-III. The general classification of DSM-III affective disorders was the most common diagnosis (74%), the agreement rates increased, and the overall kappa value was 0.69.

In an analysis of the diagnoses for each case by the three centers, it was found that the Nagasaki center tended to diagnose patients as having affective psychoses or affective disorders (65%). The Shanghai center tended to diagnose patients having neurotic disorders or anxiety disorders (73%). For the cases at the Seoul center, the preference of diagnoses between affective psychoses and neurotic disorders was not as marked as in the other two centers. Instead, there was greater variation in the types of diagnoses given (for example, schizophrenia and others).

Next, we looked at the evaluation of clinical symptoms. We considered that symptom recognition is one of the most important factors affecting

TABLE 14.1. Distribution of ICD-9 diagnosis for 15 patients from three centers.

| ICD-9 codes | Diagnoses | Nagasaki cases | | | | | Shanghai cases | | | | | Seoul cases | | | | | Total (%) |
|---|---|---|---|---|---|---|---|---|---|---|---|---|---|---|---|---|---|
| | | 1 | 2 | 3 | 4 | 5 | 1 | 2 | 3 | 4 | 5 | 1 | 2 | 3 | 4 | 5 | |
| 296 | Affective psychoses | 12 | 8 | 9 | 12 | 8 | 3 | 2 | 11 | 0 | 1 | 1 | 12 | 0 | 3 | 15 | 97 (43) |
| 298 | Other nonorganic psychoses | 2 | 2 | 0 | 0 | 0 | 0 | 0 | 1 | 0 | 0 | 0 | 0 | 0 | 0 | 0 | 5 (2) |
| 300 | Neurotic disorders | 1 | 5 | 6 | 3 | 7 | 11 | 12 | 3 | 15 | 14 | 0 | 0 | 15 | 12 | 0 | 104 (46) |
| | Others | 0 | 0 | 0 | 0 | 0 | 1 | 1 | 0 | 0 | 0 | 14 | 3 | 0 | 0 | 0 | 19 (9) |
| | Proportion of agreement | 0.64 | 0.37 | 0.49 | 0.66 | 0.47 | 0.55 | 0.64 | 0.55 | 1.0 | 0.87 | 0.87 | 0.66 | 1.0 | 0.66 | 1.0 | 225 |

Note. Overall kappa, 0.48.

TABLE 14.2. Distribution of DSM-III diagnoses for 15 patients from three centers.

| DSM-III | | Nagasaki cases | | | | | Shanghai cases | | | | | Seoul cases | | | | | Subtotal | Total |
|---|---|---|---|---|---|---|---|---|---|---|---|---|---|---|---|---|---|---|
| index code | No. | 1 | 2 | 3 | 4 | 5 | 1 | 2 | 3 | 4 | 5 | 1 | 2 | 3 | 4 | 5 | (%) | (%) |
| 6, Affective | 66 | 13 | 8 | 10 | 14 | 9 | 4 | 4 | 14 | 0 | 2 | 1 | 12 | 0 | 3 | 15 | 109 (48) | 167 (74) |
| disorders | 64 | 0 | 7 | 5 | 1 | 6 | 10 | 8 | 0 | 3 | 2 | 0 | 0 | 1 | 12 | 0 | 55 (25) | |
| | 68 | 2 | 0 | 0 | 0 | 0 | 0 | 0 | 0 | 0 | 0 | 1 | 0 | 0 | 0 | 0 | 3 (1) | |
| 0, Anxiety | 01 | 0 | 0 | 0 | 0 | 0 | 0 | 2 | 1 | 12 | 0 | 0 | 0 | 3 | 0 | 0 | 18 (8) | 28 (13) |
| disorders | 02 | 0 | 0 | 0 | 0 | 0 | 0 | 0 | 0 | 0 | 0 | 0 | 0 | 8 | 0 | 0 | 8 (4) | |
| | 00 | 0 | 0 | 0 | 0 | 0 | 0 | 0 | 0 | 0 | 0 | 0 | 0 | 2 | 0 | 0 | 2 (1) | |
| 7, Somatoform | 70 | 0 | 0 | 0 | 0 | 0 | 0 | 0 | 0 | 0 | 7 | 0 | 0 | 0 | 0 | 0 | 7 (3) | 10 (4) |
| disorders | 78 | 0 | 0 | 0 | 0 | 0 | 0 | 0 | 0 | 0 | 3 | 0 | 0 | 0 | 0 | 0 | 3 (1) | |
| X, Others | | 0 | 0 | 0 | 0 | 0 | 1 | 1 | 0 | 0 | 1 | 13 | 3 | 1 | 0 | 0 | 20 (9) | 20 (9) |
| Proportion of | 1 digit | 1.0 | 1.0 | 1.0 | 1.0 | 1.0 | 0.87 | 0.64 | 0.87 | 0.66 | 0.49 | 0.75 | 0.66 | 0.74 | 1.0 | 1.0 | 225 | |
| agreement | 2 digits | 0.75 | 0.47 | 0.52 | 0.87 | 0.49 | 0.49 | 0.33 | 0.87 | 0.66 | 0.25 | 0.74 | 0.66 | 0.30 | 0.66 | 1.0 | | |

Note. Overall kappa, 0.69.

diagnosis by a psychiatrist. To clarify and test this, we selected a case in which diagnosis varied most. This case was Nagasaki case No. 3, and was examined by comparing the results obtained from the PSE. For this case, all the researchers from Nagasaki gave the diagnosis of manic depressive psychosis, depressed type, whereas most of the researchers from Shanghai diagnosed the case as a neurotic depression. At the Seoul center, the diagnoses given to this case varied.

Figure 14.1A,B shows a comparison of the distribution of average scores formulated by 15 researchers from three centers on 47 items selected from the PSE that were mainly concerned with depressive states. There were no significant differences among the three centers. Comparisons were also made among the three centers in terms of the syndrome check list of PSE, PSE subscore, and CATEGO analysis. The CATEGO class given by most of the researchers was R+ (retarded depression), and the most frequent tentative diagnosis was either manic-depressive psychosis, depressed type, or neurotic depression.

## Discussion

Our study started with a clarification of the differences in diagnostic methods among the participating countries to investigate reasons for the reportedly low prevalence rates of depression in Asian countries. Our results showed inter-center differences, although we had selected the same kinds of cases and used standardized diagnostic methods. The Nagasaki center tended to diagnose patients as having a psychotic depression, whereas the Shanghai center tended to diagnose patients as having a neurotic depression. The Seoul center tended to make diagnoses somewhere in between those of the other two centers.

As we understand it, the factors influencing psychiatric diagnostic distribution and reliability include the following:

1. Recognition of symptoms: Our study showed only a few differences in symptom recognition. Among the cases in which diagnosis varied most, there was little difference in the evaluation of symptoms among the three centers. Only one case suggested that there were substantial differences in symptom recognition.

2. Differences in diagnostic preferences: Nakane (1988) analyzed the psychiatric history of three countries where these centers were located and suggested that the differential frequencies of the diagnosis of neurotic depression appears to be related to differences in diagnostic preferences, which in turn seem to be a function of degree of alienation with modern Western psychiatry. Flexibility in acceptance of Western psychiatry seems to be closely related to history, culture, tradition, and national traits of each country concerned. All of these elements are considered to be important in the development of diagnostic preferences.

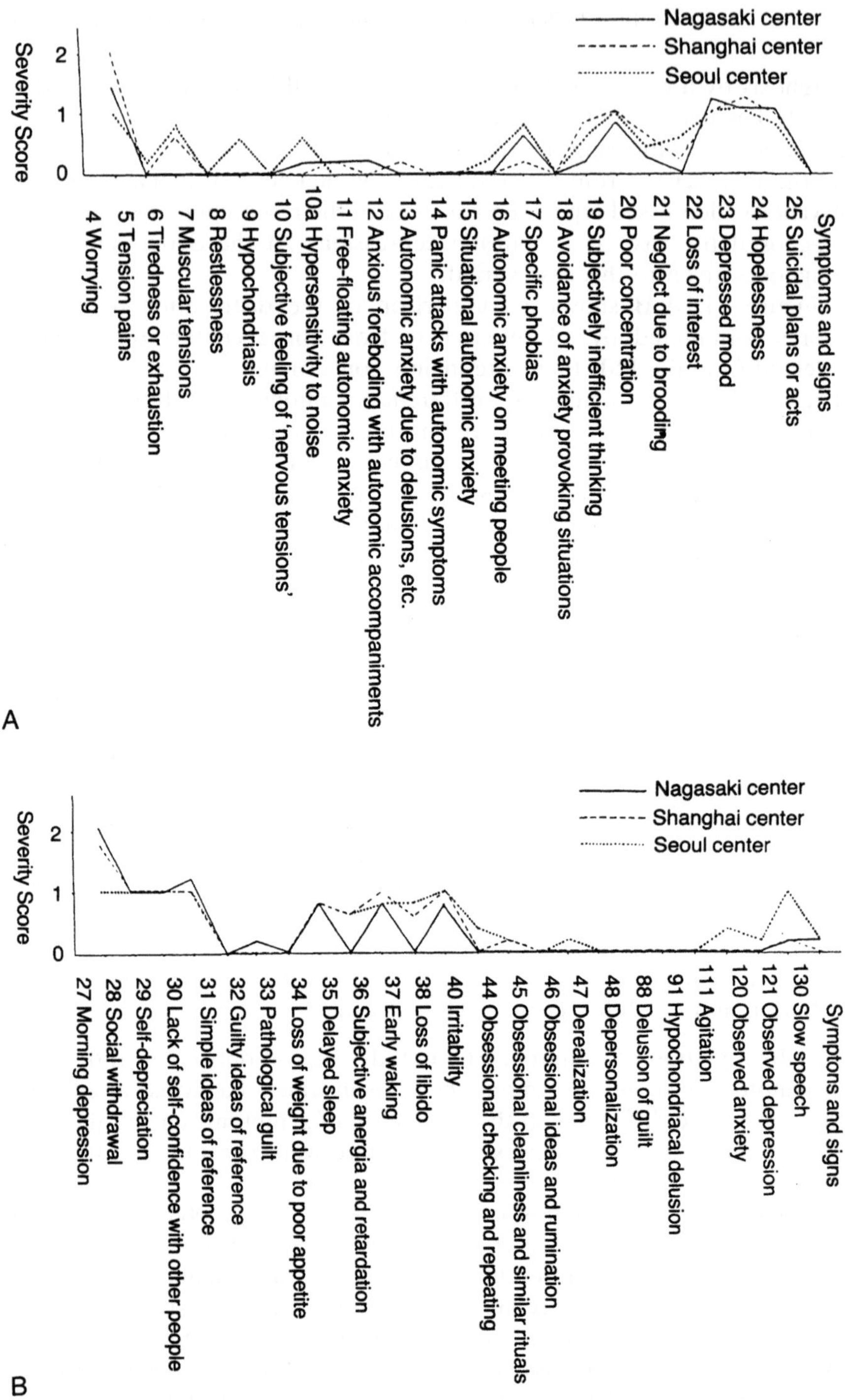


FIGURE 14.1*A*,*B*. Profiles of selected PSE symptoms and signs in the Nagasaki, Shanghai, and Seoul centers for Nagasaki Case No. 3 (103).

3. Importance of operational diagnostic criteria and classification system for making reliable comparisons: In our study, the results showed that when using DSM-III, the affective disorders were the most common diagnoses (74%), the overall inter-rater reliability kappa was 0.69, and this agreement rate was higher than that for ICD-9 (0.48), a difference that was significant. Malt (1986) has pointed out that research workers with an empirical bent tend to favor DSM-III, whereas others, more prepared to acknowledge the value of intuition for the comprehension of psychological phenomena, prefer ICD-9, which offers more flexibility.

The fact that operational diagnostic criteria attained higher agreement rates suggests that this is an important methodology for the future practice of international collaborative studies. ICD-10 has improved the diagnostic criteria or research in this regard. Correspondingly, the reports from the ICD-10 field trials have indicated the advantages of better application, satisfactory validity in diagnosis, and high acceptance and feasibility; the inter-rater reliability has also been high (Shen 1991). Another major change in ICD-10 has been that disorders with common themes or characteristics are grouped together. Cyclothymic Personality and Depressive Neurosis are placed in the Affective (Mood) Disorders group, and the differentiation between psychoses and neuroses as a fundamental organizing principle has been abandoned. Because of its greater descriptive precision, use of ICD-10 in our study may have increased the agreement rates.

We hope further progress can be accomplished in the future by following up the course and assessing the disability of these cases. But, we also submit that inconsistencies in psychiatric diagnosis may stem less from technical limitations built into diagnostic and classificatory systems than from the minds and biases of psychiatrists. Whatever one's theoretical orientation, we believe it is essential to recognize these shortcomings. The most protracted problems of diagnosis may in fact represent a challenge to psychiatric education (Cooper 1988, Guimon 1989).

## References

Cooper JE (1988). An overview of the prospective ICD-10 Classification of Mental Disorders. *British Journal of Psychiatry* 152:21–23 (suppl 1).

Guimon J (1989). The biases of psychiatric diagnosis. *British Journal of Psychiatry* 154:33–37 (suppl 4).

Malt UF (1986). Philosophy of science and DSM-III. *Acta Psychiatrica Scandinavica* 328:10–17 (suppl 73).

Nakane Y, et al (1988). Comparative study of affective disorders in three Asian countries. *Acta Psychiatrica Scandinavica* 78:698–705.

Shen Y-C, et al (1991). Results of field trials of ICD-10 in China. Technical Report, Mental Health Institute, Beijing Medical University, China.

# 15
# Empirical Comparison of ICD-10 and DSM-III-R in Peru

DANTE E. WARTHON, TALYA LANDMANN, JAVIER E. SAAVEDRA, FREDY VÁSQUEZ, PEDRO MAKABE, AND JUAN E. MEZZICH

The last three decades have been crucial for the development of psychiatry in the areas of diagnosis and classification. The Tower of Babel is giving way to the development of a language that is complex but increasingly systematic. In line with this, a series of structured interviews have been developed, such as the Present State Examination (PSE) (Wing et al 1974), the Schedule for Affective Disorders and Schizophrenia (SADS) (Endicott and Spitzer 1978), the Diagnostic Interview Schedule (DIS) (Robins et al 1981), the Initial Evaluation Form (IEF) (Mezzich et al 1981), the Composite International Diagnostic Interview (CIDI) (Robins 1985), the Structured Clinical Interview for Diagnosis (SCID) (Spitzer et al 1989). These control to a large extent one of the main sources of diagnostic unreliability, that is, dissimilar data collection (Ward et al 1962). Also, a series of classification systems such as the Research Diagnostic Criteria (Spitzer et al 1975) and the Diagnostic Criteria for Use in Psychiatric Research (Feighner et al 1972) have contributed to making more explicit the process of assigning diagnostic categories, which was another major source of unreliability (Kreitman 1961).

The *Diagnostic and Statistical Manual of Mental Disorders*, 3rd edition (DSM-III) (American Psychiatric Association 1980) has become one of the most visible of these models and it has been used in many countries across the world, as a number of studies demonstrate, (eg, Botswana (Ben-Tovim 1985), Peru (Sogi et al 1989), Spain (Lopez-Ibor 1985), Norway (Dahl 1983), and England (Gregory and Cooper 1983)). Investigations on the definition of various diagnostic categories were stimulated, and this led to the revision of DSM-III (American Psychiatric Association 1987).

On an even more international framework, the World Health Organization (WHO) and its collaborators have been actively working towards the development of the 10th revision of the *International Classification of Diseases* (ICD-10), Chapter V (WHO 1989). This chapter on mental disorders and connected developments have incorporated the major methodological features of modern diagnostic systems (i.e., a largely descriptive phenomenological organization of the catalog of mental disorders, explicit categorical definitions, and multiaxial schemas).

The objective of the present study was to explore the comparative distribution of psychiatric diagnoses formulated according to ICD-10 and DSM-III-R in a sample of Peruvian general psychiatric patients.

# Material and Methods

## *Site of the Study*

The Peruvian National Institute of Mental Health, "Honorio Delgado-Hideyo Noguchi," is one of the three major psychiatric institutions in Lima, the capital of Peru. The Institute's catchment area covers a population of about 2 million people, predominantly residing in shantytowns or "barriadas," poor urban areas where basic services are scarce. The Institute was constructed with the support of the Japanese International Cooperation Agency and has facilities to care for a wide range of psychiatric problems through outpatient clinics and 100 inpatient beds.

## *Assessment Procedures*

All the patients who come to this center are evaluated with the Initial Evaluation Form (IEF) developed by Mezzich et al (1981) at the University of Pittsburgh and adapted and translated into Spanish by Sogi et al (1982). This instrument has a phenomenological approach that permits making DSM-III-R and ICD-10 diagnoses. Its main sections are history of present psychiatric illness, history of other psychiatric disorders, mental status (with 64 items in its symptom inventory), family history, personal and social history, general medical history, and narrative assessment summary. It has a descriptive, narrative track and a standardized track running side by side.

The clinicians who took part in the present study were psychiatrists members of the Institute staff and familiar with the IEF diagnostic evaluation procedures, DSM-III-R, and the 1989 draft of ICD-10 Chapter V.

## *Clinical Sample*

For the present study, 254 adult patients were quasi-randomly selected and their IEF's were separately reviewed by two clinicians. One formulated a diagnosis according to ICD-10 and the other, independently, according to DSM-III-R.

TABLE 15.1. Demographic characteristics of 254 adult psychiatric patients in Lima, Peru.

| Demographic variables | | % |
|---|---|---|
| Age | 18–29 | 56 |
| | 30–59 | 40 |
| | >60 | 4 |
| Sex | Female | 54 |
| | Male | 46 |
| Marital status | Single | 50 |
| | Married | 41 |
| | Separated/divorced | 6 |
| | Widowed | 3 |
| Education | Elementary school | 27 |
| | High school | 33 |
| | Technical school | 4 |
| | University | 24 |
| | None | 12 |
| Occupation | Remunerated | 23 |
| | Student | 5 |
| | Housewife | 37 |
| | None | 35 |

As Table 15.1 on demographic distribution shows, 56% of the sample was between 18 and 29 years of age, 40% was between 30 and 59 years, and only 4% was over 60 years of age. This distribution reflects the population pyramid in Peru, typical of developing countries. (Of note, 12% were illiterate and 35% were unemployed, which reflects population patterns in the country.)

## Results

The distribution of diagnoses in terms of major categories is displayed in Table 15.2. According to ICD-10, the greatest number of patients (42%) were diagnosed as experiencing neurotic, stress-related, and somatoform disorders (F4). Thirty-eight percent of the patients fell into the equivalent DSM-III-R categories (ie, anxiety, somatoform, dissociative, and adjustment disorders). Thirty-five and thirty-seven percent of the sample were diagnosed as mood disorders according to ICD-10 and DSM-III-R, respectively. In both systems, 13% of the sample received a diagnosis of schizophrenia. The difference in diagnoses of adjustment disorder is worth noting: It was 15% in ICD-10 and only 6% in DSM-III-R.

Next, the degree of overlap or concordance between similarly named diagnostic groups according to ICD-10 and DSM-III-R was examined. Seventy-two percent of the DSM-III-R schizophrenic patients were also diagnosed as schiozophrenic according to ICD-10, and the reverse was true for 75% of the patients. The patients that were not concordant received diagnoses in conceptually similar categories, such as schizophreniform, schizotypal, or acute and transient psychotic disorders. Fifty-five percent of the patients diagnosed as presenting either a depressive episode or recurrent depression in ICD-10 were diagnosed as major depressive in DSM-III-R.

The patients who received a diagnosis of DSM-III-R dysthymia, were diagnosed in ICD-10 as dysthymic in 43% of the cases, as single episode or recurrent depression in 22%, and as anxiety disorders in 31%. On the other hand, the patients with ICD-10 dysthymia, were diagnosed in DSM-III-R as dysthymic in 31% of the cases, as major depression in 22%, and as generalized anxiety disorder in 16%.

Of the patients with DSM-III-R somatoform disorder diagnoses, 41% were diagnosed as having ICD-10 mood disorder, 18% as ICD-10 somatoform disorder, and 18% as ICD-10 adjustment disorder. Conversely, of the patients with ICD-10 somatoform disorder, 44% were diagnosed as presenting DSM-III-R mood disorder and 33% as DSM-III-R somatoform disorder.

Patients with DSM-III-R adjustment disorder, were diagnosed in ICD-10 as adjustment disorder in 63% of the cases and as dysthymic in 31%.

TABLE 15.2. ICD-10 and DSM-III-R distributions in 254 adult psychiatric patients in Lima, Peru.

| ICD-10 disorders | % | DSM-III-R disorders | % |
|---|---|---|---|
| Organic mental | 2 | Organic mental | 7 |
| Mental, due to substance use | 2 | Substance use | 7 |
| | | Substance-induced organic mental | 2 |
| Schizophrenia | 13 | Schizophrenia | 13 |
| Schizotypal | 2 | Schizotypal personality | 1 |
| Acute and transient psychotic | 3 | Schizophreniform | 3 |
| Mood | 35 | Mood | 37 |
| Manic episode and bipolar | 1 | Bipolar | 1 |
| Depressive episode | 10 | Single-episode major depression | 17 |
| Recurrent depressive | 4 | Recurrent major depression | 4 |
| Dysthymia | 20 | Dysthmia | 15 |
| Specific personality | 5 | Personality Dis; non-schizotypal | 10 |
| Neurotic, stress-related and somatoform | 42 | Anxiety, somatoform, dissociative and adjustment | 38 |
| Phobic and other anxiety | 20 | Anxiety | 22 |
| Generalized anxiety | 12 | Generalized anxiety | 7 |
| Panic | 3 | Panic Dis W/agor | 2 |
| Phobic | 3 | Phobias | 5 |
| Unspecified anxiety | 0 | Anxiety dis nos | 5 |
| Adjustment | 15 | Adjustment | 6 |
| Dissociative | 2 | Dissociative | 3 |
| Somatoform | 4 | Somatoform | 7 |
| Mental retardation | 2 | Mental retardation | 1 |

Somewhat differently, patients with ICD-10 adjustment disorder, were assigned DSM-III-R diagnoses of adjustment disorder in 23% of the cases, of major depression also in 23%, of anxiety disorders in 18%, and of dysthymia in 13%.

## Discussion

One of the interesting findings of the present study refers to somatoform phenomena. Clinicians participating in the study perceived an almost ubiquitous presence of somatic symptoms in the major part of the patient sample, even in those diagnosed with schizophrenia. This is reflected in part in the elevated prevalence of somatoform disorders: 4% according to ICD-10 and 7% according to DSM-III-R, which are much higher than the 0.6% of DSM-III somatoform disorder found in a US study of 11,292 general psychiatric patients using the same assessment instrument (Mezzich et al 1989). This could be in line with the trend to "somatize" often noted in traditional societies, in contrast with the trend to "psychologize" health problems experienced in technologically developed Western societies (Mezzich, Kleinman, Fabrega and Parron, in press).

An additional observation was that in some patients the somatic symptoms were accompanied by a depressive syndrome. In this regard, we should ask if these are cases of somatoform disorder where a separate depressive disorder emerges or somatoform disorders associated with the "demoralization" described by Frank (1973) as a consequence of living in socioeconomic conditions such as those often present in developing countries. Another viewpoint is that mood disorders in traditional societies should include somatic symptoms as diagnostic criteria and not only as associated features as it happens in ICD-10 and, particularly, in DSM-III-R.

Other interesting findings correspond to the diagnosis of dissociative disorders that was present in 3.1% of the cases according to ICD-10 and in 2.4% according to DSM-III-R. In contrast, in the aforementioned US study (Mezzich et al 1989) only 0.2% of the general psychiatric sample received this diagnosis. Of note, the clinicians participating in the present study observed that many patients, aside from those with a diagnosis of dissociative disorder, experienced fainting spells. These may not be necessarily pathological, as they may correspond to socially acceptable ways of seeking support, as in the case of "ataques de nervios" (Mezzich et al [in press]). These observations agree with comments made by Wig (1983) for third world countries at large. For some of these patients, an ICD-9 diagnosis of dissociative hysteria (which includes in its characterization, "a narrowing of the field of consciousness") could have been made. The diagnostic value of this experience is not clearly recognized in DSM-III-R or ICD-10.

Among the anxiety disorders, the most common ones were by far generalized and unspecified anxiety disorders (12%) rather than those involving panic or phobic disorders (6–7%), which appeared to predominate in US studies (Mezzich et al 1989).

As for dysthymia, the high frequencies found in this Peruvian clinical sample are notable: 20% according to ICD-10 and 15% according to DSM-III-R. These figures are substantially higher than the 6.2% obtained in the US study (Mezzich et al 1989). Also interesting is the superposition noted between dysthymia on the one hand, and various other depressive disorders and anxiety disorders, on the other. The presence of anxiety disorders among the dysthymic patients, according to both diagnostic systems, coincides with the clinician's observations that dysthymic patients almost invariably presented an anxiety syndrome associated with their depressive syndrome, although anxiety is not a diagnostic criterion for dysthymia in DSM-III-R. Of note, ICD-10 does have a category of mixed anxiety and depressive disorder (F41.2), which in our study had a prevalence of 4%, 50% of these patients were classified in DSM-III-R as mood disorders, and 40% as anxiety disorders.

In many of our dysthymic patients as well as in some not diagnosed with a depressive syndrome, other forms of emotional disturbance such as irritability, resentment, anger or hostility, have been observed to form the preponderant elements in their psychopathological profile. These are not adequately represented in any specific category of DSM-III-R or ICD-10. Our observations coincide with those of Wig (1983) in India who pointed out that in certain cultures an excess of any morbid emotion, such as greed, jealously, rage, or eroticism (and not only depression and anxiety), is considered abnormal.

The considerable differences in the distributions of patients diagnosed with adjustment disorder according to DSM-III-R and ICD-10 (on overall rates and, particularly, on overlap distributions) may be in part related to the criterion of duration. In many cases, the symptoms of anxiety and depression emerging in reaction to a clearly identified stressor lasted more than 6 months, which is the maximum duration permitted by both systems to qualify for a diagnosis of adjustment disorder. According to both diagnostic systems, longer illnesses should be given other diagnoses, but it is difficult not to take into account that facilities for health care are barely accessible for most people in the Peruvian population, and this may prolong the duration of all forms of psychopathology. It is also worth mentioning that in present-day Peru there are many social and economic stressors that are enduring or chronic for many people, and this may tend to perpetuate "adjustment disorders."

When the reactive symptoms are mostly anxious (and often somatic) and 6 months have passed, some patients do not present the whole set of manifestations, particularly cognitive ones, required for the DSM-III-R diagnosis of generalized anxiety disorder, which could partially explain the relatively high frequency found for the DSM-III-R diagnosis of anxiety disorder, not otherwise specified (NOS) (4.7%).

Some of the between-system differences noted for schizophrenia are probably related to different duration criteria. In DSM-III-R, only 1 week of acute symptoms is required, whereas ICD-10 specifies 1 month. For example, 13% of the patients with DSM-III-R schizophrenia were diagnosed as presenting ICD-10 acute and transient psychotic disorder, which is often used for patients who do not complete 1 month of symptoms.

## Conclusion

The present study found similar rates for most diagnostic categories formulated according to ICD-10 and DSM-III-R on a Peruvian general psychiatric sample. On the other hand, complex distribution patterns were obtained when examining the overlap between similarly named diagnostic groups formed with the two diagnostic systems. Areas were noted (such as those on anxiety and dissociative psychopathology) where DSM-III-R criteria (and to some extent also those of ICD-10), did not seem to apply well to Peruvian clinical reality. Much higher figures for dysthymic; generalized and unspecified anxiety; somatoform; and dissociative disorders were found in this Peruvian sample as compared to levels usually obtained in industrialized countries. It is hoped that increasing research in traditional societies will contribute to enhance the basis for international classification and diagnosis.

## *References*

American Psychiatric Association (1987). *Diagnostic and Statistical Manual of Mental Disorders, Third Edition, Revisid (DSM-III)*. American Psychiatric Association, Washington, DC.

American Psychiatric Association (1980). *Diagnostic and Statistical Manual of Mental Disorders* (3rd ed). American Psychiatric Association, Washington, DC.

Ben-Tovim D (1985). DSM-III in Botswana: A field trial in a developing country. *American Journal of Psychiatry* 142:342–345.

Dahl A (1983). A comparison of DSM-III and ICD-8/ICD-9 diagnosis of functional psychiatric disorders in hospitalized patients. In RL Spitzer, JB Williams, AE Skodol (eds), *International Perspectives on DSM-III*. American Psychiatric Press, Washington, DC.

Endicott J, Spitzer RL (1978). A diagnostic interview: The schedule for affective disorders and schizophrenia. *Archives of General Psychiatry* 35:837–844.

Feighner JP, Robins E, Guze SB, et al (1972). Diagnostic criteria for use in psychiatric research. *Archives of General Psychiatry* 26:57–63.

Frank J (1973). *Persuasion and Healing: A Comparative Study of Psychotherapy*. Johns Hopkins University Press, Baltimore.

Gregory S, Cooper J (1983). Comparison of ICD-9 and DSM-III diagnoses of 71 patients first presenting with severe mental illness. In RL Spitzer, JB Williams, AE Skodol (eds), *International Perspectives on DSM-III*. American Psychiatric Press, Washington, DC.

Kreitman N (1961). The reliability of psychiatric diagnosis. *Journal of Mental Science* 107:876–886.

Lopez-Ibor JJ (1985). Spanish psychiatry and DSM-III. In RL Spitzer, JB Williams, AE Skodol (eds), *International Perspectives on DSM-III*. American Psychiatric Press, Washington, DC.

Mezzich JE, Dow JT, Rich CL, et al (1981). Developing an efficient clinical information system for a comprehensive psychiatric institute. II: Initial evaluation form. *Behavioral Research Methods & Instrumentation* 13:464–478.

Mezzich JE, Fabrega H, Coffman GA, Haley R (1989). DSM-III disorders in a large sample of psychiatric patients: Frequency and specificity of diagnoses. *American Journal of Psychiatry* 146:212–219.

Mezzich JE, Kleinman A, Fabrega H, Parron D (ed.in press). *Culture and Psychiatric Diagnosis*. American Psychiatric Press, Washington, DC.

Robins LN (1985). Composite International Diagnostic Interview. Paper presented at the 138th Annual Meeting of the American Psychiatric Association, Dallas, May 21.

Robins LN, Helzer JE, Croughan J, Ratcliff K (1981). National Institute of Mental Health Diagnostic Interview Schedule: Its history, characteristics and validity. *Archives of General Psychiatry* 38:381–189.

Sogi C, Warthon D, Mezzich J, et al (1987). Traducción y adaptación del Formato de Evaluación Inicial (Versión 1982) a la lengua española (Spanish translation and adaptation of Initial Evaluation Form, 1982 Version). *Acta Psychiatrica Psicológica de Améria Latina* 33:123–130.

Sogi C, Warthon D, Mezzich JE, Valverde J, Saavedra-Castillo A, Ahn CW (1989). Comparative distributions of DSM-III diagnoses in North and South.

Spitzer RL, Endicott J, Robins E (1975). *Research Diagnostic Criteria*. Biometrics Research Division, New York State Psychiatric Institute, New York.

Spitzer RL, Williams E (1989). *Structured Clinical*. Interview for DSM-III Disorders (SCID).

Ward CH, Beck AT, Mendelson M, Mock JE, Erbaugh JK (1962). The psychiatric nomenclature. Reasons for diagnostic disagreement. *Archives of General Psychiatry* 7:198–205.

World Health Organization (1977). *Manual of the International Statistical Classification of Diseases, Injuries and Causes of Death*, Vols. I and II (9th rev). World Health Organization, Geneva.

World Health Organization (1989). *ICD-10 1989 Draft of Chapter V. Mental and Behavioral Disorders (Including Disorders of Psychological Development), Clinical Descriptions and Diagnostic Guidelines*. World Health Organization, Geneva.

Wig N (1983). A perspective from the third world. In RL Spitzer, JB Williams, AE Skodol (eds), *International Perspectives on DSM-III*. American Psychiatric Press, Washington, DC.

Wing JK, Cooper JE, Sartorius N (1974). *The Measurement and Classification of Psychiatric Symptoms*. Cambridge University Press, London.

# 16
# Relationships Between Chapter V(F) of the ICD-10 and National Psychiatric Classifications

John E. Cooper

This chapter describes the purposes and main characteristics of Chapter V(F) of the 10th revision of the *International Classification of Diseases* (ICD-10), Mental and Behavioral Disorders (including disorders of psychological development), with emphasis upon how it is, and might in the future, be related to psychiatric classifications produced by national or other professional groups.

The whole of the ICD, with chapters referring to the diseases of all the systems and parts of the body plus a variety of aspects of the use of medical services, is required for international use in: (1) communication between nations about statistics of mortality and morbidity, (2) general communication about medical care and activities, and (3) medical education and research.

To fulfill these purposes, the individual chapters of ICD-10 must be acceptable to a very wide range of users, and must be easy to understand and to use in practice. With these requirements in mind, an important new policy of "different versions for different purposes" was adopted by the Division of Mental Health of the World Health Organization (WHO), Geneva, with respect to Chapter V(F). This policy has led to the development of: (1) Clinical Diagnostic Guidelines, (2) Diagnostic Criteria for Research, (3) short and simple versions for use in primary and general health care, and (4) a multiaxial system.

The version for use by psychiatrists, now entitled Clinical Diagnostic Guidelines (World Health Organization 1992a), has been produced by means of the international collaborative work described in Chapter 11 by N. Sartorius, and a set of Diagnostic Criteria for Research (DCR-10) has been derived directly from this. The details of these two versions of ICD-10V(F) cannot be described here; it is sufficient to say that the wording of the Clinical Diagnostic Guidelines is appropriate for use by clinical psychiatrists and gives considerable flexibility in the way diagnostic decisions are made. This is particularly important when the information available under busy clinical conditions may not be complete, and it may not be appropriate for the clinician to try to work through a detailed list of specified clinical criteria. The diagnostic criteria for research are specifically designed for research projects, when it is important to have groups of patients who are as homogeneous and, therefore, as carefully selected as possible. Research workers tend to have more time and information available than busy clinicians, so it is appropriate to have a version of the classification which requires quite detailed information, and that puts greater restrictions upon the way a diagnosis is made.

In addition to these two versions, a multiaxial system is now under development for general use (see Chapter 17).

Another version of the text of Chapter V(F) has also been prepared, and has now been approved by the World Health Assembly, for publication in the official volumes of the whole ICD-10 (World Health Organization 1992b). This is much shorter than the Clinical Diagnostic Guidelines and is not intended for general use by psychiatrists. The development of these different versions, all of which are based on the same underlying classification, has been undertaken by the WHO because of the very different requirements of users in different countries and work settings.

## The Influence of Existing Classifications on the Development of ICD-10V(F)

Some examples of the way in which ICD-10V(F) has appropriately drawn on existing classification will now be given. Table 16.1 shows the overall arrangement of Chapter V(F), so that the position of the selected examples within the classification can be identified.

TABLE 16.1. List of two-character categories, F0 to F9, of ICD-10.

| Category | Disorder |
|---|---|
| F0 | Organic mental, including symptomatic |
| F1 | Mental and behavioral due to psychoactive substance use |
| F2 | Schizophrenia, schizotypal and delusional |
| F3 | Mood (affective) |
| F4 | Neurotic, stress-related, and somatoform |
| F5 | Behavioral syndromes associated with physiological disturbances and physical factors |
| F6 | Adult personality and behavior |
| F7 | Mental retardation |
| F8 | Psychological development |
| F9 | Behavioral and emotional, with onset usually occurring in childhood or adolescence (and mental, unspecified) |

One of the subdivisions of F2, Schizophrenia, Schizotypal and Delusional Disorders, is F23, Acute and Transient Psychotic Disorders. Table 16.2 shows the way in which these acute disorders have been further subdivided, depending on the clinical syndrome present and the presence or absence of clear precipitating stress. Although at first sight this arrangement may appear to be innovative, it is better described as simplistic. It is only innovative in that it makes no assumptions about necessary relationships between acute onset, type of symptoms, and precipitating stress, and it draws upon well established clinical traditions of French (Pichot 1984) and Scandinavian (Strömgren 1988) psychiatry. The French concept of *Bouffée Délirante* has been included, but under the name of Polymorphic Syndrome. To avoid assumptions about etiology and about the symptom patterns of acute psychoses, the various syndromes have been arranged so that it is possible to classify the Polymorphic Syndrome, the Acute Schizophrenic Syndrome, and the presence or absence of an obvious immediate precipitating stress, all in combination with each other, or without each other. This gets away from the unjustified assumption that all acute psychoses must have an immediate environmental cause, and that acute psychoses do not have typical symptoms of schizophrenia. There is evidence to suggest that none of these assumptions, although commonly made in clinical practice, are justified. This new arrangement should encourage descriptive research into these important disorders.

In the Section F30, Affective (Mood) Disorders, the concept of dysthymia, which first appeared in a formal classification in *Diagnostic and Statistical Manual of Mental Disorders, Third edition (DSM-III)* (American Psychiatric Association 1989) has been followed. There are still many problems in its definition and use, but in the opinion of a variety of international experts it is probably better to include it than to leave it out.

TABLE 16.2. F23, Acute and transient psychotic disorders.

| Subcategory discription |
| --- |
| F23.0, Acute polymorphic psychotic disorder (without symptoms of schizophrenia) |
| .00 Without associated acute stress |
| .01 With associated acute stress |
| F23.1, Acute polymorphic psychotic disorder with symptoms of schizophrenia |
| .10 Without associated acute stress |
| .11 With associated acute stress |
| F23.2, Acute schizophrenia-like psychotic disorder |
| .20 Without associated acute stress |
| .21 With associated acute stress |
| F23.3, Other acute predominantly delusional psychotic disorder |
| .30 Without associated acute stress |
| .31 With associated acute stress |

In the Category of F4, which has purposefully been labelled Neurotic, although without attempting to define this term, there are a number of important inclusions that rely on either a national classification, or the classificatory requirements of groups of developing countries (Wig et al 1985). Many developing countries have emphasized their need for categories that deal with the expression of psychological problems in terms of physical symptoms, and a somatoform category, again first appearing in United States literature and in DSM-III, has been included.

A special category of Mixed Anxiety and Depressive Disorder has been included, with psychiatrists in developing countries and psychiatrists working in primary care facilities in mind. This category is defined as a mixture of symptoms of anxiety and depression, but with none of them being so severe that a separate, independent diagnosis of anxiety or depression can be made. There are also mixed categories for dissociative disorders (called hysterical disorders in previous classifications), often noted as being particularly common in developing countries. The category of neurasthenia has been retained, because, although it is not used in large parts of United States and Europe, it is used in some European countries and is a very important diagnosis in China.

Category F6, Abnormalities of Adult Personality and Behavior, remains the biggest problem of all (as it always has been in psychiatric classifications). There are no particular national classifications that seem to be giving a lead in this difficult field. In view of the widespread, although still-controversial, use of the concept of borderline personality disorder, the term has been included in this section, although in a rather brief and simplified form.

Category F8, Disorders of Psychological Development, and F9, Behavioral and Emotional Disorders (with onset usually occurring in childhood or adolescence), owe a good deal to the descriptive traditions of British psychiatry (Rutter and Hersov 1985). It may well be that further extension of some of these sections is required to deal with the particular problems of developing countries, where very large proportions of the population are comparatively youthful. However, evidence about any such special requirements has been very scanty up to now, and further development or extension of these categories awaits further evidence.

These illustrations make it clear that ICD-10-V(F) has drawn, where appropriate, on a wide variety of existing classifications. Similarly, if other classifications are developed, it is appropriate for them to draw upon ICD-10-V(F). Nobody has a patent or copyright on the development or use of medical concepts and their classification, and it is up to the international scientific community to see that there is continual and productive interchange of ideas between countries and between organizations.

## The Purposes of National Psychiatric Classifications

In view of the international nature of ICD-10-V, national psychiatric organizations need to consider very carefully what role might be played by any classification they might themselves develop. To have a proliferation of national classifications with very few differences between them would be counterproductive rather than helpful. There has been a great deal of international communication in all ways on medical matters in the last few years, and particularly in psychiatry. One of the main conclusions arrived at by the large number of international experts that helped to develop ICD-10-F is that there is a surprising amount of agreement and compatibility between schools of psychiatric thought across countries. The remaining differences are comparatively small, and require to be dealt with by research rather than by attempts to set up special classifications that are incompatible with ICD-10-Chapter V(F) in its international role.

National classifications might be justified if they provide for special requirements of a country when it can be demonstrated that some psychiatric disorders that are important in that country are not adequately dealt with in ICD-10. However, this conclusion should be arrived at only after careful study of the evidence. It may well be that all that is required is for some of the categories of ICD-10-F to have additions or subdivisions made to include local service needs or research. Also at issue is that there is no point in producing a classification with a national title simply by omitting some categories of ICD-10 not considered to be particularly common in that particular country. If any condition that is present in ICD-10-V(F) is unusually rare in a particular country or location, this is an interesting and valuable observation that requires investigation. However, the converse already mentioned (ie, adding to or subdividing existing ICD-10 categories) is likely to be more common, and could produce very worthwhile results.

Special problems of language and translation may also require the development of special national sections of ICD-10 with alternative versions or extended descriptions of concept.

The existence of specially important historical traditions of psychiatry in a particular country may also be a stimulus for the development of special sections for particular countries. However, it needs to be carefully established that any existing national tradition of psychiatry can be justified by descriptive clinical data rather than by custom only.

This is perhaps a good point at which to emphasize that the fundamental principle of the development of ICD-10-V(F) has been to rely upon description as far as possible, and to avoid interpretation. In addition, etiological assumptions were also avoided as much as possible. One exception to this is the inclusion of broad classes of etiology in the main sections, such as organic etiology and the groups of disorders due to drugs, alcohol, and acute stress. However, these are general etiological assumptions that are necessary if a classification is to be reasonably attractive to clinical users, and they are etiologies attached to quite large groups of conditions.

## Future Prospects

It is to be hoped that the present arrangements for collaboration and consultation between WHO and all its member states will continue, with respect to the future of both ICD-10-V(F) and any national classifications that may be considered. The World Psychiatric Association has played an important part in the development of ICD-10-V(F), and presumably will continue to help in the future. Another good example of international cooperation is given by the close and detailed discussions that have been held between the various committees advising the WHO on the production of ICD-10-V(F), and the working parties that developed DSM-III and are now developing the future DSM-IV for the American Psychiatric Association.

Science knows no national boundaries, and if we are guided by the scientific method then we should not be faced in the future with a series of incompatible national psychiatric classifications. In this sense, science means the development of concepts of psychiatric disorders that are based on careful and detailed descriptions and observations, with constant awareness of problems of bias, reliability, and validity. Assumptions of etiology based only on theory or derived from politics or ideology have no place in the development of an international psychiatric classification.

Because of its international purposes and derivation, Chapter V(F) of ICD-10 should be studied and used by psychiatrists in all countries. Psychiatrists in countries that have produced a national classification should be familiar with both their own classification and Chapter V(F), and should be constantly discussing how both might be improved. Classifications will change as knowledge increases; they are not fixed or "true," but are temporary statements waiting for improvement.

## *References*

American Psychiatric Association (1980). *Diagnostic and Statistical Manual of Mental Disorders* (3rd ed). American Psychiatric Association, Washington, DC.

Pichot P (1984). The French approach to psychiatric classification. *British Journal of Psychiatry* 144:113–118.

Rutter M, Hersov L (1985). *Child and Adolescent Psychiatry*. Blackwell, Oxford.

Strömgren E (1988). Scandinavian approaches to psychiatric diagnosis. In JE Mezzich, M von Cranach (eds), *International Classification in Psychiatry: Unity and Diversity*. Cambridge University Press, Cambridge.

Wig NN, Kusumanto SR, Shen Y-C, Sell H (1985). Problems of psychiatric diagnosis and classification in the third world. In *Mental Disorders, Alcohol and Drug Related Problems: International Perspectives on their Diagnosis and Classification*. Excerpta Medica, Amsterdam.

World Health Organization (1992a). *ICD-10 Classification of Mental and Behavioral Disorders: Clinical Descriptions and Diagnostic Guidelines*. World Health Organization, Geneva.

World Health Organization (1992b). *International Classification of Diseases and Health-Related Problems* (10th rev). World Health Organization, Geneva.

# Part III
# Multiaxial Issues

# 17
# Multiaxial Diagnosis: Purposes and Challenges

JUAN E. MEZZICH

The multiaxial approach to comprehensive diagnosis, which constitutes one of the fundamental innovations of modern diagnostic systems, has old roots and antecedents. It can be seen as evolving from the contraposition of an analytic, textural, and experiential Aristotelian perspective to a synthetic, bold, and abstract Platonic conceptualization of disease entity as a sufficient description of a patient's clinical condition. The ontogeny of multiaxial diagnosis can be understood further, as suggested by Ojesjo (1978) following Nietzschean insights on drama, as the point of convergence between, on the one hand, an idealized and rationalistic Apollonian tradition striving for parsimonial order and clarity, and on the other, a Dionysian tradition, vitalistic, empathetic, and closer to the patient. In this scenario, multiaxial diagnosis can be perceived as an attempt at comprehensiveness and sensitivity in the description of the patient's condition through a standardized, reliable, and structurally coherent schema.

## Purposes of Multiaxial Diagnosis

The general purposes of multiaxial diagnosis, as one particular approach to the diagnostic task, are the same as those of diagnosis in general, that is, clinical description, professional communication, treatment planning, prognosis, clinical research, and professional training. Additionally and more specifically, multiaxial diagnosis has purposes that have been the actual motivation for the development of particular proposals and schemas. These purposes correspond to a given conceptualization of the appropriate scope of the clinical condition to be orderly, systematically, and succinctly described and coded (ie, diagnosed), and that have been historically referred to earlier.

The descriptive capabilities and potentialities of the multiaxial model have been applied in both psychiatric and general medicine to two subjects: Illness complexity and the patient's whole clinical condition. The articulation of these two topics has constituted over the past few decades the main purposes of multiaxial diagnosis. These perspectives are outlined sequentially below.

## *Articulating Illness Complexity*

Articulating or structuring the fundamental components of an illness was the first purpose of multiaxial diagnosis in both psychiatry and general medicine.

In psychiatry, this first purpose motivated the development of the earliest multiaxial diagnostic schemas. Essen-Möller and Wohlfahrt (1947) in Sweden (to constitute the official Swedish classification), and Lecomte et al (1947) in France (as a practical grid for clinical work), proposed that the best way to describe a psychiatric illness was to separately specify syndrome and etiology. Bilikiewicz (1951) in Poland and Leme Lopes (1954) in Brazil published triaxial systems involving general psychiatric syndromes, personality conditions, and biopsychosocial etiopathogenic constellations of the patient's illness.

For the classification of illness in general medicine, the first multiaxial proposal seems to have been the Standard Nomenclature of Pathology (SNOP) (College of American Pathologists 1965), which included the following four axes: I, topography; II, morphology; III, etiology; and IV, symptoms.

The successor of SNOP, termed Standard Nomenclature for Medicine (SNOMED) (College of American Pathologists 1977), added axes such as nosological entities or diseases, which supplemented at a different level of discourse, the elementarian and analytic approach of SNOP.

The recent International Classification of Diseases for Oncology (Percy et al 1990), developed as one specialty member of the ICD-10 family of classifications (Brämer 1988), includes two axes: Topography (which identifies the location of the tumor) and morphology (which specifies histologic type and tumor behavior and differentiation). The developers of this taxonomy considered that the use of these two axes was the only reasonable way to describe neoplasms effectively.

## *Formulating the Patient's Whole Clinical Condition*

A second major purpose or use of multiaxial diagnosis is to describe not only the illness but the patient's condition as a whole. In this regard, there has been a relatively early interest in describing the context of the illness, historically as well as cross-sectionally or environmentally. Another critical concern has been to indicate the impact of the illness on the functioning of the individual.

This second purpose has been prominently connected to the need to facilitate the preparation of a comprehensive treatment plan.

The hope has been that by bringing to the forefront of the clinician's attention and the clinical chart critical features of the patient condition, the need for certain treatment modalities (eg, medication, psychotherapy, vocational rehabilitation) and a multidisciplinary team can become clearer and more justified.

Illustrating the purpose of more comprehensively understanding and managing the patient's condition, nearly 20 multiaxial systems have been published in the psychiatric literature during the past four decades (Mezzich 1988). The following areas have been the most frequently considered: (1) psychiatric syndromes, including assessments of their severity, course and etiology; (2) personality conditions; (3) mental retardation and developmental delays; (4) physical or general medical disorders; (5) psychosocial stressors; and (6) adaptive functioning and disabilities.

One of the best-known contemporary multiaxial systems has been that developed for children and adolescents by Rutter and an international group of collaborators (1969, 1975) under World Health Organization (WHO) sponsorship. Other approaches were proposed by Ottoson and Perris in Sweden (1973), Helmchen (1975, 1980) in Germany, and Bech et al (1987) in Denmark. Williams (1987) has described the development of and experience with the multiaxial schema of the *Diagnostic and Statistical Manual of Mental Disorders*, 3rd edition (DSM-III) (American Psychiatric Association 1980). This schema has been revised for the new DSM-IV (Williams et al 1990).

Also within the objective of describing more fully the patient's condition, a multiaxial schema for general psychiatric patients is being developed as part of the *International Classification of Diseases*, 10th revision (ICD-10) family of classifications. The groundwork for the development of this schema included analyses of the worldwide literature in this field and the international surveys on ICD-10 conducted by the World Psychiatric Association (Mezzich 1988, 1990). The 1993 draft of the ICD-10 multiaxial schema (Mezzich et al 1993) has the following three axes:

I. Clinical diagnoses (mental and nonmental disorders): These are to be coded according to the 20 disease chapters in the core classification of ICD-10.

II. Disabilities: This axis is to be evaluated with a revised and shortened version of the WHO Disability Assessment Scale (World Health Organization 1985). Four major areas are to be considered: personal care and survival, occupational functioning (as remunerated worker, student, or homemaker), functioning with family (assessing both the regularity and quality of interactions with relatives), and broader social behaviors (interaction with other individuals and the community at large, and leisure activities).

III. Contextual factors: This is to be coded with selected Z-codes from ICD-10 Chapter XXI, Factors Influencing Health Status and Contact with Health Services.

In general medicine, a significant effort inscribable within the multiaxial purpose of formulating the patient's whole clinical condition is constituted by the Triaxial Classification of Health Problems for primary or general health care (Clare 1992), which contained axes on physical, psychopathological and social problems. Also relevant to this point is the multiaxial classification for primary care developed on the basis of a careful study of clinical cases seen by general practitioners in the United Kingdom (Jenkins et al 1988), which contained axes on psychological problems, social problems and supports, personality, and physical illness, all further qualified by severity and duration considerations. The family of classifications corresponding to ICD-10 contains components such as core chapters on pathology or diseases, factors influencing health status and contact with health services, and classification of impairments, disabilities and handicaps, all of which are pertinent to a more complete characterization of a patient's condition in general medicine.

Furthermore, leaders in general medicine are increasingly concerned with issues of functioning, social relationships, and quality of life as crucial for an adequate assessment of health status (eg, House et al 1988, Wenger et al 1984). On reviewing the current status of nosology in clinical medicine, Feinstein (1988) concluded that requirements for advancement include the use of standardized names, operational criteria, and multiaxial arrangements.

## Challenges for Progress

Diagnostic systems are, in part, theories of reality and as such they will always be imperfect. At the same time, it can be argued that they are improvable on the basis of advances in our observation and understanding of clinical reality, heuristic model building organizing pertinent quantitative and qualitative information, and empirical validation internationally conducted in a variety of setttings. On the road to making advances on comprehensive diagnosis, particularly with regard to multiaxial approaches, the following challenges appear prominent.

### *Biopsychosocial Reformulation of the Field*

Many well-known and authoritative textbooks, such as the *Comprehensive Textbook of Psychiatry* (Kaplan and Sadock 1989) and the *Handbook of Psychiatry* (Shepherd 1985), emphasize the multifactorial causality (from genetics to sociocultural variables) of most psychiatric disorders, and the wide range of valuable therapeutic modalities (from psychotropic medication to psychotherapy and vocational rehabilitation strategies). However, a reductionistic perspective focused on the brain and pathology has been conspicuous recently in many circles, which has led penetrating philosophical reviewers to note a paradigmatic shift of the field from biopsychosocial to biomedical (Wilson 1993).

This situation calls for a reaffirmation of the field within a biopsychosocial framework. The effort would be consistent with the humanistic ideals of psychiatry, concerned not only with illnesses but with the whole person who experiences mental problems. It would be furthermore consistent with recent development in general medicine and health care such as the broadened scope of ICD-10 as a family of classifications (Brämer 1988).

## *Efficient Structure for Multiaxial Diagnosis*

The use of multiaxial schemas in daily clinical care is challenged not only by the conceptual reductionism prevailing in many circles, but the practical issues derived from the structural innovation it represents and the unfamiliarity of many psychiatrists with it. This is compounded by the fact that, in comparison with single label uniaxial diagnosis, multiaxial formulations are more laborious and time-consuming to complete.

The difficulties call first for efforts to simplify multiaxial schemas. A conspicuous step in this direction is the ongoing development of the multiaxial presentation of ICD-10, which has only three axes, in contrast with five as the modal number in published multiaxial schemas (Mezzich 1979). Another helpful strategy for clinical practice is the use of standard recording formats (eg, those developed by Mezzich et al [1982]) for charting DSM-III. Such structures, as documented by Bassett and Beiser (1991), can enhance the implementation of multiaxial systems.

## *Cultural Sensitivity in Multiaxial Diagnosis*

A major issue in the development of international diagnostic systems is the discrepancy between the geographic distribution of psychiatric patients, 80% of whom reside in developing countries, and the overwhelming concentration within Nordic Europe and North America of the experts responsible for the conceptualization of such key professional tools. For example, in the preparation of the ICD-10 classification of mental disorders (a process which probably represented the widest and most meaningful international collaboration for any diagnostic system to date) (World Health Organization 1992) only 10% of the writers of initial drafts resided in developing countries. The limitations in cultural sensitivity suggested by the earlier observations are also noticeable intranationally, as is the case of DSM-III (American Psychiatric Association 1980), which has few references to cultural issues, despite the fact that the United States has substantial numbers of ethnically identified minorities and refugees. These restrictions are noticeable not only in the core categorization and definition of mental disorders in standard diagnostic systems, but also in their multiaxial arrangements.

Steps in the direction of greater cultural validity are being taken in the development of DSM-IV through the inclusion of cultural elements in its introduction, in the text associated with diagnostic categories, and in its multiaxial schema, in addition to a Cultural Formulation Guideline and a Glossary of Culture-Bound Syndromes in its appendix (Mezzich et al [in press]).

As part of the development of the family of classifications and educational materials for ICD-10, a cultural lexicon and a casebook containing culturally diverse cases are being prepared. Also pertinent here are the adaptations of ICD-10 to local clinical reality being generated in countries such as China, Cuba, and Japan. Much work remains to be done towards harmonizing effectively the needs for universal communication and for attention to cultural diversity.

### *Empirical Validation*

Although the results of data-based investigations are being discernibly used in the development of standard diagnostic systems, such as ICD-10 and DSM-IV, the majority of their diagnostic categories and features are not adequately validated yet and are predominantly based on the judgment of expert committees. These limitations are largely also applicable to multiaxial schemas.

The empirical substantiation of a multiaxial diagnostic system involves much more than documenting the reliability and validity of its syndromic categories. Validation is also needed for the number and kinds of axes it incorporates, as well as for the typologies or dimensional scales structuring its various axes.

In addition to reliability (reproducibility or generalizability across possible users and circumstances), pertinent validation perspectives correspond to the objectives or purposes of diagnosis. These include professional understanding of and communication about psychiatric cases, treatment planning, and prediction of course and outcome, in addition to training, clinical research, and policy development. Although some promising findings have been generated regarding the reliability (eg, Fernando et al 1986), perceived clinical usefulness (eg, Williams 1987), and predictive validity (eg, Mezzich et al 1984) of multiaxial approaches, much more work is needed, particularly for validating the newer schemas.

## Conclusion

Multiaxial diagnosis has ancient roots, including rationalistic and experiential developmental lines. Its purposes have expanded over the past few decades from an original focus on the articulation of the elements of an illness to the formulation of the patient's whole clinical condition. Challenges for the further development of multiaxial diagnosis include the need for a biopsychosocial reformulation of psychiatry, the design of efficient schemas and formats to facilitate their implementation, the consideration of cultural sensitivity, and the empirical substantiation of the reliability and validity of its architecture and individual components.

## *References*


American Psychiatric Association (1980). *Diagnostic and Statistical Manual of Mental Disorders, Third Revision (DSM-III)*. American Psychiatric Association, Washington, DC.

Basset AS, Beiser M (1991). DSM-III: Use of the multiaxial diagnostic system in clinical practice. *Canadian Journal of Psychiatry* 36:270–274.

Bech P, Jhorts S, Lund K, Vilmar T, Kastrup M (1987). An integration of the DSM-III and ICD-8 by global severity assessments for measuring multidimentional outcomes in general hospital psychiatry. *Acta Psychiatrica Scandinavica* 75:297–306.

Bilikiewicz T (1951). Próba ukladu nozograficznego etioepigenetycznego w psychiatrii. *Neurologia i Neurochirurgia Polska* 1:68–78 (in Polish).

Brämer GR (1988). 10th Revision of the International Classification. *British Journal of Psychiatry* 152:29–32 (suppl 1).

Clare A, Gulbinat W, Sartorius N (1992). A triaxial classification of health problems presenting in primary care: A World Health Organization multicentre study. *Social Psychiatry and Psychiatric Epidemiology* 27:108–116.

College of American Pathologists (1965). *Systematized Nomenclature of Pathology* (SNOP). College of American Pathologists, Chicago.

College of American Pathologists (1977). *Systematized Nomenclature of Medicine* (SNOMED). College of American Pathologists, Skokie, IL.

Essen-Möller E, Wohlfahrt S (1947). Suggestions for the amendment of the official Swedish classification of mental disorders. *Acta Psychiatrica Scandinavica* 47:551–555.

Feinstein AR (1988). ICD, POR, and DRG: Unsolved scientific problems in the nosology of clinical medicine. *Archives of Internal Medicine* 148:2269–2274.

Fernando T, Mellsop G, Nelson K, Peace K, Wilson J (1986). The reliability of the Axis V of the DSM-III. *American Journal of Psychiatry* 143:752–755.

Helmchen H (1975). Schizophrenia: Diagnostic concepts in the ICD-8. *British Journal of Psychiatry* No. 10 (special pub).

Helmchen H (1980). Multiaxial systems of classification. *Acta Psychiatrica Scandinavica* 61:43–55.

House JS, Landis KR, Umberson D (1988). Social relationships and health. *Science* 241:540–544.

Jenkins R, Smeeton N, Shepherd M (1988). Classification of mental problems in primary care. *Psychological Medicine* 12:1–69 (suppl).

Kaplan HI, Sadock BJ (eds) (1989). *Comprehensive Textbook of Psychiatry* (5th ed). Williams & Wilkins, Baltimore.

Lecomte M, Damey A, Delage E, Marty P (1947). Essai d'une statistique synoptique de médicine psychiatrique. *Techniques Hospitaliers* 18:5–8.

Leme Lopes J (1954). *As Dimensões do Diagnóstico Psiquiátrico*. Agir, Rio de Janeiro.

Mezzich JE (1979). Patterns and issues in multiaxial diagnosis. *Psychological Medicine* 9:125–137.

Mezzich JE (1988). On developing a psychiatric multiaxial schema for ICD-10. *British Journal of Psychiatry* 152:38–43 (Suppl 1).

Mezzich JE (1990). The World Psychiatric Association and the development of ICD-10. In C Stefanis, AD Rabavilas, CR Soldatos (eds), *Psychiatry: A World Perspective*. Elsevier Science Publishers, Amsterdam.

Mezzich JE, Coffman GA, Goodpastor SM (1982). A format for DSM-III diagnostic formulation: Experience with 1111 consecutive patients. *American Journal of Psychiatry* 139:591–596.

Mezzich JE, Evanczuk KJ, Mathias RJ, Coffman GA (1984). Admission decisions and multiaxial diagnosis. *Archives of General Psychiatry* 41:1001–1004.

Mezzich JE, Kleinman A, Fabrega H, Parron D (eds) (in press). *Culture and Psychiatric Diagnosis*. American Psychiatric Press, Washington, DC.

Mezzich JE, Sartorius N, Kastrup MC, Katschnig H, Lopez-Ibor JJ, Janca A (1993). Paper presented at the WHO Symposium on ICD-10: A Common Language, Annual Meeting of the American Psychiatric Association, San Francisco, May 25, 1993.

Ojesjo L (1978). Psychiatric classification and diagnosis: Some guidelines. *Nordisk Psykiatrisk Tidsskrift* 32:239–250.

Ottoson JO, Perris C (1973). Multidimensional classification of mental disorders. *Psychological Medicine* 3:238–243.

Percy C, van Holten V, Muir C (1990). *International Classification of Diseases for Oncology*. World Health Organization, Geneva.

Rutter M, Shaffer D, Shepherd M (1975). *A Multiaxial Classification of Child Psychiatric Disorders*. World Health Organization, Geneva.

Rutter M, Levovici S, Eisenberg L, et al (1969). A triaxial classification of mental disorders in childhood. *Journal of Child Psychology and Psychiatry* 10:41–61.

Shepherd M (ed) (1985). *Handbook of Psychiatry*. Cambridge University Press, Cambridge.

Wenger N, Mattson M, Furberg C, Elinson J (eds) (1984). *Assessment of Quality of Life in Clinical Trials of Cardiovascular Therapies*. Le Jacq Publishing, New York.

Williams JBW (1987). Multiaxial diagnosis. In AE Skodol, RL Spitzer (eds), *An Annotated Bibliography of DSM-III*. American Psychiatric Press, Washington, DC.

Williams JBW, Goldman H, Gruenberg A, Mezzich JE, Skodol AE, Shaffer D, Spitzer RL, Setterberg S (1990). Towards DSM-IV: The multiaxial system in progress. *Hospital and Community Psychiatry* 41:1181–1182.

Wilson M (1993). DSM-III and the transformation of American psychiatry: A history. *American Journal of Psychiatry* 150:399–410.

World Health Organization (1985). *Disabilities Assessment Schedule*. World Health Organization, Geneva.

World Health Organization (1992). ICD-10 classification of Mental and Behavioral Disorders: Clinical Descriptions and Diagnostic Guidelines. WHO, Geneva.

World Health Organization (1992). *International Classification of Diseases and Health-Related Problems* (10th rev). World Health Organization, Geneva.

# 18
# Axial Organization of Clinical Diagnoses

JUAN J. LOPEZ-IBOR

The draft of the ICD-10 multiaxial system has three axes. The first includes general psychiatric syndromes, developmental conditions (including personality disorders and mental retardation), and physical diseases. In the following, it is called Axis I (Clinical Disorders). The second deals with levels of disability associated with the pathological phenomena included in Axis I, and the third axis deals with environmental factors of relevance to the presentation and course of the clinical disorders.

Several multiaxial systems have been proposed (Mezzich 1979). The oldest ones, such as that of Essen-Möller and Wohlfahrt (1947) focused on the distinction between phenomenology and etiology. More recent systems pay attention also to onset, course, medical conditions and associated factors, intensity or severity, adaptive functioning or personal relationships, and stressful events. For comparative purposes, allusions are made only to the multiaxial schema in *Diagnostic and Statistical Manual of Mental Disorders*, 3rd edition (DSM-III), which is the best known of those published to date.

The *International Classification of Diseases*, 10th revision (ICD-10) Axis I (Clinical Disorders) is roughly equivalent to Axes I, II, and III of DSM-III and later versions of Axis I (Clinical Disorders) include (1) Psychiatric Disorders of Chapter F of the ICD-10, (2) Personality Disorders of Chapter F of the ICD-10, and (3) Other Disorders of Chapters A–E and G–Y of the ICD-10.

There are several reasons, to be outlined later in this chapter, that justify what seems to be a step backward from the DSM-III independence of Axis II (Personality) and Axis III (Physical Problems), whose purposes are to remind clinicians of the importance of their patients' personality and possible physical diseases.

Multiaxial diagnostic systems were introduced in psychiatry to take into consideration different aspects of the clinical condition. The main types or themes of the different proposals identified by Mezzich (1979) are the following:

1. Phenomenology (symptomatology, personality disorder and intellectual level/mental subnormality).
2. Etiological or associated factors (biological and psychosocial factors conceptualized and organized in various ways).
3. Time frame (onset, duration and course of the symptomatology).
4. Social functioning (work performance, interpersonal relations, and other aspects of adaptive functioning).
5. Other (psychopathological severity, certainty, and the "illness," "caseness" contrast proposed by Kato 1977).

The ICD-10 is a classification to be used in a great variety of settings, including primary care, and in both developed and developing countries. There is no consensus, much less agreed-on theory, as to the most adequate number of axes, but much speaks in favor of a simple multiaxial system. Furthermore, there is no clear definition of what an axis is or should be. Of course, multiple axes can describe clinical reality in a better way, but may also be seen as (partially) independent decision lines, reflecting the activities of different health professionals (ie, in DSM-III Axis I, Psychiatric Disorders: psychiatrists; Axis II, Personality: psychologists; Axis III, Somatic Disorders: other physicians; Axis IV, Social Adaptation: social workers). In any case, five axes may be too many to be used in clinical settings other than those in developed countries.

The relationship between the different axes of multiaxial systems is seldom clarified, which will be discussed later, when referring to specific axes. In the DSM-III, the axes are presented as independent, and the relationships between them are not always clear. In the following section, the relationships between the axes dealing with psychiatric disorders and those dealing with personality as well as with organic/somatic disorders are considered. The relationship between personality disorders and somatic illness seems to be an almost forgotten research topic.

## Hierarchical Principles Versus Multiple Diagnoses

In the past, psychiatric classifications have been guided by Jaspers hierarchical principle (Jaspers 1963), which is a principle widely used in medical diagnosis. According to this principle, the presence of a specific symptom pattern or disorder excludes the diagnosis of disorders lower in the hierarchy. For instance, the presence of panic anxiety together with the hearing of voices commenting the patient's activity is irrelevant for the actual diagnosis of schizophrenia. Today, there is a tendency to move away from this hierarchical principle, which can be done by withdrawing the exclusion criteria from a classification. This approach leads to multiple diagnoses, which is important in the description of patients and in the gathering of information. In a hierarchical system, a patient with major depression who suffers also from panic attacks, could not be distinguished from one who has never had such symptoms of anxiety. This multiple diagnosis approach does not mean that comorbidity of several disorders has to be accepted (Frances 1980). It is just a better way of describing reality.

## The Expansion of Axis I (Psychiatric Disorders)

There is a clear historical trend towards incorporating into Axis I (Psychiatric Disorders), disorders that were previously included in other axes, for instance, the personality disorders that are considered clinically relevant because of their etiology, severity or psychopathology, or the organic disorders. Ever since Bingley (1958) described epileptic traits in the personality of patients with temporal lobe tumors without epileptic fits, the epileptic personality disorder has been considered not as a variant of the personality, but as an organic disorder. Similarly, according to DSM-III, many patients who would previously have been diagnosed as suffering from some kind of affective personality disorder will now receive the diagnosis of a regular affective disorder (ie, cyclothymia or dysthymia). In the ICD-10, what used to be called schizotypal personality disorder is now named schizotypal disorder and is to be found in the section of schizophrenia and delusional disorders. Finally, there are reasons to sustain that anxious-avoidant personality disorder would be more correctly classified with categories belonging to the section on neurotic, stress-related, and somatoform disorders.

### *The Relationship Between Psychiatric Disorders and Personality Conditions*

The main reason for having an Axis II in DSM-III as separate from Axis I was to ensure that personality aspects were not overlooked in the presence of a more florid Axis I disorder (Frances 1980). Prior personality traits are considered relevant for the clinical picture and Widiger and Hyler (1987), have discussed many of the possibilities. Nevertheless, several aspects have to be considered:

1. Psychiatry has always had difficulties in the definition and classification of personality disorders, although it has always recognized them. For Griesinger (1872), psychiatric illnesses were brain illnesses, but he added that aberrations of the intelligence (psychological abnormalities in present terms) belonged also to the realm of psychiatry. The classification of the abnormal personality variants is problematic. Two main principles have been applied, both very different from the categorical classification of other psychiatric syndromes. One is prototypical (ie, Schneider's ap-

proach 1950), another is dimensional (ie, as based on Minnesota Multiphasic Personality Inventory (MMPI)). Personality disorders have often been considered as minor forms of psychosis (*psychosis mitis*) or, at least, they have been described using words that suggested a strong relationship between them. Personality is in itself an ill-defined concept, and different authors have used different notions. For Schneider (1950), personality only includes tendencies and will. Intelligence was also excluded by Jaspers (1963), who considered it an instrument of the personality.

2. The historic trend mentioned above, by virtue of which a subgroup of personality disorders is being incorporated into Axis I (Psychiatric Disorders).

3. Personality disorders as included in the DSM-III and even more so, in the ICD-10, do not include all the aspects of the personality relevant for psychiatry or medicine (type A behavior, Friedman and Rosenman 1960; typus melancholicus, Tellenbach 1980; and others are excluded).

4. The Axis I–II distinction in the DSM-III has been criticized because the differences between Axes I and II are often difficult to assess or appear arbitrary (Gunderson and Pollack 1985), because the interaction between Axis I and II is sometimes confusing and sometimes becomes a diagnostic redundancy. The association of specific personality disorders with psychiatric disorders has received considerable attention in an attempt to clarify whether there are etiological relationships, or whether it is an artifact or the expression of comorbidity. A multiple diagnostic approach, without prejudging the nature of the association, may clarify this area. The most commonly described associations have been alcohol and substance use with antisocial personality disorder or other personality disorders (although a personality disorder may be preexisting, but not necessarily be predisposing (Blume 1989)); or borderline personality disorder (Alnaes and Torgersen 1988a); schizophrenia and schizoid with schizotypal personality disorder; mood and substance abuse disorders with borderline personality disorder (Akiskal et al 1885, Gunderson and Elliot 1985, Alnaes and Torgersen 1988a), or with other personality disorders such as "eccentric" or "dramatic" or a combination of several of them (Alnaes and Torgersen 1988a, 1988b, 1989). An association of mood disorders with borderline personality disorder has been found when studying biological markers (Lahmeyer et al 1988, 1989); obsessive-compulsive disorder with anankastic personality disorder (Alnaes and Torgersen 1988a); and anxiety disorders with dependent, avoidant, and histrionic personality disorder (Mavissakalian and Hamann 1988). Relationships in the other direction are, for example, the association of personality disorders with anxiety and depressive disorders (Klass et al 1989) or other disorders. Nevertheless, these associations are difficult to interpret because, for instance, a mood disorder may increase the significance of preexisting personality traits (Joffe and Regan 1988). When associating eating disorders with borderline personality disorders (Johnson

et al 1989; Yager et al 1989) the question of what comes first may be raised.

5. The ICD-10 Chapter F includes symptoms or syndromes of clinical relevance. Earlier versions of the ICD-10 covered two kinds of personality disorders: (1) Personality variants consisting of abnormal exaggerations of specific personality traits, and (2) personality disorders in the strict sense. After the first field trials, the former categories were withdrawn for two reasons. First, the categories themselves proved insufficiently reliable; second, and more important, the decision was taken that the ICD-10 Chapter F(V) should only include disorders as such, and not social or psychologically abnormal conditions or situations which cannot be considered as clinical disorders.

The strategy of ICD-10 multiaxial approach allows the personality disorders in Axis I (Clinical Disorders) and the normal and abnormal personality variants or personal life-style on life management factors, as described in Chapter Z, in ICD-10 Axis III. Therefore, there is a clear distinction between personality disorders and personality traits or variants. The latter may be considered as a representation of individual defense systems against external psychological stressors (Millon 1981) and also against internal ones, which may manifest themselves in many aspects of the life of the individual.

Therefore, in order to make the diagnosis of a personality disorder (Axis I, Clinical Disorders) several diagnostic criteria (ie, symptoms) have to be present, while the personality of the patient is defined by the presence of specific traits or defense or coping styles. This means that the concept of a personality disorder relies on clinical diagnosis whereas the evaluation of the personality of a patient may need a different approach and the use of more specific methods for the evaluation, such as psychological tests. The methodology for the evaluation of the personality relies on particular principles (Huber 1988) that do not fully overlap with clinical methodology.

This approach will probably allow personality disorders to be more clearly defined, and at the same time, would move to ICD-10 Axis III the problem of the assessment of personality variants or traits, the dimensions to be considered in such a classification, and the evaluation of the degree of abnormality of the personality traits present.

## Somatic Disorders in Axis I (Clinical Disorders)

The somatic disorder axis in the DSM-III and other nosological systems present unsolved problems. The main one is that its relationship to general psychiatric syndromes is not always clear. A somatic disorder can be the cause or the result of a psychiatric disorder, or both can be secondary to another disorder or just a concomitant clinical phenomenon. Having psychiatric disorders and somatic disorders in one single axis could also help prevent the separation of psychiatry from general medicine (Sartorius, Chapter 11 of this volume).

Organic psychiatric disorders, as described in the ICD-10, are full-fledged disorders and not mere secondary symptoms of brain affections. Some of them are also to be found in other chapters of the ICD-10, mainly in the neurological chapter. The strategy adopted by ICD-10 prevents the splitting of a single disorder (eg, Alzheimer's dementia) into a psychopathological syndrome (chronic organic brain syndrome) and a neurological disease.

## Conclusion

The ICD-10 triaxial schema incorporates in its Axis I all clinical diagnoses, including mental and nonmental disorders. Problems in earlier proposals separating general psychiatric disorders and somatic illnesses are critically reviewed. This simplification in the ICD-10 multiaxial approach may be conceptually sounder and facilitate its implementation across the world.

## *References*


Akiskal H, Yerevanian B, Davies G (1985). The nosological status of borderline personality: Clinical and polisomnographic study. *American Journal of Psychiatry* 142:192–198.

Alnaes R, Torgersen S (1988a). DSM-III symptom disorders (Axis I) and personality disorders (Axis II) in an outpatient population. *Acta Psychiatrica Scandinavica* 78:348–355.

Alnaes R, Torgersen S (1988b). The relationship between DSM-III symptom disorders (Axis I) and personality disorders (Axis II) in an outpatient population. *Acta Psychiatrica Scandinavica* 78:485–492.

Alnaes R, Torgersen S (1989). Personality and personality disorders among patients with major depression in combination with dysthymic or cyclothymic disorders. *Acta Psychiatrica Scandinavica* 79:363–369.

Bingley I (1958). Mental symptoms in temporal lobe epilepsy and temporal lobe glioms. *Acta Psychiatrica Neurologica*:33 (suppl 120).

Blume SB (1989). Dual diagnosis: Psychoactive substance dependence and the personality disorders. *Psychoactive Drugs* 21:139–144.

Essen-Möller E, Wohlfahrt S (1947). Suggestions for the amendment of the official Swedish classification of mental disorders. *Acta Psychiatrica Scandinavica* 47:551–555 (suppl).

Frances A (1980). The DSM-III personality disorders section. A commentary. *American Journal of Psychiatry* 137:1050–1054.

Friedman M, Rosenman RH (1960). Overt behavior in coronary disease. *Journal of the American Medical Association* 173:1320–1325.

Griesinger W (1872). *Gesammelte Abhandlungen. Band I: Psychiatrische und Nervenpathologische Abhandlungen* (Reimpression [1968] EJ Bonset, Amsterdam).

Gunderson J, Elliot G (1985). The interface between borderline personality disorder and affective disorder. *American Journal of Psychiatry* 142:277–288.

Gunderson J, Pollack W (1985). Conceptual risks of the Axis I–II division, pp 81–95. In H Klar, L Siever (eds), *Biologic Response Styles: Clinical Implications*. American Psychiatric Association, Washington, DC.

Huber W (1988). Methodology of the evaluation of the personality. *Acta Neurochirurgia (Wien)* 44:48–53 (suppl).

Jaspers K (1963). *General Psychopathology*. University of Chicago Press, Chicago.

Joffe RT, Regan JJ (1988). Personality and depression. *Journal Psychiatric Research Reports* 22:279–286.

Johnson C, Tobin D, Enright A (1989) Prevalence and clinical characteristics of borderline patients in an eating-disordered population. *Journal of Clinical Psychiatry* 50:9–15.

Kato M (1977). Multiaxial diagnosis in adult psychiatry. Paper presented at the VI World Congress of Psychiatry, Honolulu, Hawaii.

Klass ET, DiNardo PA, Barlow DH (1989). DSM-III-R personality diagnoses in anxiety disorder patients. *Comprehensive Psychiatry* 30:251–258.

Lahmeyer HW, Reynolds CF III, Kupfer DJ, King R (1989). Biologic markers in borderline personality disorder: A review. *Journal of Clinical Psychiatry* 50: 217–225.

Lahmeyer HW, Val E, Gaviria FM, Prasad RB, Pandey GN, Rodgers P, Weiler MA, Altman EG (1988). EEG sleep, lithium transport, dexamethasone suppression, and monoamine oxidase activity in borderline personality disorder. *Psychiatric Research Reports/APA* 25:19–30.

Mavissakalian M, Hamann MS (1988). Correlates of DSM-III personality disorder in panic disorder and agoraphobia. *Comprehensive Psychiatry* 29:535–544.

Mezzich JE (1979). Patterns and issues in multiaxial psychiatric diagnosis. *Psychological Medicine* 9:125–137.

Millon T (1981). *Disorders of Personality: DSM-III Axis II*. Wiley, New York.

Schneider K (1950). *Psychopathic Personalities* (9th ed). Grune & Stratton, New York.

Tellenbach H (1980). *Melancholy*. Duquesne University Press, Pittsburgh.

Widiger TA, Hyler SE (1987). Axis I and II interactions. In R Michelis, JO Cavenar, A Cooper (eds), *Psychiatry* (vol 1). Lippincott, Philadelphia.

Yager J, Landsverk J, Edelstein CK, Hyler SE (1989). Screening for Axis II personality disorders in women with bulimic eating disorders. *Psychosomatics* 30:255–262.

# 19
# Multiaxial Diagnosis and Environmental Factors: Psychosocial Stressors and Supports

Marianne C. Kastrup

One of the prerequisites for a widely applicable and acceptable diagnostic system is thoroughness, that is, a classification providing a comprehensive picture of the disorder (Mezzich 1989). Analyses of the various diagnostic classifications seem to suggest that a multiaxial approach may be beneficial to achieve this. A multiaxial diagnostic system provides an opportunity for a more comprehensive view of the patient's condition, the informational support for a diversified treatment planning, and an enhancement of clinical and epidemiological research (Mezzich 1988).

Several reasons may be given to introduce a multiaxial approach (Stieglitz et al 1988) including the fact that the multiaxial classification facilitates an understanding of the complexity of psychiatric diagnoses, takes into account more fully that psychiatric diagnoses consist of different elements reflecting different qualities of the disorder, is more easily in accordance with the assumptions of a multifaceted etiopathogenesis, and improves a prognostic evaluation. The usefulness of multiaxial classifications has been demonstrated in both clinical practice and research, and since Essen-Möller and Wohlfahrt (1947) published the multiaxial scheme, proposals for such classifications have repeatedly been brought forward (eg, Rutter et al 1969, von Knorring et al 1978, Helmchen 1980).

The axes considered in published systems may be grouped according to their content (Mezzich 1979) including: (1) phenomenology, (2) etiological or associated factors, (3) time frame, and (4) social functioning.

There seems to be a general agreement that one of the axes contains information on psychosocial factors conceptualized in various ways. Thus, the domain of environmental and psychosocial factors has been included under various names in most of the multiaxial schemes proposed until now. A consideration of the environmental factors is also included in the most prevailing multiaxial systems presently, namely the *Diagnostic and Statistical Manual of Mental Disorders*, 3rd edition (DSM-III) and revised edition, DSM-III-R. In DSM-IV, the multiaxial approach, comprising an evaluation of the psychosocial stressors and social functioning is an integral part of the classificatory system.

In an overview of the prospects for the *International Classification of Diseases*, 10th revision (ICD-10), Jablensky (1988) describes the introduction of a multiaxial classification of psychiatric disorders specific to childhood as one of the major developments. The forthcoming ICD-10 shall be seen as a family of documents retaining a basic uniaxial core structure but with a key to multiaxial recording of diagnostic formulations (Jablensky 1988). Thus, ICD-10 will provide an opportunity to assess the environmental and circumstantial factors of relevance for the condition, which is consistent with WHO's expansion of the scope of the ICD-10 to encompass not only diseases but also health-related factors.

That the multiaxial approach has been well received is also reflected by the fact that 83% of a worldwide sample of 175 experts participating in a World Psychiatric Association (WPA)-sponsored study (Mezzich et al 1985) were familiar with and had experiences with the multiaxial concepts and that 67% considered them as highly useful. The limited research about these axes, however, suggests that clinicians may rate them as useful but not sufficiently practical.

In the multiaxial systems developed hitherto, the general psychiatric syndrome is the core domain. Psychosocial stressors and adaptive functioning are also central issues (Mezzich 1988), but we are witnessing an increasing recognition of social support as an important element of the environmental domain.

## Historical Development: Psychosocial Stressors

In the last decades, increasing interest has been noted and some attempts made to identify and quantify psychosocial stressors (Lloyd 1980). Environmental stressors have been found of significance in the development of depressive disorders, as depressive patients report a significantly increased frequency of life events compared to that of normal controls, particularly those reflecting loss of a significant other or an event being threatening. Stressful life events are also reported to be of importance in the precipitation of schizophrenic episodes, but recent results suggest (Dohrenwend et al 1987) that stressful life events appear to be of secondary relevance compared to factors such as class-related socialization experiences in adverse family environments.

Epidemiological community surveys have also demonstrated an association between adverse life events and the incidence of psychiatric disorders. Brown and Harris (1978), in their study on etiological factors in depressive illness recognized the importance of social difficulties and adverse life events as well as of vulnerability factors. They emphasized that what was crucial was the effect of stressors on vulnerable individuals rather than the life events alone. There is also evidence to suggest that minor daily events are independent predictors of disturbance (Monroe 1983) and that they are better predictors of subsequent symptoms than major life events.

Over the years, we have thus witnessed that the interest has shifted and the focus is now less on provocative factors than on factors influencing and modifying the course and outcome of the condition. Predispositions in an individual render the person particularly vulnerable and sensitive to the impact of life events (Harris 1989). On the other hand, coping strategies developed in the individual may change a person's susceptibility to the effects of stress, thus providing a more comprehensive understanding of the complexity of the association between stress and disorder (Monroe 1983). Further research is still needed in which the individual's vulnerability, the exposure to stress, the coping strategies and the social support systems simultaneously are taken into consideration.

## Social Support

The concept of social support has received increased attention in recent years. This interest is partly due to the shortcomings in life event research, partly because of a need for a conceptual denominator for the many aspects of the social environment believed to have an impact on individual mental health. Thus, differences in the way social support is conceptualized may explain the different results reported in the literature. Social support has been considered as a response to crisis and everyday occurrences and measures often contain items from both areas (Veiel 1985). The interaction between support and stressors is still a matter of debate (Bailey and Garralda 1987), and the relation between support and life events has been considered as a single construct, as separate variables in relation with the disorder, or as acting causally on each other (Brugha et al 1990).

The assumption of a single notion, social support, may be too simple and should perhaps be replaced by a multidimensional conceptual frame (Veiel 1985). In the codification of social support we need answers to questions of what type of support is offered, what relationship exists between the provider and recipient, and what measures are used to assess it (Veiel 1985).

Some studies claim an association between actual lack of social network and the prevalence of psychiatric disorder (eg, Henderson et al 1981). Others (eg, Brown and Harris 1978) indicate that support may protect against the emergence of a disorder in case of stressful situations.

Psychiatric patients tend to have social networks and support of limited use in stressful situations. But findings have been reported (Bailey and

Garralda 1987) of no significant relationship between factual and subjective ratings of social support, which may be interpreted as showing that it is the depth and subjective role rather than the number of contacts with family and friends that plays a role as a supportive factor (Henderson et al 1980).

## The Diagnostic Process

To be universally applicable and comparable, a rating of the influence of environmental factors needs to be based on criterion-based assessments (Schrader et al 1986), thereby reducing the subjectivity of the clinical material.

When it comes to the codification of the stressors and supports, this may be carried out separately or it may be an integrated part of the diagnostic process.

In the prevailing multiaxial systems, a codification of abnormal psychosocial situations takes place, despite the fact that the benefits of this approach are sparsely elucidated scientifically when it comes to the relationship among psychosocial stressors, social support and functioning, and psychiatric disorder.

## Experiences with DSM-III

In DSM-III (1980), Axes IV and V are concerned with psychosocial stressors and social functioning, respectively. A limited number of studies (among them, Mezzich et al 1985, Rey et al 1987b), have addressed the reliability and validity of these axes.

The reliability of the Axis IV was reported low in the DSM-III field trials. This was also the case in studies of children (Mezzich et al 1985) as well as of adolescents (Rey et al 1987b), but with the more severe events more reliably identified than the less severe ones. Validity studies of Axis IV have failed to confirm the predictive validity of its ratings. In light of the experiences with the DSM-III classification, a number of methodological issues have been raised regarding environmental factors.

A particular problem is that of assessing the etiological significance of the stressor, and hence, its importance for the exacerbation of the current mental health status (Skodol and Shrout 1989). In the implication of Axis IV in DSM-III, the judgment of the etiological significance has been a major difficulty. It has been pointed out (Schrader et al 1986) that in any assessment of stress the evaluator makes a hypothesis about the psychiatric diagnosis, and that the usefulness of a psychosocial axis may increase if there was no requirement of an etiological significance. A worthwhile alternative could be a broader delineation of a stressor as having contributed either to development of a new disorder, recurrence of a previous one, or exacerbation of an existing one; or that it is coexistent with the current psychopathological episode (Skodol and Shrout 1989).

The impact of environmental factors on an individual should always be seen in the proper sociocultural context, not only at the individual level but also in the general awareness, whether factors considered stressful in one cultural group may be so in another. Of particular concern is the codification of stressors, which is based on an assessment of an "average" person in similar circumstances and with similar sociocultural values. This generalization is difficult unless the clinician is quite familiar with the cultural background of the patient and may run the risk of becoming stereotypic (Guarnaccia 1991). An increasing understanding of the cultural and anthropological context is called for as well as a recognition by the assessing clinician of her or his own more or less overt prejudices.

Within a given cultural setting, we are faced with the problem of significance and impact of the environmental factors for the individual, particularly if these are coded according to some average standard. This individual vulnerability concerns the specific factors as well as the general strain and frustration perceived. By avoiding any interpretation of the significance of a symbolic "trauma" the rating may seem less subjective (Gyllenhammar and Wistedt 1987).

Another aspect is that of desirability of the environmental factors. In life-event research it is questioned whether it is the change these lead to or their degree of undesirability that should be rated (Zimmerman et al 1985). Identification and quantification of environmental stressors could be made in terms of their degree of undesirability for the individual. The validity might be improved if it was decided only to base the codification on the negative events, as the literature indicates that it is the undesirable factors that are associated with the psychiatric illness and not the desirable ones (Zimmerman et al 1985). For the clinician, there is a need to assess whether a specific factor can be considered undesirable or alien to a given individual, irrespective of how the clinician himself evaluates the situation.

The rating of severity is another issue of concern. It has been suggested that the severity of each stressor should be evaluated, but little seems to indicate that this will increase the reliability (Rey et al 1987a) as evaluators, despite agreeing in the identification of an event, may not agree in the rating of its severity, and similar severity ratings may be assigned to events considered of relevance (Rey et al 1987a). A global rating of severity may, however, give the notion that all types of stressors work through a single mechanism in contrast to research findings that different mechansims may be operating (Williams 1987).

In clinical practice, we are also more likely to identify stressors that we consider of clinical relevance and, therefore, a short schedule of severe events may be more useful (Rey et al 1987a). For the DSM-IV, options are considered for shifting the Axis IV from overall severity of stressors to either such a list of specific stressors or to a focus on the appraisal of support factors (Mezzich in press)

Taking into account the time available in daily clinical practice, the clinician is unlikely to get a detailed view of all possible stressors, and evidence suggests that minor events are less reliably identified (Rey et al 1987a).

The clinical importance of a severity rating of psychosocial stressors is related to its impact on prognosis (Zimmerman et al 1985). Looking at the association between severity of stressor and prognosis, it seems that the first episode of psychiatric illness is particularly associated with severe stressors (Skodol and Shrout 1989). In the DSM-III, Axis IV, the assumption is that the prognosis is more favorable if a disorder develops after a severe stressor than after a minor stressor. This hypothesis is, however, too simple and findings by, among others, Zimmerman and coworkers (1987) are not consistent with it. Similarly, Gordon and Gordon (1987) have reported that chronically ill psychiatric patients seem to have the most severe stress according to Axis IV and the lowest level of premorbid functioning according to Axis V.

A further issue is the balance between repeated but subliminal stressful events and single major stressors. Until now, particular emphasis has been put on the major, stressful discrete events and changes, whereas less research has been carried out on the effect of constant strain and minor but constant stressors. For persons living under strenuous conditions, however, even a minor stressor may lead to a need for help (Gyllenhammer and Wistedt 1987).

Similarly, interest has focused primarily on stressors of an acute nature. Such acute, well-defined incidents are relatively easy to recognizable and their impact psychologically understandable. But we have to distinguish them from the more chronic, but not necessarily major episodes. Scores have been found more highly correlated to acute rather than chronic events, and a more explicit rating of chronic stressors may be a worthwhile innovation (Zimmerman et al 1985). The latter may seem trivial from an observer's point of view but they leave the individual in a chronic tense condition. In the DSM-III-R the solution has been chosen with the possibility to rate whether stressors represent predominantly enduring or acute strain, respectively.

## ICD-10

In ICD-10 (1989) it is stated that the proposed Z-codes have been developed to give a possibility to rate other circumstances of a psychosocial nature relevant for the disease. Such occasions may arise either when a person encounters the health services for some specific purpose without being currently sick or when some circumstance or problem is present that influences the person's health status without being in itself a current illness or injury.

Environmental factors are classified in the ICD-10 multiaxial field trials according to headings covering all aspects of human life, which renders it possible to classify at different levels and with different degrees of sophistication, thereby expanding the use to cover also primary care settings or settings with few available resources.

In the ongoing work on the multiaxial aspects of ICD-10, a rearrangement and selection of the Z-codes is taking place with the aim of facilitating the coding of environmental and circumstantial factors. These are divided into (1) environmental factors including all relevant events of a psychosocial nature with a further subdivision into recent or chronic difficulties, and (2) life-style/life-management problems including problems related to the personality and life style of the individual. This proposal is at present being further evaluated in field trials.

## Conclusion

Despite the shortcomings, there is little doubt that an inclusion of environmental factors is useful in the classification of a disorder. If this is to become an integrated part of the diagnostic process it must be kept in mind that one thing is field trials and another is routine clinical assessments.

In diagnostic work we are all faced with the choice between reaching comprehensiveness and the aim of parsimony (Rey et al 1988), particularly if the diagnostic system is to be used for routine purposes in all cultural settings and with a diversity of available services. In many settings, parsimony is a virtue and a necessity, and here a condensed list of psychosocial stressors and supports may be the feasible solution. Another prerequisite in assessing the interrelationship between environmental factors and mental health is relevant, continuous training and feedback from experienced clinicians. Whereas a solid training in the classification of the psychiatric core syndromes is an essential part of any psychiatric curriculum, this is not the case for training in the psychosocial aspects. As an example, only 38% of the participating psychiatrists at the DSM-III field trials believed that Axis IV was likely to be of clinical use (Skodol 1991) and major resistance has been reported due to its complexity (Jampala et al 1986). In other words, we are without a classificatory tradition regarding these aspects and we may still find clinicians expressing resistance about the possibility of coding them properly at all. To overcome such obstacles we have to set priorities accordingly for the teaching of new generations of psychiatrists. Only in this way will the complex interaction between environmental stress, social support, and the presence of mental disorder be further elucidated.

## *References*


American Psychiatric Association (1980). *Diagnostic and Statistical Manual of Mental Disorders* (3rd ed). American Psychiatric Press, Washington, DC.

Bailey D, Garralda ME (1987). The use of the social stress and support interview in families with deviant children: Methodological issues. *Social Psychiatry* 22:209–215.

Brown G, Harris T (1978). *Social Origins of Depression*. Tavistock, London.

Brugha TS, Bebbington PE, Stuart E, MacCarthy B, Wykes T (1990). The relation between life events and social support networks in a clinically depressed cohort. *Social Psychiatry and Psychiatric Epidemiology* 25:308–313.

Dohrenwend BP, Shrout PE, Link BG, Skodol AE (1987) Social and psychological risk factors for episodes of schizophrenia, pp 275–296. In H Häfner, WF Gattaz, W, Janzarik (eds), *Search for the Causes of Schizophrenia*. Springer-Verlag, Berlin.

Essen-Möller E, Wohlfahrt S (1947). Suggestions for the amendment of the official Swedish classification of mental disorders. *Acta Psychiatrica Scandinavica* 47:551–555 (suppl).

Gordon RE, Gordon KK (1987). Relating Axes IV and V of DSM-III to clinical severity of psychiatric disorders. *Canadian Journal of Psychiatry* 32:423–424.

Guarnaccia P (1991). Cultural perspective on culture and multiaxial diagnosis. Paper presented at NIMH Conference on Culture and Diagnosis, Pittsburgh, PA, April 1991.

Gyllenhammar C, Wistedt B (1987). Life events and psychiatric disorders. *Stress Medicine* 3:239–245.

Harris T (1989). Implications of a vulnerability model for the prevention of affective disorder, pp 207–227. In B Cooper, T Helgason (eds), *Epidemiology and the Prevention of Mental Disorders*. Routledge, London.

Helmchen H (1980). Multiaxial systems of classification. *Acta Psychiatrica Scandinavica* 61:43–55.

Henderson S, Byrne DG, Duncan-Jones P (1981). *Neurosis and the Social Environment*. Academic Press, Sydney.

Henderson S, Duncan-Jones P, Byrne DG, Scott R (1980). Measuring social relationships: The interview schedule for social interaction. *Psychological Medicine* 10:723–734.

Jablensky A (1988). An overview of the prospects for ICD-10, pp 343–364. In JE Mezzich, M von Cranach (eds), *International Classification in Psychiatry*. Cambridge University Press, Cambridge.

Jampala VC, Sinles FS, Taylor MA (1986). Consumer's views of DSM-III: Attitudes and practices of US psychiatrists and 1984 graduating psychiatric residents. *American Journal of Psychiatry* 143:148–153.

Lloyd C (1980). Life events and depressive disorder reviewed. *Archives of General Psychiatry* 37:541–548.

Mezzich JE (1979). Patterns and issues in multiaxial psychiatric diagnosis. *Psychological Medicine* 9:125–137.

Mezzich JE (1988). On developing a psychiatric multiaxial schema for ICD-10. *British Journal of Psychiatry* 152:38–43 (suppl 1).

Mezzich JE (1989). Structural methodology for designing diagnostic systems, pp 298–305. In JE Mezzich, M von Cranach (eds), *International Classification in Psychiatry*. Cambridge University Press, Cambridge.

Mezzich JE (in press). Culture and multiaxial diagnosis. In JE Mezzich et al (eds), *Culture and Psychiatric Diagnosis*. American Psychiatric Press, Washington, DC.

Mezzich JE, Fabrega H, Mezzich AC (1985). An international consultation on multiaxial diagnosis. In P Pichot, P Berner, R Wolf, K Thau (eds), *Psychiatry—The State of the Art* (vol I). Plenum Press, London.

Mezzich AC, Mezzich JE, Coffman GA (1985). Reliability of DSM-III vs DSM-II in child psychopathology. *Journal of the American Academy of Child Psychiatry* 24:273–280.

Monroe SM (1983). Major and minor life events as predictors of psychological distress: Further issues and findings. *Journal of Behavioral Medicine* 6:189–205.

Rey JM, Plapp JM, Stewart G, Richards I, Bashir M (1987b). Reliability of the psychosocial axes of DSM-III in an adolescent population. *British Journal of Psychiatry* 150:228–234.

Rey JM, Stewart GW, Plapp JM, Bashir MR, Richards IN (1987a). Sources of unreliability of DSM-III Axis IV. *Australian and New Zealand Journal of Psychiatry* 21:75–80.

Rey JM, Stewart GW, Plapp JM, Bashir MR, Richards IN (1988). DSM-III Axis IV revisited. *American Journal of Psychiatry* 145:286–292.

Rutter M, Lebovici S, Eisenberg L, Sneznevskij AV, Sadoun R, Brooke E, Lin TY (1969). A triaxial classification of mental disorders in childhood. *Journal of Child Psychology and Psychiatry* 10:41–61.

Schrader G, Gordon M, Harcourt R (1986). The usefulness of DSM-III Axis IV and Axis V assessments. *American Journal of Psychiatry* 143:904–907.

Skodol AE (1991). Axis IV: A reliable and valid measure of psychosocial stressors? *Comprehensive Psychiatry* 32:503–515.

Skodol AE, Shrout PE (1989). Use of DSM-III Axis IV in clinical practice: Rating etiologically significant stressors. *American Journal of Psychiatry* 146:61–66.

Stieglitz RD, Fähndrich E, Helmchen H (1988). AMDP in multiaxial classification, pp 180–204. In JE Mezzich, M von Cranach (eds), *International Classification in Psychiatry*. Cambridge University Press, Cambridge.

Veiel HOF (1985). Dimensions of social support: A conceptual framework for research. *Social Psychiatry* 20:156–162.

von Knorring L, Perris C, Jacobsson L (1978). A multi-aspect classification of mental disorders. *Acta Psychiatrica Scandinavica* 58:401–412.

Williams JBW (1987). Multiaxial diagnosis, pp 31–36. In AE Skodol, RL Spitzer (eds), *An Annotated Bibliography of DSM-III*. American Psychiatric Press, Washington, DC.

World Health Organization (1989). *International Classification of Diseases* (10th rev). World Health Organization, Geneva.

Zimmerman M, Pfohl B, Coryell W, Stangl D (1987). The prognostic validity of DSM-III axis IV in depressed inpatients. *American Journal of Psychiatry* 144: 102–106.

Zimmerman M, Pfohl B, Stangl D, Coryell W (1985). The validity of DSM-III Axis IV (severity of psychosocial stressors). *American Journal of Psychiatry* 142:1437–1441.

# 20
# Disabilities in a Multiaxial Formulation

HEINZ KATSCHNIG

Interest in systematically assessing disabilities in mental patients has slowly grown over the last decades. Approximately a decade after the "mother scale" of all standardized rating scales for the assessment of psychiatric symptoms, the Hamilton Depression Rating Scale, was introduced (Hamilton 1960), more and more instruments were developed for assessing in a standardized way the functioning in social roles of persons suffering from such psychiatric symptoms. Weissman et al (1981) listed 27 different assessment instruments for social adjustment and functioning they could identify in the literature.

The Hamilton Depression Rating Scale contains one item from functioning at work, although incorrectly integrating it with symptoms into one global score. Most of these social functioning instruments assess an individual's functioning in several life domains, such as work, family, and social, and require more or less lengthy interviews of the subject.

The majority of these instruments were developed for research projects about psychiatric patients living in the community and it is probably the deinstitutionalization movement that is mainly responsible for this growing interest in the social functioning of psychiatric patients (Katschnig 1983).

In 1980 the World Health Organization (WHO) published its *International Classification of Impairments, Disabilities and Handicaps* (ICIDH) (World Health Organization 1980), a gigantic list of all kinds of impairments, disabilities, and handicaps, which was to be used for all types of diseases, not only for mental disorders. However, probably because of its clumsiness, it has not been used widely.

In the last decade the social functioning field incorporated a new aspect through the introduction of the concept of quality of life (Bergner and Rothmann 1987, Spilker 1990, Walker and Rosser 1993, Testa et al 1993). For instance, for chronic diseases such as cancer and hypertension, a person's functioning and life satisfaction became a focus of interest, thereby stressing more the subjective side of a person evaluating his or her life experiences. The number of articles published annually on quality of life increased from 207 in 1980 to 846 in 1990 (*Lancet* 1991). The concept has also spread to psychiatry. For instance, Lehman and Burns (1990) identified seven assessment instruments published between 1978 and 1988 for measuring the quality of life of severely ill psychiatric patients living in the community.

The WHO is about to release its own quality of life instrument, the WHOQOL (World Health Organization 1993a). Also, a task force is working on a revised version of the earlier-mentioned ICIHD. Furthermore, health economists tend to measure the costs of illness not only in terms of mortality or work days lost but also in terms of loss or gain of quality of life years (QALYs) (Williams 1985). Finally, as a culmination of this growing interest, a scientific journal, *Quality of Life Research* was founded in 1992.

## The Impact on Diagnostic Systems in Psychiatry

The impact of this development on diagnostic systems in psychiatry has been relatively small so far. The first structured interview for psychiatric diagnoses, the Present State Examination (PSE), developed in the 1960s but published in a usable form in its 9th revision in 1974, contained a standardized item on the patient's impairment status with a 3-point global rating scale (Wing et al 1974). However, this item was not regarded as being diagnostically important.

When the *Diagnostic and Statistical Manual of Mental Disorders*, 3rd edition (DSM-III) (American Psychiatric Association 1980) was published some years later, one of its five axes was devoted to rate a patient's adaptive functioning (on a seven-point scale, ranging from superior to grossly impaired), thus conspicuously giving special weight to the field of social functioning and its impairments. However, similar to the PSE item, this axis was not regarded as a required element for the evaluation of a patient but as a supplement to the official diagnosis. Just the fact that several hundred pages are devoted in the DSM-III and its successors to the description of clinical syndromes, and only a handful of pages to disabilities, shows where the emphasis is. This has not changed in the forthcoming revision, DSM-IV (American Psychiatric Association [in press]). It is, therefore, not surprising that Axis V of DSM-III and DSM-III-R (American Psychiatric Association 1987) have not been widely used (Goldman et al 1992).

Furthermore, in a review prepared by Mezzich (1988) on multiaxial diagnostic systems proposed in the literature up to 1988, adaptive functioning was suggested as a separate axis by only 5 of 20 proposals (Strauss 1975, Mogensen et al 1986, APA 1980, 1987, Bech et al 1987).

Recently, a WHO working group, preparing a multiaxial addendum to the psychiatric chapter of ICD-10, decided that only two axes should be added to the ICD-10 clinical diagnoses, and that one of these should be a disability axis (Mezzich et al 1993).

Why this discrepancy between the interest in recording social disabilities in research projects—documented in an abundance of assessment instruments for research—and the practical lack of use of the concept of disability in routine diagnostic systems? One clue to understanding this discrepancy is probably the difficulties inherent in the routine use of methods for assessing disabilities.

In fact, the assessment of disabilities is beset by a number of problems, which have to be considered both when developing and using assessment instruments for research projects and when designing a disability axis in a multiaxial diagnostic system. The difference between research and clinical practice is that the resources, in terms of both time and staff, to resolve these problems are available for research but not for clinical practice. The problems include the following: (1) terminological issues, (2) separation of disabilities from symptoms, (3) heterogeneity of the concept of disability, (4) time relatedness, (5) dependence from environment, (6) subjective versus objective evaluation, and (7) physical versus psychiatric cause.

The implementation of a disability axis within a multiaxial diagnostic system depends on whether these problems can be resolved in a simple way.

## Problems in Assessing Disabilities

### *Terminological Issues: Disability, Impairment, Handicap, Social Functioning, Quality of Life, or What?*

In the ICIDH (World Health Organization 1980), currently under revision, the terms impairment, disability and handicap are defined as follows (italics by the author):

> An impairment is any loss or abnormality of psychological, physiological, or anatomical *structure* or *function*. A disability is any restriction or lack of ability (resulting from an impairment) to perform an *activity* in the manner or within the range considered normal for a human being. A *handicap* is a disadvantage for a given individual, resulting from an impairment or a disability, that limits or prevents the fulfillment of a *role* that is normal (depending on age, sex, and social and cultural factors) for that individual.

Such definitions have their merits, but if translations into non-English languages are attempted, it becomes clear that these terms are not as independent from each other as they are suggested to be in the ICIDH.

TABLE 20.1. Terms used in the literature for social adjustment or aspects of it.

| Term | | |
|---|---|---|
| Positive | Neutral | Negative |
| Social adjustment | Social performance | Social handicap |
| Social role adjustment | Role performance | Social maladjustment |
| Social skills | Social behavior | Social impairment |
| Social competence | Social functioning | Social disability |
| Social effectiveness | Adaptive functioning | Social disablement |
| Social attainment | Environmental adaptation | Social dysfunction |
| Social integration | | Social ineffectiveness |
| | | Social inadequacy |

For psychiatric patients, it is especially the aspect of social disability that matters. Unfortunately, there are many synonyms for social disability. A selection of terms used in the literature has been compiled by Katschnig (1983) (Table 20.1). Besides the fact that some of the terms have a positive, negative, or neutral connotation, some of the terms put more emphasis on the social skills of the individual, while others (eg, social adjustment) clearly underline the relationship between the individual and his or her environment, pointing out the fact that social disability also depends on the demands from the environment (see later).

Disability, impairment, and handicap are negative terms, stressing the lack of abilities, whereas the term quality of life is a more neutral term that allows also for a better than normal life. In addition, although disabilities usually require evaluation by experts, quality of life is often regarded as being assessable by the patient (Slevin et al 1988).

As confusing as the field might be terminologically, this multitude of terms and meanings have one common message: It is not only symptoms that matter in psychiatry, but also the capacity of the individual to function in a satisfactory way.

## *Separation of Disabilities from Symptoms*

One reason for introducing a multiaxial diagnostic system is the assumption that assessments on different axes vary independently from each other, and there is evidence both from clinical practice and from research (eg, Goering et al 1983, Merikangas et al 1983) that psychiatric symptoms and disabilities are not strictly correlated, except perhaps for severe symptoms.

In contrast, Axis V of DSM-III-R, which consists of the Global Assessment of Functioning Scale (GAF) contains a mixture of symptoms and disabilities, as can be exemplified by the following anchor point definition: "Moderate symptoms (eg, flat affect and circumstantial speech, occasional panic attacks) OR moderate difficulty in social, occupational, or school functioning (eg, few friends, conflicts with coworkers)." With such definitions, the GAF is certainly not a clear indicator of the person's functioning, but more a measure of the severity of the disorder. Therefore, Goldman et al (1992) have suggested a revised version of the GAF to eliminate the symptoms from the definitions.

On the other hand, in DSM-III a number of definitions of clinical syndromes contain impairment in a person's functioning as a required element for the presence of a diagnosis (eg, schizophrenia, obsessive–compulsive disorder, social phobia). This is a confusing situation within a multiaxial diagnostic system that provides a separate axis for disabilities.

If a disability axis is to make any sense, disabilities must be kept clearly separate from symptoms.

## *Heterogeneity of the Concept of Disability*

A person may be functioning well in one respect but not in another. She or he may be able to live independently, but not to hold a job in the labor market. The research instruments mentioned earlier have thus, as a rule, divided the field into different areas of functioning. Typical areas are housing, occupation/social role, economic situation, leisure/social activities, family and domestic relationships, and marital, which are assessed in the Standardized Interview to Assess Social Maladjustment and Dysfunction (Clare and Cairns 1978) or work, social and leisure, extended family, marital as spouse, parental, and marital family unit as contained in the Social Adjustment Scale (Paykel et al 1971). Mellsop et al (1987) observed specific relationships between preadmission adaptive functioning in specific areas and the prognosis of psychiatric inpatients. Other studies (eg, Trzepacz et al 1989) did not find any advantage of such component ratings over a global score.

When trying to assess the disabilities of a given patient in clinical practice, one is often confronted with the situation that the patient is functioning well in one area and not so in another, and that patients who are severely disabled in one area may have specific skills in another area. It is, therefore, cognitively difficult in clinical practice—although it might seem less complicated—to make a global rating of disabilities, as is suggested in Axis V of DSM-III and Axis V of DSM-III-R.

## *Time Frame*

If disabilities are included in a multiaxial diagnostic scheme, a special difficulty arises regarding a time frame for assessment. Although diagnosis of psychiatric and general medical disorders tend to be considered as time-independent, the assessment of disabilities necessarily refers to specific time periods. Therefore, when disabilities are included in a multiaxial diagnostic scheme, careful consideration has to be given to the question of *at what point in time and to what time period* the disability axis refers.

If, as is usual in hospitals, a final diagnosis is given at the end of the treatment episode, the time frame for disability assessment may be unclear. Does it refer to the time of discharge (when disabilities might still be present despite a remission of symptoms), to when the patient entered treatment, or to the illness episode before treatment started?

A multiaxial diagnostic scheme that includes a disability axis may be most effective when formulated at the time the patient comes for care. Treatment planning requires specification of clinical disorders but also an assessment of disabilities.

## *Dependence from Environment*

Disabilities in psychiatric patients are clearly dependent on the environment, both in terms of different cultural or subcultural norms and values (which may render the same behavior acceptable in one culture and unacceptable in another) and in terms of different environmental demands and supports. The relative weight of these demands and supports may determine whether disabilities develop at all as well as their severity.

An example may be given in connection to the symptom of indecision, which tends to be much more disabling in Australia than in Japan, because people in Japan are quite likely to allow authority figures to make decisions for them. Another example comes from the International Pilot Study of Schizophrenia of the WHO, where it was found that schizophrenia has a more favorable course in developing countries. One interpretation of this finding is that demands in everyday life are not so strict in developing countries. It is well known that for schizophrenic patients, an environment that is not so demanding is more conducive to recovery.

Finally, quality of life means something quite different to a British middle-class person and to an Indian on the streets of Bombay. A multiaxial diagnostic system that is to be used around the world has to take such contextual factors into consideration.

## *Subjective Versus Objective Evaluation*

Quality of life is often defined as the subject's evaluation of his or her own happiness or well-being (Slevin et al 1988). In psychiatry, such a purely subjective evaluation by the patient himself is not appropriate in many instances. A manic patient might experience extreme well-being while he is not functioning at all and is provoking negative attitudes in his environment. On the other hand, a depressed patient's view of the world is usually bleak and her or his evaluation, for example, of the availability of social support might substantially deviate from its actual availability. Therefore, with mental patients, an "objective" evaluation of the quality of life and social functioning by others (the clinician and members of the patient's cultural reference group) might be very important in addition to the patient's subjective evaluation.

### *Physical or Psychiatric Cause?*

The DSM-III and DSM-III-R disability axes ask for the exclusion of disabilities due to physical causes. Such a restriction is not necessarily the intention of those who want multiaxial diagnostic systems to be used in daily practice. A disability interferes with the patient's life regardless of its cause. Goldman et al (1992) have, therefore, suggested the assessment of social and occupational functioning due to the combined effects of mental and nonmental medical problems.

## Ease of Handling and Completeness of Information in Psychiatric Diagnosis

In a medical context, a diagnosis is a shorthand for an illness condition, which necessarily omits many details. The very fact of brevity allows it to fulfill many purposes. A diagnosis of a psychiatric disorder can serve as quick and easy communication of complex information when a problem has to be handled by many different people or by large organizations; it can serve as a tool for preparing statistics; or as a basis for decision making (eg, about reimbursement for medical procedures or about treatment planning).

A diagnosis represents one extreme in handling complex information; the other is writing a narrative about the patient's condition. Although such a narrative may be complete, its ease of handling tends to be very low.

Structuring information by defining specific areas of interest and then assessing these areas with research instruments can be called *multidimensional assessment*. For instance, in applying many rating scales to a psychiatric patient, as is frequently the case in clinical drug trials, we obtain large amounts of information that are, however, structured in a way that makes communication easier than just narration. Information is less complete than in a narrative, but its amount may be too large for ease of communication.

A *multiaxial diagnosis* holds a position between a simple uniaxial, categorical diagnosis and an intricate multidimensional assessment. It should have some of the advantages of both—the ease of handling of a multiaxial diagnosis and the fuller description of the patient's condition offered by multidimensional assessment.

TABLE 20.2. Ease of handling and completeness of psychiatric information.

| Clinical formulation | Ease of handling | Completeness |
|---|---|---|
| Narrative | Very low | Very high |
| Multidimensional assessment | Low/high | High/low |
| Multiaxial diagnosis | High/low | Low/high |
| Uniaxial diagnosis | Very high | Very low |

Table 20.2 presents a comparative view of these clinical formulations with regard to ease of handling and completeness of information.

Those who advocate a multiaxial diagnostic scheme that includes disability as an axis argue that such a scheme forces the practitioners to think not only in terms of medical conditions and their symptoms but also in terms of the person's quality of life and functioning in a social environment. In contrast, a uniaxial psychiatric diagnosis, which encompasses just a clinical syndrome, often reflects reductionistic thinking and leads to a reductionistic management approach.

The problem of those who want to include disabilities in a multiaxial diagnostic system is that both the evaluation of disabilities and their recording must be as simple as possible to be accepted by those who use diagnosis in daily practice.

A working group of WHO (Mezzich, Katschnig, Kastrup, Lopez-Ibor, Sartorius, and Janca) has recently proposed a multiaxial addendum to ICD-10, including a disability axis, with the specific intention of making it simple enough to facilitate its widespread use in the regular care of patients.

## The Disability Axis in the Multiaxial Addendum to ICD-10

This working group has prepared a triaxial diagnostic scheme, including ICD-10 clinical diagnoses in the first axis (see Lopez-Ibor, Chapter 18) and an environmental axis (see Kastrup, Chapter 19). For the disability axis, the problems mentioned in the preceding section were approached in the 1993 version in the following way:

1. Terminology. The term disability was used because it seems to be the most global term and the one most easily translates into other languages. The WHO Disability Axis is a short version of the WHO Disability Assessment Schedule (WHO/DAS) (World Health Organization 1988) and is called the WHO Disability Diagnostic Scale (WHO–DDS). "Disablement" has been proposed more recently as an alternative.

2. Separation of disabilities from symptoms. The 1993 WHO–DDS has anchor point definitions in a scale ranging from 00 (no dysfunction) to 99 (maximal dysfunction) which, in contrast to Axis V in DSM-III, DSM-III-

R and the forthcoming DSM-IV, does not include symptoms. For example, a rating of 40 (obvious dysfunction) is to be given if "the deviation from the norm is conspicuous and dysfunctions interfere with social adjustment. Dysfunction in at least one activity/role persists nearly all the time. More severe dysfunction may appear only for a few days." Alternative rating modes are being tested.

3. The heterogeneity of the concept of disability. In contrast to the DSM solution—one global score for functioning—in the WHO–DDS ratings would be conducted on the following four specific areas of functioning, in addition to a global rating: (1) Personal care and survival; (2) occupational functioning (performance of expected role as remunerated worker, student, or homemaker); (3) functioning with family (interaction with spouse, parents, children, and other relatives); and (4) broader social behavior (functioning in other roles and activities: interaction with other individuals and the community-at-large, leisure activities).

4. Time frame. The experimental version of the WHO–DDS that is currently being field tested does not contain specific instructions for coding the time period. More explicit guidelines are to be developed on the basis of the experience obtained.

5. Context dependence. In the WHO proposal for a disability axis the difficult issue of considering the social and cultural context of the patient is taken care of by instructions stating that the rating "should represent the best estimate of the degree of dysfunction—in relation to the maximum level of expected functioning in the socio-cultural context of the patient."

6. Subjective versus objective evaluation. To make an appropriate rating in the WHO–DDS it is suggested that all available information—case notes, reports from relatives or staff, observation and interview of the patient—be taken into consideration. There might be discrepant views from these different sources, but it is the task of the clinician to integrate them.

7. Physical or psychiatric cause? In the WHO disability axis, the opportunity is offered to specify if the source of disabilities is mainly psychiatric, mainly somatic, or both somatic and psychiatric.

International, multicentric field trials are currently being carried out with the Multiaxial Presentation of the ICD-10 Classification of Mental and Behavioral Disorders, using both live patients and a set of internationally generated case vignettes.

## Conclusion

At the turn of the century the Swiss–American psychiatrist Adolf Meyer stated that "an orderly presentation of the facts alone is a real diagnosis" (Meyer 1906, quoted in Lief 1948). No doubt, attempts to construct a multiaxial diagnostic system have to be understood along the lines of Adolf Meyer's diagnostic philosophy.

However, the crucial question is how many types of facts should be presented in an orderly way? If a multiaxial diagnostic system contains too many axes, it will not be used in the daily practice it is supposed to upgrade. If the axes are formulated in too simplistic a way, their usefulness will be questioned by clinicians. Whether the WHO proposal for a multiaxial formulation of ICD-10 is an adequate solution remains to be seen.

## *References*

American Psychiatric Association (1980). *Diagnostic and Statistical Manual of Mental Disorders* (3rd ed, rev). American Psychiatric Association, Washington, DC.

American Psychiatric Association (1987). *Diagnostic and Statistical Manual of Mental Disorders* (3rd ed, rev). American Psychiatric Association, Washington, DC.

American Psychiatric Association (1994). *Diagnostic and Statistical Manual of Mental Disorders* (4th ed). American Psychiatric Association, Washington, DC.

Bech P, Hjorts S, Lund K, Vilmar T, Kastrup M (1987). An integration of the DSM-III and ICD-8 by global severity assessment for measuring multidimensional outcomes in general hospital psychiatry. *Acta Psychiatrica Scandinavica* 75:297–306.

Bergner M, Rothman ML (1987) Health status measures: An overview and guide for selection. *Annual Review in Public Health* 8:19.

Clare AW, Cairns VE (1978). Design development and use of a standardized interview to assess social maladjustment and dysfunction in community studies. *Psychological Medicine* 8:589–604.

Goering P, Wasylenki D, Lancee W, Freeman SJJ (1983). Social support and post-hospital outcome for depressed women. *Canadian Journal of Psychiatry* 28:612–618.

Goldman HH, Skodol AE, Lave TR (1992). Revising Axis V for DSM-IV: A review of measures of social functioning. *American Journal of Psychiatry* 149: 1148–1156.

Hamilton M (1960). A rating scale for depression. *Journal of Neurology Neurosurgery and Psychiatry* 23:56–62.

Katschnig H (1983). Methods for measuring social adjustment, pp 205–218. In T Helgason (ed), *Methodology in Evaluation of Psychiatric Treatment.* Cambridge University Press, Cambridge.

Lancet H (1991). Quality of life. *Lancet* 338:350–351.

Lehman AF, Burns BJ (1990). Severe mental illness in the community, pp 357–366. In B Spilker (ed), *Quality of Life Assessments in Clinical Trials.* Raven, New York.

Lief A (1948). *The common sense psychiatry of Dr. Adolf Meyer*, pp 153–169. McGraw-Hill, New York.

Mellsop G, Peace K, Fernando T (1987). Pre-admission adaptive functioning as a measure of prognosis in psychiatric inpatients. *Australia and New Zealand Journal of Psychiatry* 21:539–544.

Merikangas KR, Bromet EJ, Spiker DG (1983). Assortative mating, social adjustment, and course of illness in primary affective disorder. *Archives of General Psychiatry* 40:795–800.

Mezzich JE (1988). On developing a psychiatric multiaxial schema for ICD-10. *British Journal of Psychiatry* 152:38–43 (suppl 1).

Mezzich JE, Sartorius N, Kastrup MC, Katschnig H, Lopez-Ibor JJ, Janca A (1993). Multiaxial classification and ICD-10. Paper presented at the WHO Symposium, ICD-10: A Common Language, Annual Meeting of the American Psychiatric Association, San Francisco.

Mogensen JT, Simonsen E, Mellergaard M (1986). Multiaxial diagnosis in a department of adult psychiatry. *Ugeskrift for Laeger* 148:2869–2872.

Paykel ES, Weissman M, Prusoff BA, Tonks CM (1971). Dimensions of social adjustment in depressed women. *Journal of Nervous and Mental Disorders* 152:158–172.

Slevin ML, Plant H, Lynch D, Drinkwater J, Gregory WM (1988). Who should measure quality of life, the doctor or the patient? *British Journal of Cancer* 57:109–112.

Spilker B (ed) (1990). *Quality of Life Assessments in Clinical Trials*. Raven, New York.

Strauss JS (1975). A comprehensive approach to psychiatric diagnosis. *American Journal of Psychiatry* 132:1193–1197.

Testa MA, Anderson RB, Nackley JF, Hollenberg NK, Quality-of-Life Hypertension Study Group (1993). Quality of life and antihypertensive therapy in men. *New England Journal of Medicine* 328:907–913.

Trzepacz PT, Brenner R, Van Thiel DH (1989). A psychiatric study of 247 liver transplantation candidates. *Psychosomatics* 30:147–153.

Walker SR, Rosser RM (eds) (1993). *Quality of Life Assessment: Key Issues in the 1990s*. Kluwer, Lancaster, UK.

Weissman MM, Sholomskas D, John K (1981). The assessment of social adjustment. An update. *Archives of General Psychiatry* 38:1250–1258.

Williams A (1985) Economics of coronary artery bypass grafting. *British Medical Journal* 291:326–329.

Wing JK, Cooper JE, Sartorius N (1974). *The Measurement and Classification of Psychiatric Symptoms*. Cambridge University Press, London.

World Health Organization (1978). *International Classification of Disease* (9th ed, rev): *Mental Disorders: Glossary and Guide to their Classification*. World Health Organization, Geneva.

World Health Organization (1980). *International Classification of Impairments, Disabilities, and Handicaps. A Manual of Classification Relating to the Consequences of Disease*. World Health Organization, Geneva.

World Health Organization (1988). *WHO Psychiatric Disability Assessment Schedule (WHO/DAS)*. World Health Organization, Geneva.

World Health Organization (1992). *The ICD-10 Classification of Mental and Behavioural Disorders: Clinical Descriptions and Diagnostic Guidelines*. World Health Organization, Geneva.

World Health Organization (1993a). *Proceedings of the WHO/Ipsen Meeting on Quality of Life Assessment in Health Care Settings, Paris, 28–30 June 1993.*
World Health Organization (1993b). *Informal Consultation on Classification and Assessment of Mental Impairments, Disabilities, and Handicaps, Mannheim 28–30 June 1993.*

# 21
# Multidimensional Diagnosis of Depressive Disorders

Yomishi Kasahara

Almost two decades ago, Kasahara and Kimura (1975) proposed a multidimensional diagnostic system for depressive disorders based on five dimensions: (1) psychiatric symptoms (current conditions), (2) premorbid personality features, (3) psychosocial stressors before onset, (4) levels of social functioning prior to onset, and (5) attitudes toward psychiatric treatment (including course).

When we compared our system with the multiaxial evaluation in *Diagnostic and Statistical Manual of Mental Disorders*, 3rd edition (DSM-III) that came out several years later, we found, interestingly, that the first four dimensions were nearly the same. However, there were significiant differences between these two systems. The multiaxial evaluation advocated by DSM-III was devised to promote common understanding for all professionals in psychiatric practice and to cover all psychiatric disorders, whereas our system was to assist experienced psychiatrists to make proper diagnoses and to better treat depressed patients. Furthermore, our multidimensional system attempted to classify several clinical subtypes of depressive disorders according to combinations of the five dimensions as shown in Table 21.1.

Type I depression is most frequently seen among patients suffering from affective disorders in the outpatient clinics in urban areas of Japan. It is characterized by the following features:

Dimension I (current symptoms): Typical unipolar features, almost identical to endogenous depressive symptoms including somatic as well as mental symptoms.

Dimension II (personality): Cohesive personality or immobilithymia (Shimoda), typus melancholicus (Tellenbach), obsessoid personality (Kasahara).

Dimension III (psychosocial stressors): (1) Changes in life-style (eg, transfer to a new position, promotion, mild physical illness or injury,

TABLE 21.1. Multidimensional classification of depressive states.

| | Type I | Type II | Type III | Type IV | Type V | Type VI |
|---|---|---|---|---|---|---|
| I Present state | Depressive episode, unipolar, mild severity | Depressive episode, bipolar, recurrent | So-called neurotic, chronic | Atypical features (dysphoric, apathetic, impulse dyscontrol) | Repetitive thought of "loss" or "event" | Unspecified (organic depressive syndrome, depressive states in childhood, adolescence, and in senile persons, and in others) |
| II Premorbid personality | "Cohesive personality" (Shimoda), "typus melancholicus" | Cycloid (Kretschmer) (plus) cohesive personality | Depressive personality (Schneider) dependent, histrionic (DSM-III) | Avoidant, borderline, schizotypal (DSM-III) | Unspecified | |
| III Outbreaking situations (stressor) | Changes in way of life (new career, promotion) | Unclear, often no stressors | Persisting inner conflicts | Identity problems | Loss of close relatives, unusual psychic trauma | |
| IV Premorbid social functioning | Very good or good (businessmen or housewives of middle age) | Good or fair (from adolescence to middle age) | Fair or poor (young and middle age) | Fair or poor (late adolescence and young adults) | Unspecified | |
| V Attitudes toward treatment | Good relationship, good response to pharmacotherapy | Almost good, but sometimes unstable relationship | Poor response to pharmacotherapy | Poor response to pharmacotherapy, unstable relationship | Rarely visits psychiatrists | |
| Levels of severity | I-1<br>I-2<br>I-3<br>I-4 | II-1<br>II-2<br>II-3<br>II-4 | III-1<br>III-2<br>III-3<br>III-4 | IV-1<br>IV-2<br>IV-3<br>IV-4 | V-1<br>V-2<br>V-3<br>V-4 | |

Kasahara and Kimura 1975.

sudden increase or diminution of responsibility, change of residence, going abroad, etc); (2) No psychosocial stressor.

Dimension IV (social functioning): Good or excellent functioning as business person or homemaker of middle age to presenile age, upper-middle or middle class.

Dimension V (attitude toward therapist and treatment): Constant and good relationship with therapist, coping ability against distresses, good response to pharmacotherapy.

The cohesive personality or immobilithymic personality in Dimension II was proposed by M. Shimoda (1885–1980) in 1932 as premorbid personality for manic–depressive illness, particularly of unipolar depression. According to Shimoda's description (1941, 1950), those who have cohesive personality suffer from neither dysphoric nor pessimistic mood when they are functioning normally. Shimoda described people with this personality type as possessing above-average ability or as being an ideal worker or model soldier. Therefore, this personality is not a personality disorder but a depression-prone "normal" personality among Japanese.

Cohesive personality was summarized by Yamashita (1981) as a union of the following three personality tendencies: (1) zealous, devoted, persistent, stable; (2) conscientious, upright, dutiful, reliable; and (3) orderly, perfectionistic, meticulous, scrupulous.

Shimoda's conceptualization was not well accepted in his day, but in the 1960s, when a milder form of unipolar depression began to increase among outpatients, his theory started to be reevaluated. According to my experience, it seems that no less than 50% of the depressive patients visiting my clinic possessed cohesive personality traits during the years in the 1980s. This concept roughly corresponds to the concept of typus melancholicus proposed by Tellenbach in 1961 in Germany as premorbid pesonality for unipolar depression. According to Tellenbach, the most fundamental component of typus melancholicus lies in "love of orderliness" or "fixation on orderliness." Typus melancholicus was well accepted in Japan because of its resemblance to Shimoda's concept of the cohesive personality.

If we were to convert cohesive personality to DSM-III-R terminology, it would possibly be classified under Obsessive–Compulsive Personality. As compared with the typical obsessive–compulsive personality disorder, obsessive–compulsive symptoms and aggressiveness and egocentric stubbornness are not seen overtly. Rather, people with this type of personality show tendencies to avoid conflicts and try to seek harmonious and comfortable relationships with others. I proposed calling such an ego-syntonic and nonaggressive type of obsessive–compulsive personality disorder an obsessoid personality (1987) and described its characteristics as follows: (1) orderly, perfectionistic, duty-bound, achievement-oriented; (2) longing for comfortable social relationships; (3) quiet, nonaggressive.

Type II depression corresponds almost exactly to classical endogenous bipolar disorder.

Dimension I (current symptoms): Less typical and comprehensive than symptoms of Type I, episodes of mania or hypomania, sometimes pyknic body habitus.
Dimension II (premorbid personality): Cycloid or cyclothymic personality (Kretschmer), sometimes cohesive personality, typus melancholicus, obsessoid personality.
Dimension III (psychosocial stressors): Unclear, sometimes a physical condition, for example, menstruation, seasonal factors, physical exhaustion.
Dimension IV (social functioning): Good or fair, sometimes difficult to evaluate because of insufficient social experiences in adolescents and young adults.
Dimension V (attitude toward therapist and therapy): Possibly an unstable relationship, moderate response to pharmacotherapy, prolonged course and tendency to relapse.

Both III and IV types of depression could be classified as neurotic according to traditional concepts. Studies of borderline conditions or borderline personality disorder and of mild or oligosymptomatic schizophrenia since the 1960s were a stimulus to discriminate between these two types of depression. The discrimination between these two types can be made on the basis of their multiaxial features.

The clinical picture of Type III corresponds with so-called neurotic symptoms. Type IV includes atypical clinical features such as dysphoric, apathetic or pan-neurotic, sometimes impulse–noncontrol symptoms. As for premorbid personality for Type III, depressive psychopath (Schneider), dependent personality disorder (DSM-III) and Shinkeisitsu (nervosity) of Morita (1922) are prominent, whereas in Type IV, avoidant personality disorder, borderline personality disorder, and schizotypal personality disorder (DSM-III) are often evident. As for triggering situations or psychosocial stressors prior to onset, persistent inner conflicts are observed in Type III, whereas identity crisis is present among adolescents and young adults in Type IV.

Type V depression corresponds to grief reaction, adjustment disorders with depressive mood or post-traumatic stress disorders with depressive mood. Type VI is a residual category for any kind of depressive state that cannot be classified according to the five dimensions (eg, organic depressive syndromes, depressive states occuring in childhood, early and middle adolescence, and in the senium).

In summary, these six types of depression could be termed as follows: Type I, Personality-situation type; Type II, Circular type; Type III, Conflict-reaction type; Type IV, Schizoid-borderline type; Type V, Grief-reaction type; and Type VI, Miscellaneous.

Levels of severity add another aspect to this diagnostic table. Four levels of severity in Type I are as follows: I-1, mild severity, including masked depression or depressive equivalents; I-2, moderate severity, including a single 1- or 2-week hypomanic episode in the final stage of pharmacotherapy; I-3, chronic cases including secondary manifestations of neurotic conflicts resulting from the chronic nature of the illness; I-4, transient psychotic features including mood-incongruent psychotic states or atypical psychoses.

Needless to say, Use of the international system is advantageous for statistical and epidemiological studies. On the other hand, local classifications such as our six-subtype diagnosis could help clinicians to make precise selection of therapeutic maneuvers for each patient. Our next plans for this system are to learn from excellent studies on multidimensional or multiaxial characteristics of depressive disorders in the literature. According to Mezzich et al (1987), nine aspects are important for a comprehensive description of depressive patients: symptoms, course, severity, personality, physical illness, psychosocial stressors, etiology, social functioning, and demographics. Among these items, symptoms, course, and personality attract the most attention of researchers. When Akiskal (1981) classified three subtypes of chronic depression, he adopted seven aspects: onset, course, personality, developmental history, family history, rapid eye movement (REM) latency, and pharmacological response. The addition of one or two aspects concerning biological markers such as REM latency in Akiskal's table to my classification system would be desirable. Plasma biopterin levels in patients with affective disorders (Hashimoto et al 1987, 1988) would be another likely addition for us.

# Conclusion

The comprehensive diagnosis of complex conditions such as those of depressive patients has been attempted through several multiaxial schemes. These have been reviewed with particular focus on a proposed system that includes five dimensions (current symptoms, personality, psychosocial stressors, social functioning, and attitude towards therapist and treatment) plus a severity axis. On the basis of this scheme, several prototypes of depression were outlined. Promising lines for future development were identified.

## *References*

Akiskal HS (1981). Chronic depression. *Journal of Affective Disorders* 3:297–315.

Hashimoto R, Ozaki N, Ohta T, et al (1987). Total biopterin levels of plasma in patients with depression. *Neuropsychobiology* 17:176–177.

Hashimoto R, Ozaki N, Ohta T, et al (1988). Plasma biopterin levels of patients with affective disorders. *Neuropsychobiology* 19:61–63.

Kasahara Y, Fujita O, Sakai K (1987). Industrialization and mental health in Japan. Mental health of large enterprise employees in their 40s and 50s. *Japanese Journal of Psychiatric Neurology* 41:179–185.

Kasahara Y, Kimura B (1975). Zur Klassifizierung depressiver Zustaende. *Psychiatric Neurologic Japonica* 77:715–715–735 (in Japanese).

Mezzich JE, Fabrega H, Coffman GA (1987). Multiaxial characterization of depressive patients. *Journal of Nervous and Mental Disease* 175:339–346.

Morita M (1922). *Shinkeishitsu*. Hakusuisha, Tokyo (in Japanese).

Shimoda M (1941). Premorbid Charakter der mainisch-depressiver Irreseins. *Psychiatric Neurologic Japonica* 45:101–103 (in Japanese).

Shimoda M (1950). Ueber manisch-depressiver Irresein. *Yonago Medical School Journal* 2:1–5 (in Japanese).

Tellenbach H (1961). *Melancholie*. Springer, Berlin.

Yamashita I (1981). *Depression in Japan*, pp 89–93. In TA Ban, et al (eds), *Prevention and Treatment of Depression*. New Port Press, Baltimore.

# 22
# Multiaxial Issues on Personality Disorders

YUTAKA ONO, SATOKO EZOE, AND KEIGO OKONOGI

A psychiatric classification system must satisfy the following two objectives: First, it must serve as a basis from which to clarify individual psychiatric disorders. Because most psychiatric disorders currently discussed are syndromes, they are only tentatively considered a disorder concept. To examine the validity of the classification, research must be conducted from empirical, clinical, and biological viewpoints. Based on the observations obtained, the classification system is then revised, after which more studies are performed and classifications further revised. Through procedures such as these, we gradually gain understanding of the disorder.

Second, the classification must be clinically useful. Even if psychiatric disorders are tentative concepts, clinicians, for the time being, diagnose and treat patients based on the classification system. As far as we clinicians are concerned, the value of the classification system is determined by the appropriateness of the indices provided at treatment.

An example of diagnostic criteria that meets these requirements is the American Psychiatric Association's *Diagnostic and Statistical Manual of Mental Disorders*, 3rd edition, revised (DSM-III-R) (1980), because it is atheoretical, sets clear-cut criteria, is polythetic and prototypic to certain disorders, and enables multidiagnosis.

Of particular significance is the concept of multiaxial classification. It is especially noteworthy that DSM-III-R divides the classification system into five axes, and makes sure that attention is paid not only to the so-called state disorders such as schizophrenic disorder and mood disorder, but also to the patient's personality, physical state, stress, and adaptability. In addition, as was pointed out by Frances (1980, 1982), DSM-III-R should be acclaimed for positioning personality disorders in Axis II, which prompted clinicians and researchers to see the patient as a whole person. Moreover, because the classification cri-teria centered on behavior assessments, it helped to enhance inter-rater reliability. Ideas such as these are also incorporated in the *International Classification of Diseases*, 10th revision (ICD-10) formulated by the World Health Organization (1992).

At the same time, however, some limitations of DSM-III-R's Axis II have been pointed out. One is the confusion of the following three concepts: "Pure" personality disorders, a chronic subtype and residual symptoms of Axis I disorders, and the so-called personality traits or styles that are uniformly observed whether the patient is sick or not. These limitations are probably due to the lack of consistency of classifications with different theoretical and clinical backgrounds. For this and other reasons, substantial redundancy is found in Axis II diagnoses.

This chapter is based on our research in Japan and investigates personality disorders from a multiaxial diagnostic viewpoint to study the significance of multiaxial diagnosis and the characteristics of personality disorders unique in Japan.

## Subjects and Methods

*Study 1.* Subjects of our study were 66 patients with suspected personality or neurotic disorders and comprised 30 males (mean age, 29.9) and 36 females (mean age, 28.8), a majority of whom lived in Tokyo or its suburbs. Personality disorders were diagnosed using the Japanese version of the International Personality Disorder Examination (IPDE) developed by Loranger (1989) and Lorarger et al (1991).

*Study 2.* Another study targeted 995 computer engineers and administrative employees of an electrical manufacturing company, aged 20 to 49. Using a questionnaire based on the Structured Clinical Interview for DSM-III-R Personality Disorders II (SCID II) Questionnaires (Spitzer et al 1989), we studied the patients' personality traits. Questions were taken from those in the SCID II with the exception of two questions (one related to the diagnostic criteria of antisocial personal disorder, and the other was deemed unappropriate) and were arranged in random order. The rating system was changed from the two-point scale (yes–no) to a three-point scale (0–1–2). Zung's Self-Report Depression Scale (SDS) and the 30-question version of the General Health Questionnaire (GHQ) were used simultaneously to assess psychiatric disorders.

## Results

Study 1 diagnosed 24 patients as having the following DSM-III-R personality disorders: avoidant personality disorders (eight patients); borderline personality disorders (six patients); histrionic, passive–aggressive and dependent personality disorders (three patients each); paranoid, narcis-

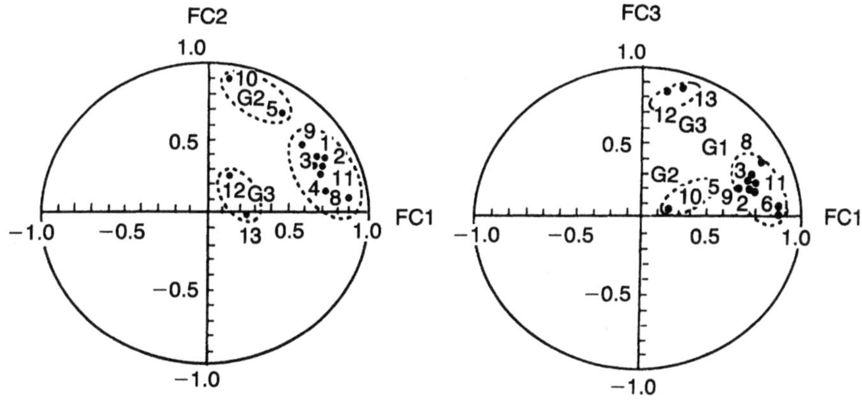


FIGURE 22.1. Display of personality traits on factors 1 and 2 and 1 and 3, respectively, extracted from a study of 781 male computer engineers and 214 male clinical workers.

sistic, and obsessive–compulsive (two patients each); and schizotypal and self-defeating personality disorders (one patient each). In addition, four patients were diagnosed with personality disorders not otherwise specified (NOS). Of these 24 patients, eight (36%) were diagnosed as having overlapping personality disorders; twelve (55%) had just a single symptom. Of those diagnosed as having personality disorders, 12 (50%) had either overlapping personality disorders or NOS.

Factor analysis (Figure 22.1) conducted in Study 2 to examine the distribution of personality traits, extracted the following three common factors: (1) A factor relating to instability, including histrionic, narcissistic, borderline, paranoid, self-defeating, dependent, passive aggressive, obsessive–compulsive, and schizotypal traits; (2) a factor related to withdrawal, such as schizoid and avoidance; and (3) a factor related to depression diagnosed by the SDS and the GHQ.

## Discussion

Of the 24 patients diagnosed in our study as having personality disorders, 50% were found to have overlapping diagnoses or NOS. Needless to say, having an overlapping personality disorder is, by itself, not always problematic. It is possible for a patient to have several personality disorders at the same time. However, if half of the subjects are found to have overlapping personality disorders as well as unspecified personality disorders, the validity of this categorical classification becomes questionable.

Once the confusion of concepts has been corrected and several personality disorders shown to be a single clinical entity or pathology, it is possible to place personality disorders in line with Axis I state disorders as ICD-10 does.

Notwithstanding these problems, it is particularly significant that avoidant personality disorder is the symptom that appeared most frequently in our study. This observation agrees with many reports that indicate fear of interpersonal situations as a symptom commonly seen in Japan. Many patients in Japan suffering from this condition would benefit greatly from future studies in this field. Another research possibility is to study the relation between personality disorders characterized by avoidance and Japan's society/culture.

Another important discussion, in addition to one that focuses on personality disorders, is how to position patients' personality characteristics or traits within the classification system (Ono 1988). This is important because to become involved with a patient as a whole person, it is essential to understand both her or his personality disorder and personality traits and characteristics. This understanding becomes particularly significant when considering the patient's involvement in psychotherapy.

In regard to treatment method and treatment process, clinicians and participating family members can be guided in part by the presence of specific personality traits.

It has often been pointed out that the dimensional classification of personality traits (studies of which have thus far been mainly developed by psychologists rather than psychiatrists) can provide a valuable hint. It is possible to use individual DSM-III-R personality disorders dimensionally. However, having thirteen axes makes the process much too cumbersome. Moreover, because each disorder overlaps with other symptoms, using it as a dimension is not always recommended.

DSM-III-R's cluster classification may also be used. However, in our Study 2, targeting nonpatients to examine their personality traits, two factors were identified: object-seeking and withdrawal. One reason may be the bias of our subjects, all of whom were employees of a computer-related company. It is also doubtful if the DSM-III-R cluster classification can adequately classify personality characteristics. Furthermore, it might be unreasonable to consider dimensional classification, which also has continuity with normal people, based on the categorical classification of abnormal personality disorders. Thus, to describe personality traits, it is necessary to create a new classification linked with general personality traits.

Many psychologists have already begun research on this topic and include models by Eysenck and Eysenck (1985), Eysenck (1987), Widiger et al (1987), Tellegen (1985), Wiggins (1982), Millon (1981), Kiesler (1986), Cloninger (1987), and Costa (1990), among others. They are, however, yet to be incorporated into the classification criteria because their differences are currently highlighted but still relatively unknown among clinicians.

These studies nevertheless share some common concepts. For example, most of these models attempt to represent personality traits with three axes. By grouping similar dimensions of each of the models mentioned above, personality traits can be divided into the following tridimensional models. First is the closeness (close/dependent vs distant/independent) dimension, which is characterized by the tendency to move toward or away from others and referred to by terms such as social involvement, reward dependency, affiliation, and dependence. Second is the power (controlling/alloplastic vs submissive/autoplastic) dimension, which is characterized in other models by the tendency to a higher or lower position to others and referred by terms such as lack of assertion, harm avoidance, submission–dominance. Third is the activity (active/implusive vs passive/inhibited) dimension, which is characterized by too little or too much control over one's drive/behavior and referred to by terms such as tendency to act out and novelty-seeking vs anxious rumination. Focusing attention on these common factors may trigger the development of the current classification system to become more clinically useful.

## Conclusion

It is clinically important to understand and to grasp not only the categorical classification of personality disorders but also that of personality traits. It is also useful to differentiate "pure" personality disorders, personality traits, and subtypes of Axis I disorders. It should be noted that personality traits include aspects that are variable, and that these may change any time under the influence of psychiatric disorders or environment/culture. There are even some cases in which completely contrasting personality traits are seen within one person, although the degree differs among individuals.

Therefore, studies must be conducted, from a clinical, epidemiological, and biological perspective to come up with an appropriate and clinically useful classification of personality characteristics. Further research is also necessary to investigate the relationship between psychiatric disorders and sociocultural environment to personality disorders and personality traits, as well as the relationship between the patient's self-assessment obtained through questionnaires and the clinician's assessment.

*Acknowledgment.* Our research was partially supported by grants from the Mental Health Okamoto Memorial Foundation and the Takeda Foundation for Psychoanalysis.

## *References*


American Psychiatric Association Committee on Nomenclature and Statistics (1980). *Diagnostic and Statistical Manual of Mental Disorders* (3rd ed). American Psychiatric Association, Washington, DC.

Cloninger CR (1987). A systematic method for clinical description and classification of personality variants: A proposal. *Archives of General Psychiatry* 44: 573–588.

Costa PT, McCrae RR (1990). Personality disorders and the five-factor Model of Personality. *Journal of Personality Disorders* 4:362–371.

Eysenck H (1987). The definition of personality disorders and the criteria appropriate for their description. *Journal of Personality Disorders* 1:211–219.

Eysenck HJ, Eysenck MW (1985). *Personality and Individual Differences*. Plenum Press, New York.

Frances A (1980). The DSM-III personality disorder section: A commentary. *American Journal of Psychiatry* 137:1050–1054.

Frances A (1982). Categorical and dimensional systems of personality diagnosis: A comparison. *Comprehensive Psychiatry* 23:516–527.

Kiesler D (1986). The 1982 Interpersonal Circle: An analysis of DSM-III personality disorders. In T Millon, G Klerman (eds), *Contemporary Issues in Psychopathology*. Guilford, New York.

Loranger A, Hirschfeld N, Sartorius D, Reigier DA (1991). The WHO/ADAMHA international pilot study of personality disorders: Background and purpose. *Journal of Personality Disorders* 5:296–306.

Loranger AW (Ono, Sueoka, Ezoe, Okonogi, trans) (1989). Personality Disorder Examination with PDE Scoring Manual. White Plains, NY (in Japanese).

Millon T (1981). *Disorders of Personality—DSM-III: Axis II*. Wiley & Sons, New York.

Ono Y (1988). Diagnostic classification of personality disorders—in search of a new system. *Journal of the Japanese Psychoanalytic Association* 32:1–22 (in Japanese).

Spitzer RL, Williams E (1989). Structured Clinical Interview for DSM-III Disorders (SCID).

Tellegen A (1985). Structures of mood and personality and their relevance to assessing anxiety, with an emphasis on self-report. In AH Tuma, JD Maser (eds), *Anxiety and the Anxiety Disorders*. Erlbaum, Hillsdale, NJ.

Widiger TA, Trull TJ, Hurt WS, et al (1987). A multidimensional scaling of the DSM-III personality disorder. *Archives of General Psychiatry* 44:557–563.

Wiggins J (1982). Circumplex models of interpersonal behavior in clinical psychology. In P Kendall, J Buthcher (eds), *Handbook of Research Methods in Clinical Psychology*. Wiley & Sons, New York.

World Health Organization (1992). *ICD-10 Classification of Mental and Behavioral Clinical Disorders: Clinical Descriptions and Diagnostic Guidelines*. World Health Organization, Geneva.

# Part IV
## Impact of Psychiatric Diagnosis on Health Care

# 23
# The Validity of Diagnostic Systems for Treatment

Hanfried H. Helmchen

The ultimate purpose of diagnosis is prognostic information and successful treatment of the individual patient. However, current diagnostic systems in psychiatry are far from serving this purpose.

The American Psychiatric Association (APA) Task Force Report on treatments of psychiatric disorders (Karasu 1989) makes this very clear, although it is specifically related to the DSM-III-R which is currently the most developed psychiatric diagnostic system in terms of operationalization, comprehensiveness, and acceptance. Caution and warnings against using the described treatments as obligatory standards for specific psychiatric disorders can be found running like a red thread throughout the whole report. In almost all chapters there are statements such as "there can be no correct treatment for an individual who suffers from one variant or another of a heterogeneous disorder" as schizophrenia is assumed to be (p 1485), or "the concept of therapeutically and prognostically valid patient subtypes within the general class of individuals with alcoholism remains an area in need of further study" (p 1071), or, "in discussion of treatment of a condition . . . a clinician must be able to consider each clinical problem at several conceptual levels in designing the most appropriate treatment program" (p xii).

These warnings are justified not only to combat the misuse of today's preliminary knowledge as though it were definitive, but also because in principle a class in a diagnostic system can at best serve to indicate more or less specifically a therapeutic principle, but not a specific application in an individual case. In any case, nowadays such a global therapeutic impact of diagnostic classes seems to be rather low.

An example of less specification is the currently predominant conviction that the Kraepelinian triadic system may serve as a framework for the focal point of treatment of so-called minor psychiatric disorders, reactive or maladaptive or adjustment disorders, and personality disorders primarily for psychotherapeutic or social treatments; endogenous psychoses basically for drug treatments; and organic mental syndromes for treatment of the causes, if known. Somewhat greater specification may be exemplified by drug treatment in psychotic disorders (eg, antidepressant drugs in depressive disorders, and MAO-inhibitors in atypical depression).

However, although these examples refer to established indications of treatment principles, their specificity to certain diagnostic classes remains to be validated. This implies the risk of neglecting other indications, for example, the relevance of social treatments in schizophrenic disorders, especially in residual states with negative symptoms, or the efficacy of antidepressant drugs in some anxiety disorders, particularly in panic disorders. The latter example may also illustrate the impact of treatments on the classification of psychiatric disorders. In general, the specificity of the relationship between diagnostic classes and distinct treatments is fairly limited. In other words: the more individualized the treatment goal, the less useful the psychiatric diagnosis is, and vice versa. And it should be added: The less severe the condition, the more individually responsive it is both to personality and environment.

## Functions of Psychiatric Diagnosis with Regard to Treatment

Psychiatric diagnosis serves as an instrument to organize epidemiologic data for administrative use, especially for planning quantity of service (eg, the rapid increase of dementias) and improving quality of service settings (eg, for schizophrenic patients, as a framework for specific treatments [Helmchen 1981]).

In some cases, psychiatric diagnosis regulates financing of care and service use, for example, the 1984 financing recommendation of the selection of the treatment with the most specific efficacy in a given special psychiatric condition, then specificity of both psychiatric diagnoses and treatments must be elaborated further to improve treatment planning. This is discussed for psychiatric diagnoses and for psychiatric treatments in the following sections.

### *Psychiatric Diagnoses*

Treatment-specific disadvantages of psychiatric diagnoses and systems are the following:

*Heterogeneity.* First of all, this means that psychiatric diagnoses and their classification are a nonsystematic mixture of different aspects of psychiatric disorders (eg, phenomenology, etiology), and furthermore, of different concepts (eg, in the case of schizophrenia that of a course-related entity by Kraepelin, or that of a group of disorders by Bleuler). Thus, the problem of heterogeneity of nosological groups arises due to the polythetic approach of many diagnostic categories.

Heterogeneity *sensu strictu* means a class of several genetically different psychiatric disorders under the same diagnostic term. Diversity, in contrast, means the fact that different aspects, for example, stages or sections of the course of one disease can be found under different diagnoses. Diversity also results from concepts such as that of vulnerability insofar as under a longitudinal perspective it differentiates more or less time-invariant trait factors for disposition from time-dependent state factors for precipitation or persistence of a current disorder. A consequence may be the need for multiple diagnosis in the same patient.

But do multiple diagnoses help overcome a simple addition of single treatments for each partial diagnosis and indicate an integrated treatment based on a Task Force Report of the US Department of Health and Human Services to remove limitations of Medicare coverage on services of Alzheimer's disease and related disorders (Karasu 1989).

In the individual case, the impact of any timely diagnosis on treatment is the challenge to treat (eg, to diagnose a beginning dementive process against so-called normal aging, or to differentiate a sluggish schizophrenic process from a nonpsychotic personality disorder).

But does the diagnosis of schizophrenia in an individual case really help to indicate whether and which drug treatment should be given, alone or in combination or sequence with a psychosocial treatment? I think it does, but only in the following sense: Psychiatric diagnoses such as schizophrenia, hypochondriasis, body dysmorphophobic disorder, or any other specific diagnosis can be used as a *key* to a more or less adequately organized knowledge, conceptual as well as empirical, and as an *instrument* to organize and document individual evaluation data.

Again however, this knowledge is not well organized with regard to specific treatments: In general there can either be found multimodal and vastly overlapping treatments for each psychiatric diagnosis (eg, Karasu 1989, Reid 1983), or each treatment is indicated for a bulk of diverse psychiatric diagnoses, as most textbooks on psychiatric treatments show (eg, American Psychiatric Association 1984, Benkert and Hippius 1986, Meltzer et al 1987).

The last observation points to principal restrictions in using psychiatric diagnosis for individual treatment planning.

## Limitations and Solutions

Psychiatric diagnoses are not specifically designed or even empirically proven as instruments for treatment planning, and psychiatric treatments are mainly symptomatic and unspecific to the existing psychiatric diagnoses. This applies if treatment planning is defined as scientifically proven knowledge of interactions and sequences of single treatments?

*Arbitrariness.* Changing and unregulated predominance of various aspects in the definition of psychiatric diagnoses and their classification from author to author, or from one panel to another, revealed their arbitrariness and their nature as conventions: Frequently, there is neither theoretical substantiation nor empirical basis. Examples are the change of time criteria or the grading of severity of depression (Möller 1990). The existing diagnostic systems are tentative and have to be modified or extended on the grounds of cumulative knowledge based on empirical findings.

*Inflation of Diagnostic Systems.* Robins and Guze (1970) and Kendell (1975, 1985) have made the case of determining the quality of psychiatric diagnoses in terms of reliability, validity, specificity, and sensitivity by empirical research. Such proof of the quality of psychiatric diagnoses, particularly as instruments for treatment planning, has yet to be obtained. This is perhaps due to the fact that more time is needed to produce scientifically sound and representative results rather than just to attenuate the disadvantages of existing diagnostic systems. Thus, the last 15 years have brought an inflation of diagnostic assessment systems: At least 10 major systems now exist (Berner et al 1983, Philipp and Maier 1987, Stieglitz et al 1990) related to special purposes (eg, research or treatment, or care in different world or geographic regions—developing vs developed, Eastern vs Western; rural vs urban, etc), and primarily to improve the reliability of diagnoses and systems by more operationalization. Various reviews were able to substantiate this (eg, Grove 1987). However, an improvement in reliability does not necessarily mean an increase in validity. Substantiating the latter requires extensive validity studies, especially with regard to predictive validity.

*Lack of Predictive Validity.* One way in which this multiplicity, heterogeneity, and rapid change of assessment systems negatively influence habits and behavior of treating psychiatrists may be the loss of confidence in any classification system without the gain of insight into the instrumental nature of psychiatric diagnoses. Another negative consequence is an increasing difficulty in comparing the results of empirical research, including therapy research, based on different diagnostic systems. Therefore, it is necessary to demand longer intervals of time between the revisions of individual systems because it is difficult to compare results, and also because the continued development of systems is not necessarily linked to an increase in validity (Coryell and Zimmerman 1987). For example, it is necessary to evaluate the relevance of the individual criteria (eg, sensitivity, specificity) which define the diagnostic categories.

It remains to be proven whether relevant results for treatment planning can be provided by the polydiagnostic approach—the process of applying various diagnostic systems for the same disorder to find homogeneous groups of patients as the overlap of all systems (Berner et al 1983). In any case, the predictive validity of psychiatric diagnoses remains to be proven.

*Further Difficulties.* The following restrict the usefulness of the currently accepted psychiatric diagnoses for individual treatment planning:

1. Psychiatric diagnoses do not indicate the severity of the disorder although this may justify different treatments (Klein 1989).
2. Psychiatric diagnoses say almost nothing about the developmental stage of the disorder. However, in view of the theoretical background for the differentiation of a disorder's development into states and time-invariant traits as well as the further differentiation of the latter into dispositional and residual traits, it can be assumed that a differential therapy response is also influenced by the dynamic of the disease process. Post et al (1986) tried to explain the development of affective psychosis up to and including rapid cycling by models of kindling and sensitization and concluded that different developmental stages of an apparently unitary phenomenon such as kindling are differentially responsive to treatment.
3. Psychiatric diagnoses give no hint as to neuronal systems or receptor types through which biological treatments (for example, psychotropic drugs) may be effective. This is quite apart from the fact that these drug therapy-relevant neuronal systems are not necessarily those that are decisive for the pathogenesis of the disorder and thus relevant to diagnosis. Thus, the dopaminergic mechanism of the antipsychotic efficacy of neuroleptics is no evidence for the so-called dopamine hypothesis of schizophrenia (Carlsson 1987). This is because the primary disturbance may be in other systems, for example, the glutamatergic system (Kornhuber et al 1989), the psychopathogenic effects of which may be mediated exclusively—but just mediated—by the dopaminergic system.

Therefore, treatment-specific improvements of psychiatric diagnoses and assessment systems may be expected if the following is considered: Most psychiatric diagnoses contain at most only a small segment of the plethora of indicators that a treating psychiatrist must observe in making treatment choice: Timing, intensity/dosage, duration, combination, sequence, etc. Major indicators, as suggested by Frances et al (1984), are the following:

1. Psychopathological syndromes or symptoms, specifically known as target symptoms.
2. Severity of symptoms/syndromes.
3. Course of the disorder: Age at onset, duration, stage, etc or, in a broader sense, morbid developments (eg, premorbid traits [transient or persistent insufficient coping capacity due to transient or persistent stress and/or personality disorder or psychiatric disorder] lead, via the maladaptive state of alcohol abuse, to the morbid state of alcohol dependence and

directly or consequentially to secondary morbid states as organic mental disorders).

4. Causal factors, for example, in somatogenic psychic disorders or organic mental disorders.

5. Risk or conditional factors for a disposition (eg, antisocial personality disorder in male alcoholics or pre- and perinatal brain lesions in schizophrenics), or for precipitation and persistence (eg, somatic diseases and handicaps in depression of the aged, or lowered capacity of coping and compliance).

6. Pathoplastic factors of gender and age (eg, multimodal long-term treatment for developmental disorders of infancy, childhood and adolescence, or multiple treatments for the often multimorbid states of the aged).

Last, but not least, are *unknown factors*, related to the openness of individual human development, eg, peculiarities of life-style.

7. Responses to therapeutic interventions by anamnestic experiences of the individual (and first-degree relatives), and by standardized short-term treatments as probes of the dynamic capabilities of such systems.

All of these treatment indicators could be comprehensively assessed through a multiaxial diagnostic system (Mezzich 1988, Stieglitz et al 1988). This, of course, does not mean that each individual case should comprise a class in a system, because this would constitute a nonsystem. However, such a multiaxial diagnostic system may organize knowledge on the treatment-relevant functions of psychiatric diagnosis. Since the introduction of the *Diagnostic and Statistical Manual of Mental Disorders*, 3rd edition (DSM-III), the concept of a multiaxial diagnostic system, as conceptualized in the 1920s by Kretschmer (1919) and Birnbaum (1919) and later developed by Essen-Möller and Wohlfahrt (1947), has been a goal of the major diagnostic systems. However, a number of unsolved problems still exist (Stieglitz et al 1990); for example, there are no rules for making decisions about establishing the necessary number of axes for a comprehensive description. Furthermore, there is no software for easy handling of the data with practical useful results; most axes have not been sufficiently elaborated by systematic empirical research, and in practice, only the first axis of the revised version (DSM-III-R) (American Psychiatric Association 1987) is used. For example, Axis I should not be used as a system of nosological diagnoses named as syndromes, but actually as treatment-relevant psychopathological syndromes or psychopathological basic disturbances (eg, the dynamic basic disturbances by Janzarik [1959] or the positive/negative distinction by Crow [1985]). Furthermore, the diagnostics of Axis II—personality as a real dimensional axis and not as a group of categories of personality disorders—should be developed in the psychological (Zerssen and Pössel 1990) as well as in the biological direction. Not least of all, major emphases should be laid on aspects such as those corresponding to DSM-III-R axes III and IV, especially with regard to the development of standardized short-term treatment interventions and systematic evaluation of treatment responses.

## Psychiatric Treatments

Diagnosis-specific efficacy of psychiatric treatments does not exist for the following reasons:

The main indicators are either: (1) psychopathological syndromes or target-symptoms, both for biological treatments (drugs, ECT, sleep deprivation) and for behavioral psychotherapy, or (2) supposed causal factors, for somatic treatment as well as for psychodynamic therapy. These indicators are not, or at least are not unanimously believed to be linked to psychiatric diagnoses. Therefore, the capacity of the latter to serve for treatment planning is rather limited.

There is no evidence of nosological specificity of treatments. This may be due to the fact that available psychiatric treatments have more than one effect and that their efficacy may be related to their effects on more than one psychological or biological system. The same psychotherapeutic treatments may be applied in the case of diverse minor and some major psychiatric disorders corresponding to different psychiatric diagnoses. For example, neuroleptics are effective in acute schizophrenia as well as in mania and in delirious states. The curative efficacy of carbamazepine has been demonstrated in epilepsies, neuralgias, and manic and depressive states, whereas its prophylactic efficacy has been shown in manic-depressive and schizoaffective disorders.

This, among other reasons, led to the postulates of denosologization of (biological) psychiatry (Praag et al 1987) and of cross-diagnostic or trans-nosological comparisons of treatments (Helmchen 1984, 1990, Benkert 1990, Klein 1989, Klieser 1990). Early steps in this direction have shown that defined drug treatments have specific efficacy against defined biological disturbances such as those of the serotonin system, which are related to different psychopathological syndromes or diagnoses such as depression, suicidality, aggressiveness, lack of impulse control, and even obsessive–compulsive disorder (Insel and Winslow 1990, Zohar and Insel 1987). This corresponds to the concept of serotonin system-related syndromes (SRS) (Cassano and Akiskal 1990). Other examples are the recent proposal of Hudson and Pope (1990), who identified through responses to antidepressant treatment a family of "affective spectrum disorders." Benkert (1990) proposed as "minor psychiatric disorder" the concept of a number of disorders (eg, panic disorder, generalized anxiety, phobic disorders, dysthymia, hyposomnia, pain (migraine), and various psychosomatic disorders), defined by response to the same antidepressant treatment. Therefore, such disorders may share a common pathophysiological anomality.

However, treatment response may not only identify comparable pathophysiological mechanisms in morbid states with different diagnoses, but also different pathophysiological mechanisms under the same diagnosis. Illustrative of this is the early observation of the efficacy of the antidepressant drug imipramine against a distinct type of anxiety disorder, later termed panic disorder (Klein 1964), but possibly not against generalized anxiety. Another example is the neuroleptic response of Type I schizophrenia as compared to the lack of response of Type II schizophrenia (Crow 1985, Brown and Herz 1990). (For further examples see Helmchen 1990, 1991.)

The apparent discrepancy between these concepts with regard to anxiety disorders may remind the reader that Klein (1989) emphasized the possibility that differences in drug response may be due not to different underlying disorders but to different states of severity of the same disorder ("severity gradient"), for example, MAO-I responsiveness is often seen in generalized (severe) social phobias but rarely in discrete (mild) social phobias.

Therefore, distinct treatments should be comprehensively compared with each other and in regard to different psychiatric states or diagnoses to establish whether they have a differential predictive validity (Klein 1989). In that case, treatment response may indicate a specific disturbance of biological or psychological mechanisms and their specific relationship to basic psychopathological disturbances. Thus, efforts seem promising to develop the concept of treatment response as one dimension of diagnostic systems in psychiatry that are more valid for treatment planning than the existing systems.

## Conclusion

If the ultimate purpose of diagnosis is prognostic information and successful treatment of the individual patient, then the current diagnostic systems in psychiatry are far from ideal. At best, they currently may (1) serve to organize epidemiological data for administrative use in service planning as a framework for specific treatments; (2) regulate in some cases the financing of treatment, care and service use (eg, in Alzheimer's disease); and (3) be used for each specific diagnosis as a key to knowledge, an instrument to organize and document the individual evaluation, and a challenge for decision making.

Thus, the impact of existing diagnostic systems in psychiatry on treatment planning is fairly small. Reasons for this involve the following: (1) Psychiatric diagnoses are heterogeneous and diverse, with a predominance of their conventional nature, and therefore, arbitrariness and lack of empirical scientific proof of their quality, particularly their differential predictive validity, and inflation of diagnostic systems and revisions. (2)

Psychiatric treatment indications are mainly based on target symptoms with equivocal or no relationship to psychiatric diagnosis, and there is a lack of comparative evaluation with regard to both other treatments and other diagnoses: nosology-independent or "transnosological" evaluation.

Future solutions may be facilitated by the following: (1) A moratorium on the development and revisions of diagnostic systems until sufficient empirical validation can be obtained; (2) Empirical and systematic elaboration of the multiaxial DSM-III-R model, for example, especially that in Axes III and IV; and (3) Comprehensive and comparative evaluation of treatment responses.

## *References*

American Psychiatric Association (1987). *Diagnostic and Statistical Manual of Mental Disorders* (3rd ed, rev). American Psychiatric Association, Washington, DC.

American Psychiatric Association Commission on Psychiatric Therapies (1984). *The Psychiatric Therapies*. American Psychiatric Association, Washington, DC.

Benkert O (1990). Functional classification and response to psychotropic drugs, pp 255–163. In O Benkert, W Maier, K Rickels (eds), *Methodology of the Evaluation of Psychotropic Drugs*. Springer, New York.

Benkert O, Hippius H (1986). *Psychiatrische Pharmakotherapie*. Springer, Berlin.

Berner P, Gabriel E, Katschnig H, Kieffer W, Koehler K, Lenz G, Simhandle CH (1983). Diagnosekriterien für schizophrene und affektive Psychosen. Weltverband für Psychiatrie, Wien.

Birnbaum K (1919). Der Aufbau der Psychose. Ein klinischer Versuch. *Allgemeine Zeitschrift für Psychiatrie* 75:455–502.

Brown W, Herz L (1989). Response to neuroleptic drugs as a device for classifying schizophrenia. *Schizophrenia Bulletin* 15:123–129.

Carlsson A (1987). Overview of dopamine mechanism: Neurochemical and pharmacological evidence, pp 283–298. In H Helmchen, FA Henn (eds), *Biological Perspectives of Schizophrenia*. John Wiley, New York, Chichester.

Cassano GB, Akiskal HA (eds) (1990). Serotonin–system-related syndromes (SRS). Psychopathological and Therapeutic Links, Symposium in Venice, 29–31 March 1990.

Coryell W, Zimmerman M (1987). Progress in the classification of functional psychoses. *American Journal of Psychiatry* 144:1471–1474.

Crow TJ (1985). The two-syndrome concept: Origins and current status. *Schizophrenia Bulletin* 11:471–486.

Essen-Möller E, Wohlfahrt S (1947). Suggestions for the amendment of the official Swedish classification of mental disorders. *Acta Psychiatrica Scandinavica* 47:551–555 (suppl).

Frances A, Clarkin J, Perry S (1984). *Differential Therapeutics in Psychiatry: The Art and Science of Treatment Selection*. Brunner/Mazel, New York.

Grove WM (1987). The reliability of psychiatric diagnosis, pp 99–119. In CG Last, H Hersen (eds), *Issues in Diagnostic Research*. Plenum, New York.

Helmchen H (1981). Functions and consequences of psychiatric diagnoses, pp 99–105. In J Agassi (ed), *Psychiatric Diagnosis*. Proceedings of an International

Interdisciplinary Interschool Symposium, Bielefeld University 1978. Balaban International Science Services, Philadelphia.
Helmchen H (1984). Zur Problematik diagnostischer Kriterien für biologisch-psychiatrische Untersuchunger, pp 50–53. In A Hopf, H Beckmann (eds), *Forschungen zur biologischen Psychiatrie*. Springer, Berlin.
Helmchen H (1990). Psychiatrische Diagnostik ex juvantibus? *Nervenarzt* 61: 148–152.
Helmchen H (1991). Psychopharmakotherapie und Ätiologie, pp 57–66. In F Schneider, K Bartels, H Foerster, J Gaertner (eds), *Perspektiven der Psychiatrie*. Fisher, Stuttgart.
Hudson J, Pope H Jr (1990). Affective spectrum disorder: Does antidepressant response identify a family of disorders with a common pathophysiology? *American Journal of Psychiatry* 147:552–564.
Insel TR, Winslow JR (1990) Neurobiology of OCD. In M Jenike, L Baer, M Minichiello (eds), *Obsessive-Compulsive Disorders: Theory and Management*. Yearbook, Littleton, MA.
Janzarik W (1959). *Dynamische Grundkonstellationen in endogenen Psychosen*. Springer, Berlin.
Karasu B (ed) (1989). *Treatments of Psychiatric Disorders. A Task Force Report of the American Psychiatric Association*. American Psychiatric Association, Washington, DC.
Kendell RE (1975). *The Role of Diagnosis in Psychiatry*. Blackwell, Oxford.
Kendell RE (1985). Which schizophrenia? pp 145–156. In G Huber (ed), *Basisstadien endogener Psychosen und das Borderline-Problem*. Schattauer, Stuttgart.
Klein DF (1964). Delineation of two drug-responsive anxiety syndromes. *Psychopharmacology* 5:397–408.
Klein DF (1989). The pharmacological validation of psychiatric diagnosis, pp 203–214. In LN Robins, JE Barrett (eds), *The Validity of Psychiatric Diagnosis*. Raven, New York.
Klieser E (1990). *Psychopharmakologische Differential therapie endogener Psychosen*. Thieme, Stuttgart.
Kornhuber J, Mack-Burkhardt S, Riederer P, Hebenstreitz GS, Reynolds GP, Andrews HB, Beckmann H (1989). (3H) HK-801 Binding sites in postmortem brain regions of schizophrenic patients. *Journal of Neuralogy Transmitters* 77:2131–2135.
Kretschmer E (1919). Gedanken über die Fortentwicklung der psychiatrischen Systematik. *Zeitschrift Neurologie* 48:370–377.
Meltzer H (ed) (1987). *Psychopharmacology. The third generation of progress*. Raven Press, New York.
Mezzich JE (1988). Structural methodology for designing diagnostic systems, pp 298–305. In JE Mezzich, M von Cranach (eds), *International Classification in Psychiatry: Unity and Diversity*. Cambridge University Press, Cambridge.
Möller HF (1990). Personal communication.
Philipp M, Maier W (1987). *Diagnosesysteme endogener Depressionen*. Springer, Berlin.
Post RM, Rubinow DR, Ballenger JC (1986). Conditioning and sensitization in the longitudinal course of affective illness. *British Journal of Psychiatry* 149: 191–201.

Praag HM, Kahn RS, Asnis GM, Wetzler S, Brown SL, Korn ML (1987). Denosologization of biological psychiatry or the specificity of 5-HT disturbances in psychiatric disorders. *Journal of Affective Disorders* 13:1–8.

Reid WH (1983). *Treatment of the DSM-III Psychiatric Disorders*. Brunner/Mazel, New York.

Robins E, Guze SB (1970). Establishment of diagnostic validity in psychiatric illness: Its application to schizophrenia. *American Journal of Psychiatry* 126: 983–987.

Stieglitz R-D, Fähndrich E, Helmchen H (1988). AMDP in multiaxial classification, pp 180–204. In JE Mezzich, M von Cranach (eds), *International Classification in Psychiatry: Unity and Diversity*. Cambridge University Press, Cambridge.

Stieglitz R-D, Helmchen H (1990). Recent inquiries on standardized assessment and comprehensive diagnosis, pp 71–76. In CN Stefanis, AD Rabavilas, CR Soldatos (eds), *Psychiatry: A World Perspective*, vol 1. Excerpta Medica, Amsterdam.

Zerssen DVV, Pössel J (1990). A case history analysis of the "manic type" and the "melancholic type" of premorbid personality in affectively ill patients. *European Archives of Psychiatry and Neurological Sciences* 239:347–355.

Zohar J, Insel TR (1987). Obsessive-compulsive disorder: Psychobiological approaches to diagnosis, treatment and pathophysiology. *Biology Psychiatry* 22: 667–687.

# 24
# Psychiatric Diagnosis and Mental Health Services in Japan

Kunihiko Asai

Psychiatric care in Japan has emphasized hospitalization. When the Mental Hygiene Law was enacted in 1950, the number of beds occupied by "mentally ill" people was low, at 2 per 10,000 general population in the aftermath of World War II. Following Japan's rapid industrial development beginning in 1951, a nationwide compulsory Health Insurance System was instituted in 1958. The government then decided to increase the number of psychiatric hospitals, and in 1961, to restrict the number of public hospital beds and to promote private hospital beds. These policies brought an increase in the number of private psychiatric beds, which are characteristic of Japanese mental health care (Table 24.1).

Roughly speaking, 350,000 psychiatric patients are treated in 1640 mental hospitals, and nearly 1 million patients are treated on an outpatient basis. As of 1988, the number of psychiatric beds reached a peak of 28 per 10,000 general population. It is important to note that more than 85% of these beds are in the private sector (most of them are incorporated and nonprofit).

In 1965, the Mental Hygiene Law was partially revised to encourage outpatient services and other mental health services at the community level. The revised law provided that each prefecture establish the Prefectural Mental Health Center, and that public financial assistance for the outpatient psychiatric services be established. But, no plan or budget has yet been set forth for community psychiatric care. Although a system of outpatient care has been developed, the percentage of the expenses of the system in ratio to total psychiatric care expenses has stayed the same since 1965. This means that the basic pattern of psychiatric care delivery has not changed and psychiatric hospitals are still the major locus of care in Japan. (Asai 1984, 1991)

TABLE 24.1. Psychiatric hospitals and beds in Japan.

| Type of psychiatric hospital | No. of hospitals (%) | No. of beds (%) |
|---|---|---|
| Private | 1341 (81.8) | 310,868 (88.5) |
| Incorporated (nonprofit) | 977 | 249,256 |
| Private | 364 | 61,612 |
| Governmental | 249 (15.1) | 34,457 (9.8) |
| National | 91 | 9,276 |
| Local governmental | 158 | 25,181 |
| Other (established by Red Cross, etc) | 51 (3.1) | 6,033 (1.7) |
| Total | 1641 | 351,358 |

Source: Ministry of Health and Welfare, June 30, 1988.

## Demographic Data Relevant to Mental Health

The number of patients with long hospitalizations is increasing every year. Now, more than 50% of inpatients have been in the hospital for more than 5 years. The age of hospitalized patients has increased every year and reached a current peak between 45 and 55 years of age. Patients over 65 years of age accounted for 19.6% of all psychiatric patients in 1988.

According to statistics of the Ministry of Health and Welfare in 1987, using ICD-9 (Figure 24.1), in 345,000 hospitalized patients, schizophrenic psychoses top the list at 61.0%, affective psychoses, 4.2%; senile and presenile organic psychotic conditions, 9.3%; neurotic disorders, 6.2%; alcoholic psychoses, 6.0%; mental retardation, 4.4%; epilepsy, 3.5%; and other psychoses, 5.0%. But among outpatients, schizophrenic psychoses decreased to 18.2%, neurotic disorders topped the list at 33.1%, and affective psychoses were at 12.7%.

According to the fact-finding survey of mental health carried out by the Ministry of Health and Welfare in 1983, more than 30% of hospitalized patients could leave hospitals immediately if there were enough social support systems in the community. Actually 60% of all families said that they could not afford to care for discharged patients because support services were lacking (Ministry of Health and Welfare 1988a).

The stigma of mental illness that has been traditionally prevalent in Japanese society still prevails, but seems to have diminished in the last decade.

But even now, some of the diagnoses or labels such as schizophrenia (*Bunretsu-sho*) are inhibitory factors for the rehabilitation of the patients (Asai 1983, 1987).

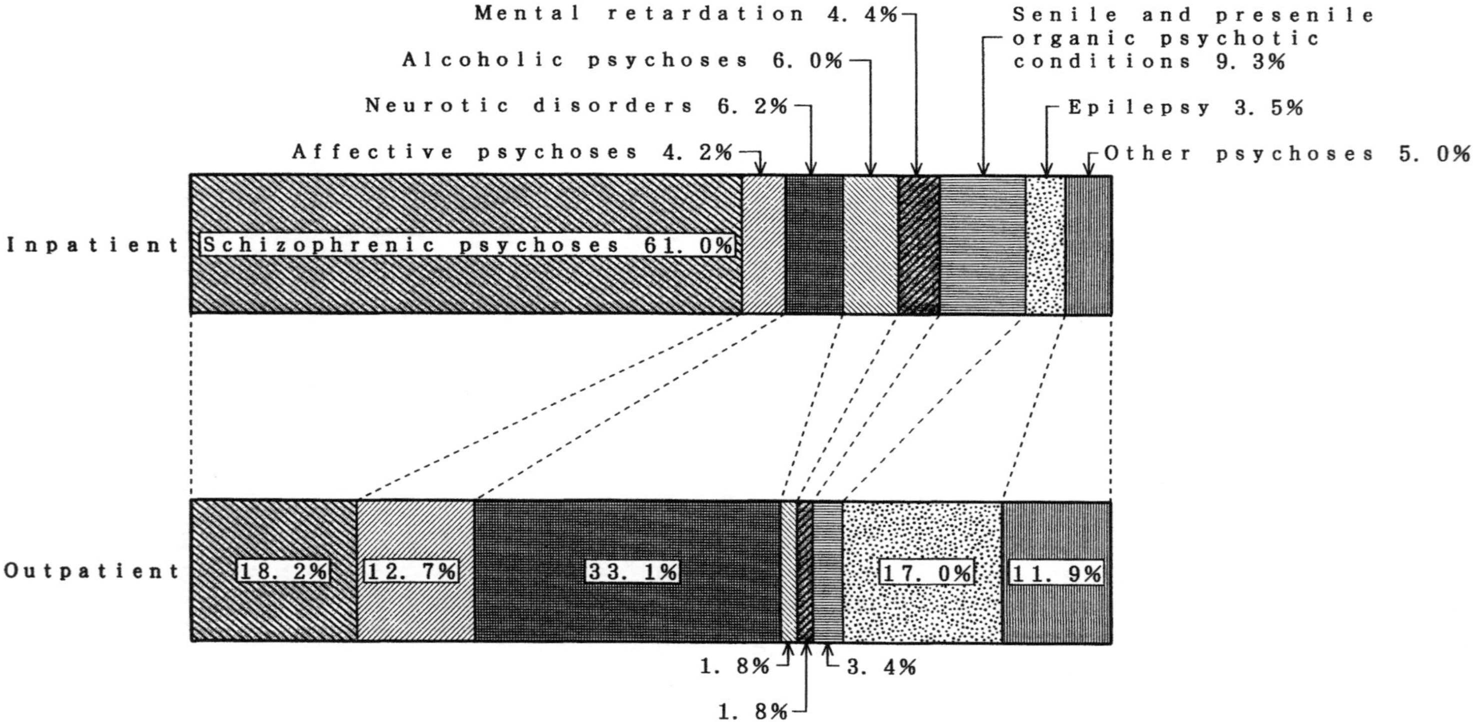


FIGURE 24.1. Distribution of Clinical Diagnosis. (Reprinted with permission from STAT. M.H.W., 1987.)

## Legislation Protecting Patient's Rights

After improper management of inpatients at Utsunomiya Hospital was reported in 1984, there were many protests domestically and internationally, suggesting that mentally ill people in Japan were being subjected to violations of human rights, and this led to the Government of Japan declaring an amendment to the Mental Hygiene Law in August 1985.

There were some confrontations in the course of the investigation between psychiatrists and jurists in reference to the best way to ensure patient's rights. After two years of investigations and discussion, the newly revised Mental Health Law was legislated in 1987, and it has been in operation since July 1988 (Ministry of Health and Welfare 1988).

The basic concepts in the amended Mental Health Law were as follows:

1. The protection of the human rights of the patients.
2. The promotion of social rehabilitation for the mentally disordered persons.
3. The establishment of the Psychiatric Review Board to protect the patient's rights.
4. Principal types of admission, as reformed, are voluntary admission, admission for medical care and custody, involuntary admission by the Prefectural Governor, and emergency admission.
5. The Designated Physician of Mental Health was recently legislated.

After the enforcement of the recently revised Mental Health Law, the newly prescribed voluntary admission already accounts for more than 50 percent of all admissions in 1989. The Psychiatric Review Board reviews the needs for involuntary admission and for its continuation on the basis of regular reports of the patient's condition and requests. More than 200 cases were discharged on the basis of such reviews in 1989.

The new law introduced designated Physicians of Mental Health to make judgments on legal procedures associated with a limitation of human rights.

According to an investigation carried out by the Japanese Association of Psychiatric Hospitals in 1989, 70% of the newly admitted patients were discharged from the hospital within 3 months, 83% within 6 months and 95% left the hospital within 1 year (Japanese Association of Psychiatric Hospitals 1990).

In Japan, community care programs for psychiatric patients have gradually developed since 1970. These community care programs include: (1) Day services at community mental health centers and public health centers (monthly or weekly), (2) day care services in private or public hospitals (but in 1988, in all of Japan, there were only 186 approved day care services [58% of them in private hospitals]), (3) an aid system for employers of ex-mental patients (the only system for vocational rehabilitation for mental patients), (4) small-scale sheltered workshops (almost 500), and (5) community residence programs.

Although day services and the aid system for employers of ex-mental patients are programs of the Japanese government, the sheltered workshops and community residence programs are run either by patient's family associations or by voluntary mental health personnel.

Recently, the national government and local self-governing bodies have given small subsidies to some of the small-scale sheltered workshops. However, there are not enough social support systems in the community to accept hospitalized patients.

The psychiatric rehabilitation system in Japan is extremely underdeveloped compared with psychiatric rehabilitation facilities in other developed countries. Many chronic psychiatric patients hesitate to leave the hospital and live in a community because of the lower cost for psychiatric hospital admission and the lack of rehabilitation facilities.

There are only 44 prefectural community mental health centers and 852 public health centers in Japan. The activities of community mental health services of these public health centers are not well coordinated with psychiatric hospitals in the community.

In terms of rehabilitation, the 1988 law set forth a policy which had been neglected since the 1965 amendment. Psychiatric rehabilitation was included in the purpose of the Law stated in Article 1 and Article 2, which prescribe that the completion and increase of rehabilitation facilities is a duty of national and local governments. The kinds of social rehabilitation facilities for mentally disordered persons, designated under the law are Activities of Daily Living training facilities and Sheltered Workshops.

Day care, small-scale workshop and group homes (by self-help groups or private) have been already started, but they are now in short supply. Therefore, most of the chronic patients in mental hospitals are unable to transfer to the community (Ministry of Health and Welfare 1990).

Schizophrenic psychosis is the most frequent primary diagnosis of mental disorders for admission and outpatient medical care. Most of the programs for social rehabilitation are designed for patients with these psychoses, working toward the idea of normalization.

## Field Trial of ICD-10 Chapter V

In Japan, *The International Classification of Diseases*, 9th revision (ICD-9) (World Health Organization 1977) has been applied for developing official statistics. National mental health policy has largely relied on statistical and epidemiological data. For example, according to these data, the government enforced the Law for the Health of the Aged in 1982 and set the policy of health care, medical care, and welfare measures for the demented elderly. The Ministry of Health and Welfare established a Task Panel for the Demented Elderly in 1986, and the Panel made a report in 1987.

In (1990), the government established a system for financing the treatment and care of elderly patients very similar to the Diagnosis-Related-Groups (DRG) system in the USA. Recently, the Ministry of Health and Welfare started countermeasures against the epidemic of alcoholic psychoses and drug psychoses.

In research settings, most Japanese clinicians now systematically refer to the *Diagnostic and Statistical Manual of Mental Disorders*, 3rd edition (DSM-III) or the revised edition (DSM-III-R). In addition, we have been interested in the ICD-10 Draft of Chapter V. This is because ICD-10 contains many more categories than ICD-9, and a multiaxial system is being prepared. Until now, we have used ICD-9 and DSM-III-R in our usual clinical practice.

In our preliminary study, using the 1988 Draft of ICD-10 Chapter V, Clinical Descriptions and Diagnostic Guidelines, we tried to apply ICD-10 to psychiatric disorders in three populations by 30 clinicians. The first population involved patients who were admitted to Asai Hospital from 1987 to 1989 (Asai Hospital is a private mental hospital located in suburban Tokyo). The second encompassed outpatients who visited Asai Hospital for the first time in 1989. The last involved outpatients who in 1989 visited the Hospital of Tokyo Medical and Dental University (a general hospital in Tokyo).

## Results

1. Frequency of patients by ICD-10 (two-digit category in F code) (Figure 24.2): F2, Schizophrenia, Schizotypal, and Delusional Disorders top the list at 44% among the inpatients of Asai Hospital. But, F2 and F3, Mood Disorders, are almost equal at 23% among the outpatients of Asai Hospital. As for the outpatients of Tokyo Medical and Dental University, F4, Neurotic, Stress-Related, and Somatoform Disorders top the list at 40%; F2, Schizophrenic, 24%; and F3, Mood Disorders, 17%.

2. Frequency of patients by three-digit category in F3 code, Mood Disorders (Figure 24.3): F31, Depressive Episode accounted for 70% of outpatients of Asai Hospital; and for 59% of Tokyo Medical and Dental University. As for the inpatients of Asai Hospital, F31, Depressive Episode accounted for 37%, and F32, Bipolar Affective Episode, 35%.

3. Frequency of patients by four-digit category within the F2 code, Schizophrenia (Figure 24.4): Many research studies in Japan reported that among subcategories of Schizophrenic Psychoses, based on ICD-9, Hebephrenic Type topped the list from 30 to 68%. As can be seen in Figure 24.4, F20.0, Paranoid Schizophrenia tops the list at 45 to 74%, and F20.1, Hebephrenic Schizophrenia is at 9 to 32%.

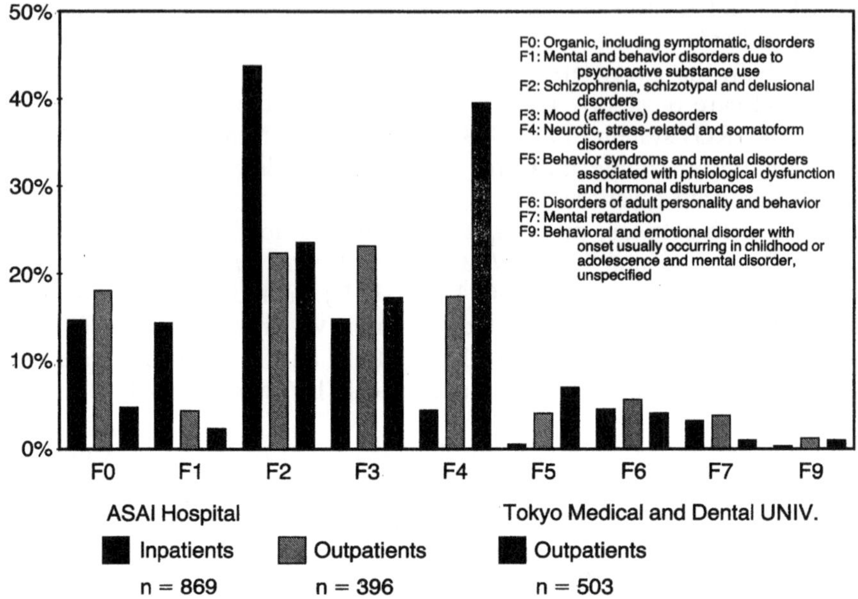


FIGURE 24.2. Frequency of Patients by ICD-10 Two-Digit Categories within the F code.

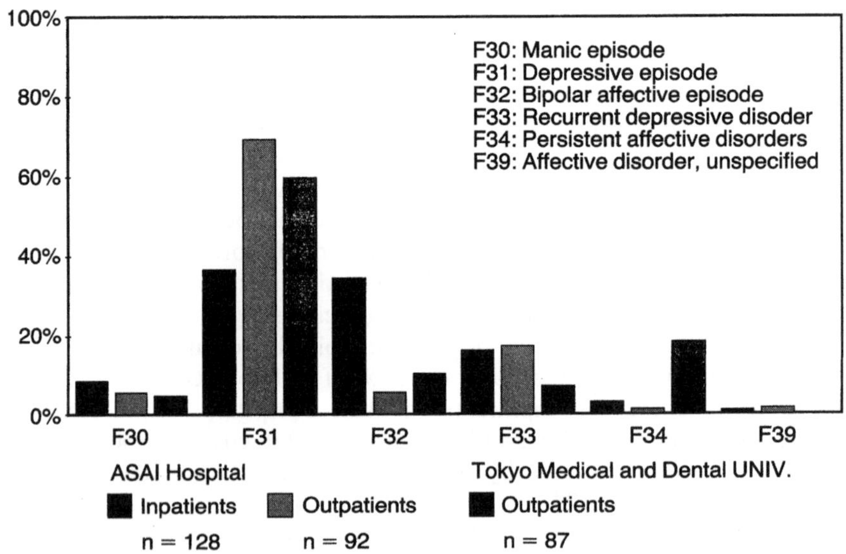


FIGURE 24.3. Frequency of Patients by ICD-10 Three-Digit Categories within the F3* code.

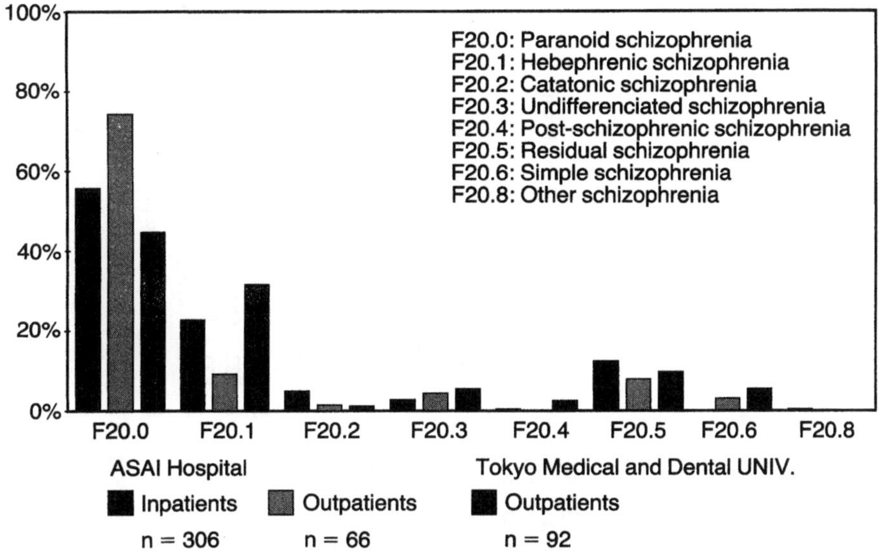


FIGURE 24.4. Frequency of Patients by ICD-10 Four-Digit Categories within the F20* code.

4. Diagnostic conversion of ICD-9 Schizophrenic Psychoses, in ICD-10 F2, Schizophrenic, Schizotypal, and Delusional Disorders (Figure 24.5).

As for the inpatients of Asai Hospital, there were several patients whose diagnosis changed from Hebephrenic Type in ICD-9 to Paranoid Schizophrenia in ICD-10.

Most of the psychiatrists said that the concept of Paranoid Schizophrenia in ICD-10 was broader and that of Hebephrenic was narrower than our conventional concepts.

5. Frequency of patients by three-digit categories within the F4 code, Neurotic, Stress-Related, and Somatoform disorders. F45, Somatoform Disorders accounted for 40% of inpatients of Asai Hospital, and for 26% of outpatients of Tokyo Medical and Dental University. As for the outpatients of Asai Hospital, F43, Reaction to Severe Stress and Adjustment Disorder accounted for 35%; F41, Other Anxiety Disorders was 21%. As for the outpatients at the University, F45, Somatoform Disorders; F41, Other Anxiety Disorders; and F43, Reaction to Severe Stress and Adjustment Disorder together ranged between 26 and 23% (Figure 24.6).

6. Diagnostic conversion of ICD-9, Affective Psychoses, in ICD-10 F3, Mood Disorders. Manic-depressive psychoses branched into many subcategories of ICD-10 (Figure 24.7). I think these subcategories of Mood Disorders of ICD-10 are more complicated for clinical use.

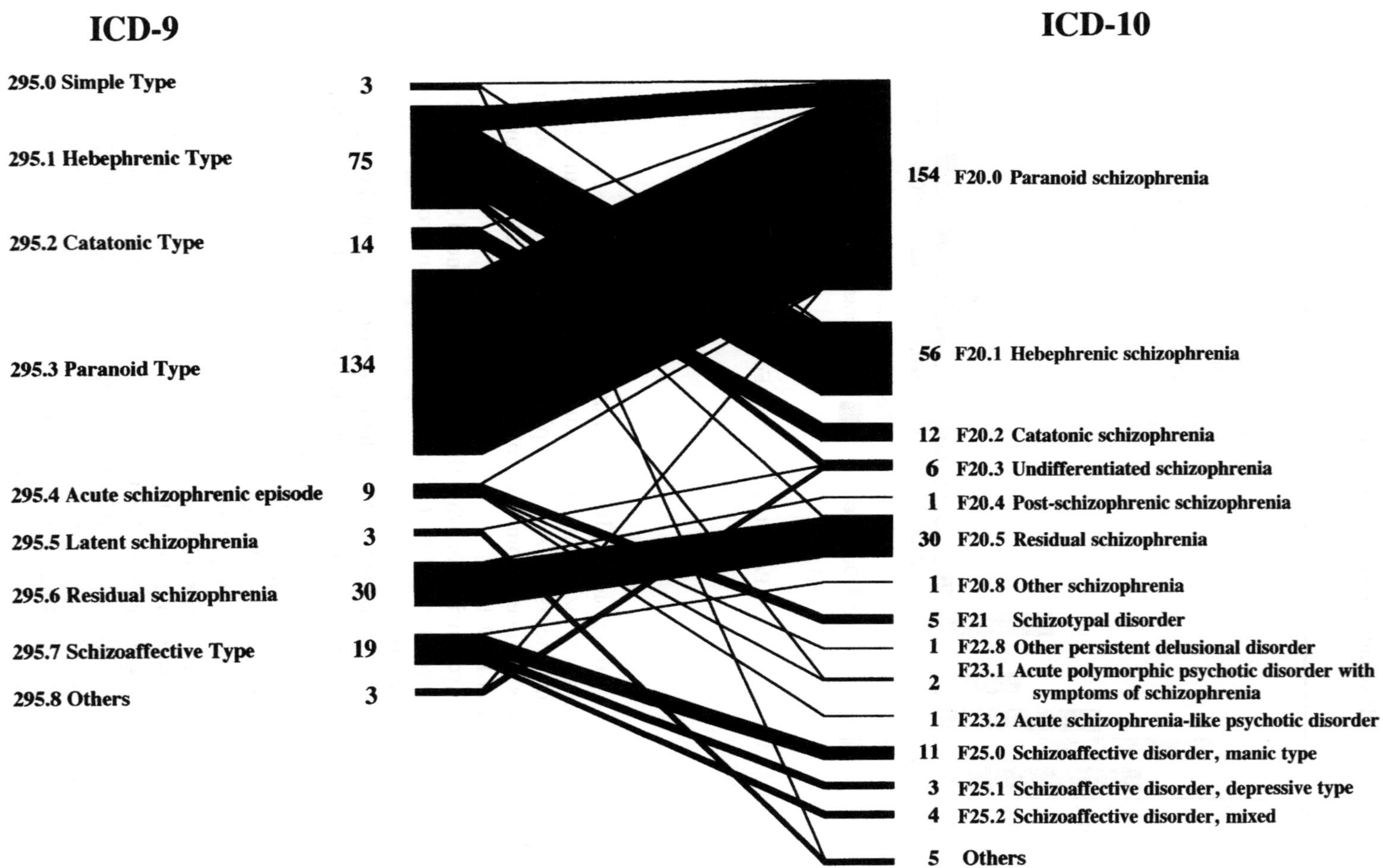


FIGURE 24.5. Changes of diagnosis from ICD-9 to ICD-10 for schizophrenia and related disorders.

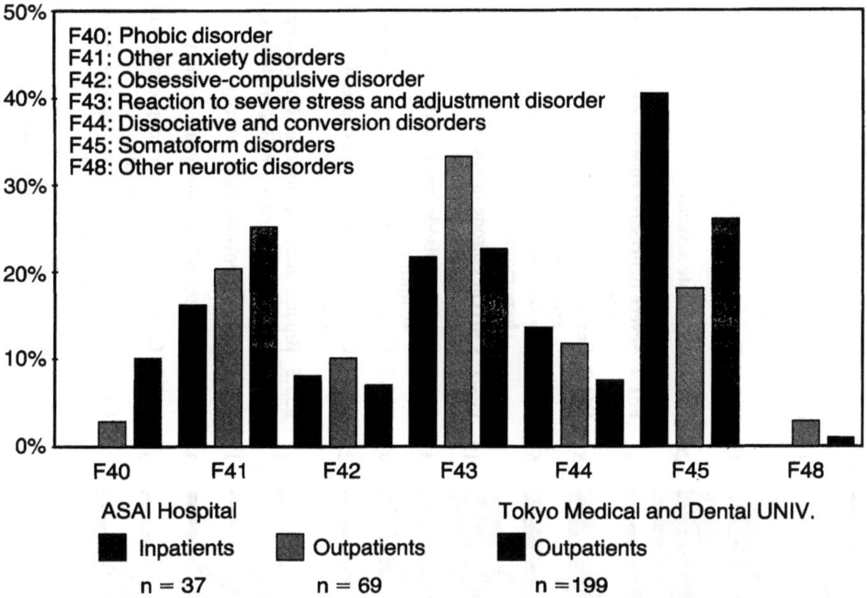


FIGURE 24.6. Frequency of Patients by ICD-10 Three-Digit Categories within the F4* code.

7. Diagnostic conversion of ICD-9, Senile and Presenile Organic Psychotic Conditions to ICD-10 F0, Organic Including Symptomatic Disorders. Dementia, Alzheimer-Type tops the list and Multi-Infarct Vascular Dementia amounts to almost half (Figure 24.8).

As for the assessment of the diagnostic categories by psychiatrists, some difficulties were found in using the same subcategories of F23, Acute and Transient Psychotic Disorders; F25, Schizo-Affective Disorders; F45, Somatoform Disorders; and F60, Specific Personality Disorder.

## Conclusion

ICD-10 Chapter V is very useful not only for clinical practice but also for educational and research purposes. Furthermore, we are expecting that the multiaxial diagnostic system, and a simplified classification for use in primary health care will be completed soon. They should play a very important role as a common language all over the world. A good psychiatric classification should have an effective impact not only in forming mental health policy in Japan but also on management and insurance. There is the hope that deep-rooted, traditional attitudes to

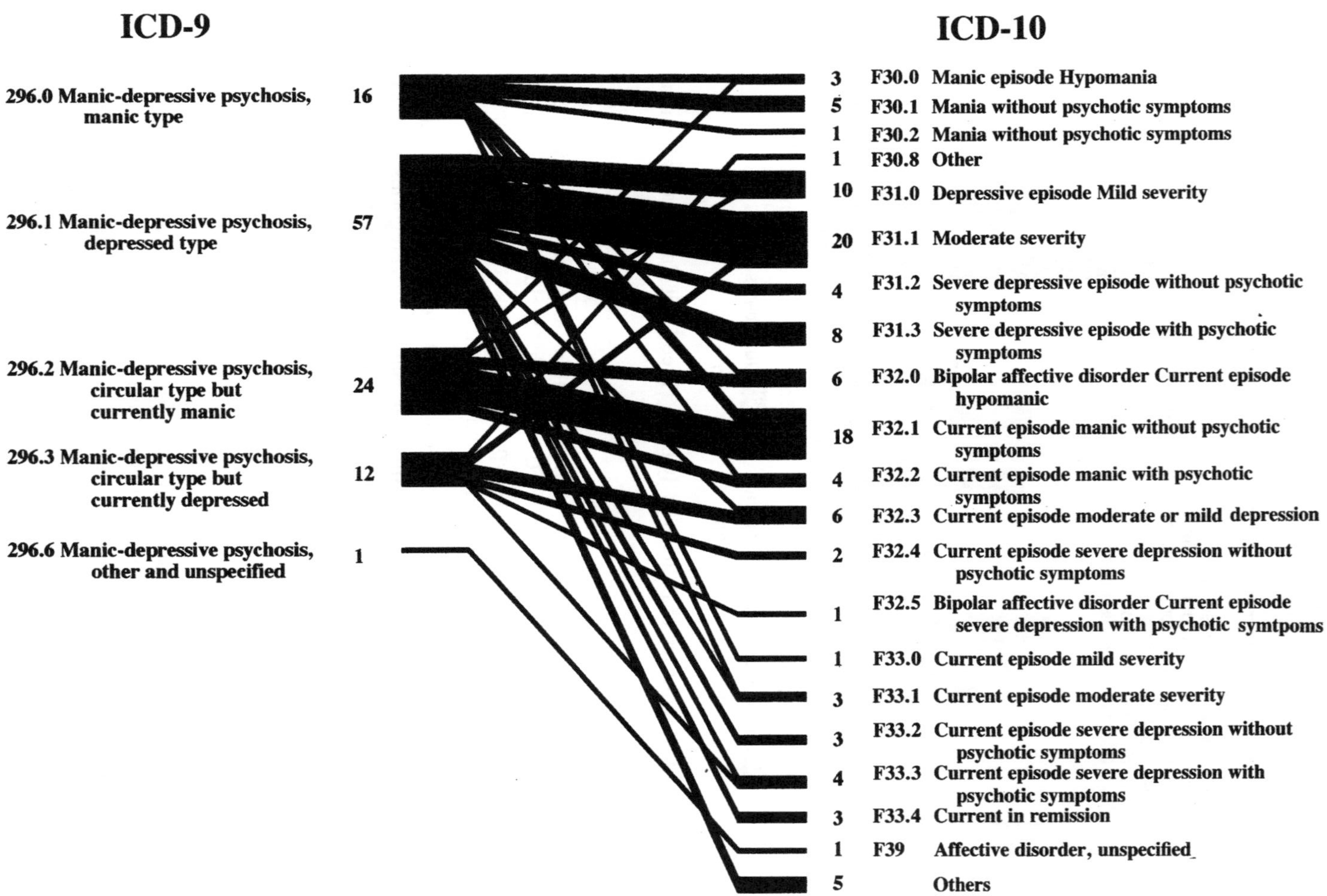

FIGURE 24.7. Changes of diagnosis from ICD-9 manic-depressive psychoses to pertinent ICD-10 categories

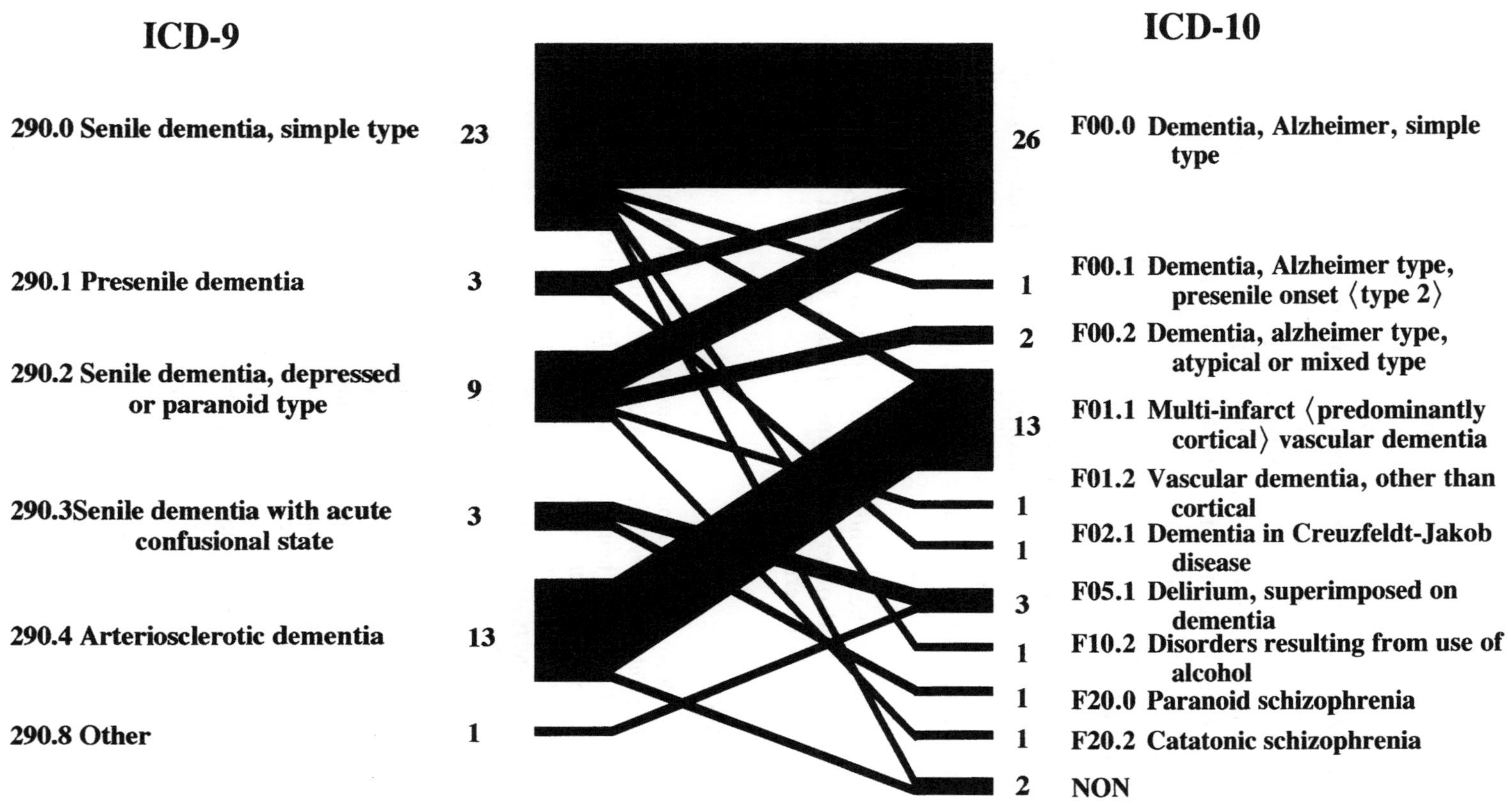


FIGURE 24.8. Changes of diagnosis from ICD-9 dementias to pertinent ICD-10 categories.

mental illness can change if the providers of mental health services demonstrate therapeutic skill and establish a trusting relationship with patients, families, and the community.

Today, Japan needs a community psychiatry system suitable to our culture and social needs. Japan also needs a policy that does not impose a financial burden on those willing to undertake community psychiatric services. Without legislation for financial support, rehabilitation services for former mental patients will almost inevitably incur a heavy deficit.

The Mental Health Law says that the National, Prefectural, and Local Governments shall endeavor to enable mentally disordered persons to adapt themselves to society by expanding and improving the facilities needed for medical care, social rehabilitation, and other welfare purposes and education. But until now, no notable change has been made in the social rehabilitation of mentally disordered persons. Requests need to be made for more subsidies and legal support to promote the rehabilitation and community care of mentally ill people in Japan.

*Acknowledgment.* The author thanks Yoshiro Okubo, MD, Akihiko Watanabe, MD, and other physicians of Asai Hospital and Tokyo Medical and Dental University.

## References

Asai K (1983). Responses of Japanese families to mental disorder. *International Journal of Social Psychiatry* 29:257–263.

Asai K (1984). Pathways of help-seeking of psychiatric patients in Japan. *American Journal of Social Psychiatry* 4:38–44.

Asai K (1987). Schizophrenic patients and their families in Japan. *International Journal of Family Psychiatry* 8:1–7.

Asai K, Takahashi T, Lin T-Y (1991). Mental hospitals as a base for community mental health in Asian cultures. *Keimei Publishing*, Tokyo (in Japanese).

Japanese Association of Psychiatric Hospitals (1990). *Journal of the Japanese Association of Psychiatic Hospitals* 9:12 (in Japanese).

Ministry of Health and Welfare (1988a). National health administration in Japan, vol II. Koken Shuppan, Tokyo (in Japanese).

Ministry of Health and Welfare (1988b). The Mental Health Law. Koken Shuppan, Tokyo (in Japanese).

Ministry of Health and Welfare, Mental Health Division of Health Service Bureau (1990). Koken Shuppan, Tokyo (in Japanese).

World Health Organization (1977). *Manual of the International Classification of Diseases*, 9th Revision (ICD-9). Author, Geneva.

# 25
# Psychiatric Diagnosis and Mental Health Care in Korea

Bou-Yong Rhi

In the history of psychiatry, diagnostic concern has been focused on the psychopathological phenomena shown by individual persons. But what are psychopathological phenomena? As Karl Jaspers pointed out in his *General Psychopathology*, it is extremely difficult to define what is normal and what is not, because, in the realm of the psyche in contrast to that of the physical, this definition is not only concerned with the concept of the average but also with the concept of the norm, the value system (Jaspers 1923).

The nature of some mental illness is too complex to be comprehended with a single diagnostic term without mentioning the personality profile of the patient and the predisposing or contributing factors to the illness. To a certain degree this is also true of some physical illness.

On the other hand, to keep the subjectivity of the examiner away from interfering with the process of diagnosis, the examiner may try to maintain absolute objectivity and rely on his object-directed perception, that is, the function of extroverted sensation among many other specific psychic functions of the examiner (Jung 1960).

During the process, however, the subjective experiences and many other intrapsychic aspects of the person are entirely excluded in the diagnostic system in spite of the clear definition of the objective signs of psychopathology. The diagnostic process should, in my opinion, be integrated with the total personality function of the psychiatrist to reach the best possible understanding of the patient as a whole.

Especially for those psychiatrists who maintain the psychodynamic viewpoint, the classification and labeling of a patient according to one strict external criterion often causes frustration because the diagnostic nomenclature does not satisfactorily explain the patient's intrapsychic states and the individual characteristics of personality problems. Therefore, they frequently rely on another diagnostic system in addition to the official one, namely, the psychological diagnosis or the phenomenological diagnosis.

Psychiatric diagnosis can play a powerful role, especially in the case of a unified international classification, because such a classification is usually regarded as being absolute, and thus is believed to always indicate the same specific treatment.

Inadequate classification, therefore, may restrict the view of mental health care professionals to narrow aspects of the psychic phenomena, which may also lead to one-sided treatment. Good classification and guidelines may be a powerful tool for a comprehensive treatment based upon a comprehensive understanding of the patient.

From these considerations, I assume that there is at present no classification of mental disorders that we can claim to be absolute and complete. With our present knowledge about mental illness, that classification always remains tentative and hypothetical, and it is only based on an agreement among mental health professionals.

The basic philosophy of mental disorders classification shown in the preface of the *International Classification of Diseases*, 10th revision (ICD-10) Draft Chapter V, seems to be quite reasonable although neither perfect nor absolute. The diagnostic guidelines maintained their clarity without being too rigid, and it was also wise to prepare a diagnostic criteria for research in addition to the one for clinical use (World Health Organization 1988).

## The Changing Concept of Mental Illness and Psychiatric Diagnosis

In traditional Korean medicine, there was no discrimination between the mental and the physical disorders, as in the archaic medical principles of other cultures. Classification of illness was based on the empirical observations as well as the theory of Yin and Yang and the five evocative systems. Psyche and soma were regarded as the two aspects of life, and emotional aspect of life was regarded as closely related to physiological function; consequently, there have been numerous descriptions of psychosomatic and somatopsychic syndromes under the heading of *Shim Sang Chung* (hurt heart syndrome) and many other labelings.

The major psychoses manifested by stuporous state, psychotic excitation, or disorganized hallucinatory behavior were designated as *Chun*, *Kwang* and *Sasu* under the chapter of internal medicine category and miscellaneous diseases. Febrile delirious states and various affective disorders have been also identified. The treatment mainly consisted of herbal medicine and accupuncture, but there is evidence of the practice of psychological or behavioral approaches of treatment, which are comparable in their techniques to modern psychotherapy and behavior therapy, respectively (Rhi 1973a, 1973b, 1976, 1986).

It is noteworthy to mention the typological classification of the character traits. The organs and viscera were regarded as the symbolic system indicating psychosomatic concordance, and the constitutional factors were seen to be closely interwoven with the character traits and physiological pattern of the individual. It was on this hypothesis of Chinese medicine that Yi Je Ma, a Korean physician of the early 20th century developed *Sasang Uihak* (Medicine of four Images) and an attempt was made to establish a typological classification of illness/character/physiology interaction.

Along with this medical diagnostic system there have been since early times, the demonologic, religious concept of mental illness and corresponding ways of healing with a shamanistic world view, as well as the theories of illness of Buddhism, Taoism, and more recently, Christianity. A certain dissociative and hallucinatory excitation with or without somatic disturbances was regarded in Korean shamanism as the signs of a call for initiation, as in universal shamanistic folk custom. Apart from this teleological view of mental illness in religious cultures, the major cause of mental disorders has been attributed to demonic possession as the result of a breach of taboo (Rhi 1983, Kim 1972).

With the introduction of Western medicine in the late 19th century into Korea, modern concepts of mental disorders also began to be introduced. The major trends of Korean psychiatry remained a Kraepelinian descriptive one until the late 1950s. After the Korean War, however, American psychiatry began to influence Korean psychiatrists. It was in the late 1950s that modern clinical psychiatry was actively taught in medical schools and that Adolf Meyer's dynamic psychiatry and psychoanalytic concepts became popular. At the same time the American Psychiatric Association's classification of mental disorders was introduced for the first time, according to which the majority of mental illness were regarded as "reactions" of the personality. The *Diagnostic and Statistical Manual of Mental Disorders* (DSM) from its first edition through the current revised third edition (DSM-III-R) (American Psychiatric Association 1980) has been cautiously followed by Korean psychiatrists and was introduced in psychiatric education for medical students and psychiatric residents.

Since the introduction of the residency training system and specialist board from the United States in the 1960s, the DSM classifications have been the subject of specialty board examinations. Nevertheless, the World Health Organization's *International Classification of Diseases* has always been the official criteria of classification for the psychiatric record and statistical use by the Korean government and hospitals.

## The Impact of Psychiatric Diagnosis on Mental Health Care

In contrast to the concern of Korean psychiatrists in training hospitals with the international classification of mental disorders and DSM classification, and in spite of the official request of the government to use the 9th revision of the ICD (ICD-9) for the medical record, the actual application of these systems for mental patients by the nonpsychiatric physician seems to be quite poor.

According to a recent survey on the opinion of 75 nonpsychiatric physicians who referred their patients for psychiatric consultation to a hospital of tertiary care, it has been revealed that the majority (93.3%) experienced difficulties in psychiatric diagnosis due to a lack of knowledge and experience about psychiatric classification. Among 56 respondents, 82.1% answered that they use ICD-9 when asked about the use of any diagnostic criteria. But 70.3% answered that they are used to describing problems instead of using any official nomenclature system in their referral sheet. And 41.3% of the respondents said that they absolutely need simpler and more appropriate classification for primary care, whereas 50.7% regarded it as being not that urgent although they admitted the necessity of such a classification. ICPC (International Classification of Primary Care) (Lamberts and Wood 1987) was used only in 1.8% of the group (Rhi et al 1990).

Public health physicians, who are obliged to work for a period of time (instead of military services) at rural health centers after graduation from medical school, have great difficulties, according to a recent survey, in diagnosing mentally ill patients. And their scope of knowledge of the classification was restricted to less than 10 names of mental disorders.

The medical insurance system introduced in the 1970s, urged every Korean physician to apply ICD code in their practice, but in reality, the tight budget in medical insurance allocated to psychiatric treatment and condition of payment for mental disorders can influence the physician in private practice. For example, nonpsychiatric physicians tend to prefer physical diagnoses to psychogenic ones when they request insurance because they cannot request fees for psychotherapy.

Psychiatric diagnosis holds imperative importance in legal situations involving the mentally ill who, by the law of social protection in Korea, must receive custodial treatment instead of punishment. But, the legal terminology in Civil Law indicating feeblemindedness (*Shim shin mo yak*) and loss of mind (*Shim shin sang shil*) is far from the scope of modern concepts of mental status.

National health policy largely relies on the epidemiological data of mental disorder. The type of measuring tools and the underlying classification system may enormously influence the results of the investigation and, inevitably, the mental health policy as well. Recent data on the prevalence of alcohol abuse in Korea was surprisingly high according to the Diagnostic Interview Schedules (DIS) when compared to previous data. This can be partly attributed to the ways of asking about alcohol use according to specific diagnostic tools (Lee et al 1987a, 1987b).

In reality, however, the Korean situation in mental health care does not seem to be much affected by the system of psychiatric diagnosis. The crucial element in mental health care seems to be not diagnostic classification but the basic philosophy underlying the efforts of classification and the attitude of the psychiatrist toward the mentally ill patient during the diagnostic process.

Especially for the layperson, the difficult nomenclature of mental illness and the ring of such terms as Schizophrenia are rather strange and threatening. They seem to prefer terms like *shin gyong song* (neurogenic) to indicate psychophysiological disturbances, or terms like neurosis, stress, or *hwa byung* (rage reaction), to academic terms.

Most Koreans are willing to help sick people with opinions and advice for health and their own prescriptions of treatment; they also have a tendency to use every possible healing method and remedy, ranging from archaic religious healing or herbal medicine to very modern psychiatric treatment, though the majority of the population are well aware of modern Western concepts of mental illness and treatment (Kim 1983, Kim et al 1989).

Although the prevailing tendency in health-seeking patterns of mental patients and their families was a combined one of multiple healing remedies (Chung et al 1975, Rhi et al 1989), the concept of mental illness and the attitudes of the laypeople toward mental illness are gradually changing from nonscientific to scientific (Kim 1983, Kim et al 1988, Lee 1988a).

According to the studies using vignettes of the attitudes of community leaders toward mental disorders, differences were found in their opinions about the severity, cause, and treatment of mental disorder among Protestant ministers, Roman Catholic priests, Buddhist monks, shamanistic healers, the families of the patients, and medical and nursing students. The opinions of Roman Catholic priests and community leaders were the most scientific and closest to the modern psychiatrist's concept, whereas other groups were inclined to appreciate religious concepts of disease and healing. Shamanistic healers were much more optimistic about the prognosis of psychotic cases than the others (Rhi and Lee 1988, Son and Rhi 1983). There was, however, one common tendency in those studies: The more educated respondents were in psychiatry, the more pessimistic they were about the outcome of psychotic disorders (Ahn et al 1986, Lee et al 1988a). We must ask whether such an attitude will be favorable for the treatment of psychotic patients.

## Academic Interest in Psychiatric Diagnosis and Classification

As for the academic interest of Korean psychiatrists in the classification of mental disorders, one should mention the first symposium on DSM-III held by the Korean Neuropsychiatric Association in 1983. The aim of that symposium was to review DSM-III and to compare it with the classification system of German psychiatry in the hope of drafting a Korean model of classification (Rhi 1983, Kim 1983, Lee 1983).

One cannot claim that systematic research in nosology has been active in Korea. Only sporadic efforts have been made in published articles on studies of illness such as schizophrenia, affective disorders, and organic brain syndromes (Oh 1977, Hahn 1979). Some folk designation of several syndromes as shaman diseases (also called *Mu Byung* or *Shin Byung*) and a folkloristic illness, *Hwa Byung*, have been the object of study in an effort to find out if there is any culture-specific syndrome in Korea (Rhi and Kwon 1986, Kim 1972, Min et al 1986). But these proved to be either a psychophysical symptom complex of various origins for the common purpose of initiation or merely the culture-specific designation for a known disorder that can be defined according to the current classification system.

Social phobia recently became the focus of academic discussion and was a main theme at the East Asian Academy of Cultural Psychiatry organized as the first joint academic meeting between Japan and Korea (Rhi and Kim 1984).

A preliminary study on ICD-10 Draft Chapter V (1986 version) was published in 1988 (Lee et al 1988b), and a renewed interest in developing a Korean model of classification has arisen.

A group of investigators was recently organized in Korea for an extensive, nationwide study on ICD-10 Draft Chapter V as well as on Diagnostic Criteria for Research. And the Korean Society for Psychopathology and Psychiatric Classification has also recently been founded.

## Conclusion

Psychiatric classification and diagnostic process inevitably elicit several problems that should be seriously taken into consideration, as mentioned in the introduction of this chapter. The reason for this lies first of all in our lack of complete knowledge of the complex nature of many mental disorders. In comparison with physical illness, mental disorders should be regarded as a total reaction of personality in its biopsychosociocultural aspects and thus, the understanding of the phenomena cannot be complete if the subjective experiences of the individual patient are not considered as well as objective manifestations of the illness.

Historical review of the concept of mental disorders and their classification in Korea has shown the unique philosophy of classification adopted by traditional medicine. This we may designate as a symbolic and typologic system of diagnosis based on the principles of psychophysical parallelism. In religious, particularly shamanistic concepts of mental illness, we have also noted the teleological viewpoint of a certain mental disorder.

The historical changes from DSM-I to DSM-III-R also reflect changing patterns in the concept of mental disorders and philosophy of classification—the interaction between the dynamic psychiatric standpoint and the descriptive one. All of these underlying viewpoints for psychiatric classification should be carefully examined without hastily abandoning the old one for the sake of the "new" classification.

In spite of the official use of international classification in Korea and the deep concern of Korean psychiatrists with DSM, these psychiatric classifications are not much used by nonpsychiatric physicians. Laypeople seem to prefer simpler terms for mental conditions and they show more of a tendency toward the folk concept of mental illness.

The reason why the official classification of mental disorders does not enjoy popularity among nonpsychiatric physicians and laypeople can be drawn from several possible factors. The classification is too complicated and contains too many categories to be comprehended by nonpsychiatric physicians and laypeople. The diagnostic classification for mental disorders has less immediate usefulness in deciding specific treatment by users than that of physical disorders, due partly to the lack of explanation about the nature of illness and prognosis. Furthermore, the classification is sometimes used carelessly even by psychiatric specialists because the nomenclature does not fit into the condition of patient and personality as a whole. This may be due partly to the lack of modern mental health education for nonpsychiatric physicians and laypeople, or due to their traditional or folkloristic ways of looking at mental illness. We may ask, "Why should we have such a large number of illnesses and disorders?" paradoxically when the whole picture of a person can be lost while wandering in an enigmatic castle of disorders.

A Korean proverb says, To know too much is illness (*Anun koshi tarida*). It apparently is rooted in the term *wuwei* of Lao-tzu, the famous Chinese sage. However, in making an ideal classification of mental disorders using our best knowledge, we have to accept the limitations of our knowledge, and should be cautious not to injure the humanity of the patient with our intellectual arrogance. At the same time, along with the academic search for the ultimate nature of mental illness, we should continue developing more appropriate classifications of mental disorders without being contaminated by commerciality, nationalistic ambition, and political or diplomatic influences. ICD-10 Chapter V (World Health Organization 1992) is a step toward this ideal goal. The recent organization of the Korean Society for Psychopathology and Psychiatric Classification and the systematic investigation of ICD-10 in Korea will contribute to international collaboration and further development of the field.

## References

Ahn DH, Rhi BY (1986). Community leaders' reactions to mental disorders. *Seoul Journal of Psychiatry* 11(4):281–297.

American Psychiatric Association (1980). *Diagnostic and Statistical Manual of Mental Disorders* (3rd ed). American Psychiatric Association, Washington, DC.

Chung KC, Rhi BY (1975). The attitudes of rural people toward the folk treatment—A sociopsychiatric study of rural society in Korea (V). *Neuropsychiatry* 14:405–416.

Hahn HM (1979). Classification of organic brain syndromes. *New Medical Journal* 22(11):18–22.

Jaspers K (1923). *General Psychopathology* (J Hoenig and Marian W Hamilton, trans). Manchester University Press, Manchester.

Jung CG (1960). *Psychologische Typen.* Gesammelte Werke Bd. 6. Rascher, Zürich.

Kim JS, Kim YS, Ha KS, Yang IH, Rhi BY (1989). The attitudes of psychiatric patients' families toward mental disorder. *Seoul Journal of Psychiatry* 14(2): 71–87.

Kim KI (1972). *Shin byung*: A culture-bound depersonalization syndrome. *Journal of the Korean Neuropsychiatric Association* 11:223–234.

Kim KI (1983). Classification of mental disorder: Theoretical and practical problems. *Journal of the Korean Neuropsychiatric Association* 22(4):9–18 (suppl).

Kim KI (1984). Clinical study of phobic disorder. *Mental Health Research* 11: 110–135.

Kim YS, Hong IK, Yang IH, Kim CY, Ha KS, Rhi BY (1988). A preliminary study of attitudes toward mental illness. *Seoul Journal of Psychiatry* 13(1): 27–36.

Lamberts H, Wood M (1987). *International Classification of Primary Care (ICPC).* Oxford University Press, Oxford.

Lee CK, Han JH, Choi JO (1987b). The epidemiological study of mental disorders in Korea (IX)—Alcoholism, anxiety and depression. *Seoul Journal of Psychiatry* 12(4):183–191.

Lee CK, Kwak YS, Rhee H, Kim YS, Han JH (1987a). The nationwide epidemiological study of mental disorders in Korea. *Journal of Korean Medical Science* 2(1):19–34.

Lee CY, Kim YS, Rhi BY (1988a). The effect of psychiatric education upon the attitudes toward mental disorder. *Journal of the Korean Neuropsychiatric Association* 27(1):96–107.

Lee HY, Chung YK, Lee MH, Min SK, Oh BH, Kim BW, Shin SC (1988b). A preliminary study on the classification of mental disorders in ICD-10: Focused on the goodness of fit and diagnostic reliability of major diagnostic categories in ICD-10. *Journal of the Korean Neuropsychiatric Association* 28(1):67–77.

Lee SH (1983). Diagnostic classification of mental illness in Korea. *Journal of the Korean Neuropsychiatric Association* 22(4):30–34 (suppl).

Min SK, Lee MH, Shin JH, Park MH, Kim MK, Lee HY (1986). A diagnostic study on *hwa byung*. *Journal of the Korean Medical Association* 29(6):653–661.

Oh SW (1977). A study on the diagnosis of schizophrenia. *Journal of Busan Medical College* 17(2):167–177.

Rhi BY (1973a). A preliminary study on the medical acculturation problems in Korea. *Neuropsychiatry* 12:97–109.

Rhi BY (1973b). The concept of mental illness according to *Dong-Ui Bo-Gam*—A Korean text of Oriental medicine from the 17th century. *New Medical Journal* 16:1–7.

Rhi BY (1976). On the treatment of mental disorders in the book of Korean medicine, *Dong-Ui Bo-Gam*, with special reference to the 5 examples of psychological treatment. *Neuropsychiatry* 15:20–27.

Rhi BY (1983). Classification of mental disorders—A historical review. *Journal of the Korean Neuropsychiatric Association* 22(4):3–7 (suppl).

Rhi BY (1986). Pathogenesis of mental illness in traditional korean medicine, pp 93–112. In Grawa T (ed), *History of Pathology*. Taniguchi Foundation, Tokyo.

Rhi BY, Kim SA, Lee SI (1990). Patterns of psychiatric diagnoses and opinions about classification of mental disorders in neuropsychiatrist physicians. *Seoul Journal of Psychiatry* 15(3):191–203.

Rhi BY, Kwon TS (1986). The shamanistic healers' reactions to mental disorders in the southern area of Seoul. *Seoul Journal of Psychiatry* 11(4):298–314.

Rhi BY, Lee JH, Kim SA (1989). A preliminary study about health—care-seeking behavior of psychiatric patients. *Journal of Korean Neuropsychiatric Association* 28(2):307–323.

Rhi BY, Lee NM (1988). The opinions and responses of three religious groups to mental disorders. *Journal of the Korean Neuropsychiatric Association* 27(2): 333–345.

Son JW, Rhi BY (1983). Opinions of Protestant pastors and Catholic fathers about the cause and treatment of the mental illness. *Neuropsychiatry* 22:57–66.

World Health Organization (1988). *International Classification of Diseases* (10th rev), 1988 Draft of Chapter V Categories F00–F99. World Health Organization, Geneva.

World Health Organization (1992). *ICD-10 Classification of Mental and Behavioral Disorders*. World Health Organization, Geneva.

# Part V
# Psychiatric Classification and Primary Care Around the World

# 26
# Simplified Versions of ICD-10 Chapter V(F) for Primary and General Medical Care

JOHN E. COOPER

The World Health Organization (WHO) has now completed the first stages of work on the new revision of Chapter V(F), "Mental and Behavioral Disorders (including disorders of psychological development)" of the *International Classification of Diseases*, 10th revision (ICD-10). It is the policy of the Division of Mental Health of WHO Geneva to provide different versions of this new classification for different purposes because the various users do not all have the same requirements in terms of the number of diagnostic categories and amount of detail. The WHO has to take a worldwide view of the needs of health workers of different types for ways of describing and recording psychiatric disorders, and in this context, the production of short and simple versions of ICD-V(F) for use in primary and general health care by health workers who are not trained as psychiatrists is of great importance.

This chapter describes the beginnings of work on such simplified versions of ICD-10 V(F), with health workers who may have had only brief training courses kept very much in mind. The status of the draft classifications and associated management flowcharts that are described here is that they are suggestions that will be put to the Division of Mental Health of WHO Geneva for consideration and possible development.

The work setting for which these short versions of the new classification are designed dictates that they must be reasonably quick and easy to use. They must have properties such as the following:

1. Brevity: They must contain a much smaller number of diagnostic categories than the version designed for psychiatrists (Clinical Diagnostic Guidelines).
2. Ease of understanding: It should be possible to comprehend the whole of the short classification at a glance.
3. Use of familiar terms: Knowledge of recent research or new fashions in terminology should not be required.

4. Attractiveness: A user should be able to see at once some benefit from the use of the classification, such as help in the management of the patient.

Two levels of the classification are envisaged: First, at an intermediate level suitable for use by any type of physician (with undergraduate but not postgraduate psychiatric experience), and second, at a simple level suitable for any mental health worker (with a professional but not medical training). It is the second and most simple classification of seven categories that is the main subject of discussion in this chapter.

From the start, the aim has been to try to ensure that the classification be presented in a way that will engage the interest of the users. There is little prospect of a classification being used by busy health care workers unless they can see some advantage in its use. The approach described here is to present the classification for use as a set of simple questions whose answers are related to unavoidable issues of management (and which can also be related to management flowcharts already in the literature for primary health care workers (Essex and Gosling 1982)).

It must also be remembered that only a provisional categorization of a patient can be expected from the decisions to be described. Provisional, probable, or temporary diagnoses expressed in broad—and therefore often not well-defined—groups are all that is required. What follows assumes that any physical disorder present has already been identified, or that any necessary physical investigations have already been arranged.

An overview of the content of both ICD-10 V(F) and *Diagnostic and Statistical Manual of Mental Disorders*, 3rd edition, revised (DSM-III-R) (American Psychiatric Association 1987) suggests that both these classifications contain about 16 or 17 major groups of disorders that are clinically familiar and, therefore, likely to be acceptable and useful. Table 26.1, column A, shows this list, which is the starting point for what follows. Examination of this list with the likely knowledge and experience of different types of primary and general health care workers in mind has produced the two levels of condensation shown in columns B and C. (It should be noted that epilepsy is not included as a psychiatric disorder in these lists. For countries where most epileptics are treated by psychiatrists, epilepsy needs to be added.)

This arrangement of diagnostic categories contains only one exception to the important principle of keeping the shorter forms of Chapter V(F) compatible with the full version (it is important because it involves a common disorder). To anyone familiar with problems of psychiatric classification, it is a predictable exception, involving the less-severe varieties of depressive disorder (or depressive neuroses). From the point of view of primary care, in particular, it is easier for the users to separate these from the severe affective disorders and to put them in the same group as anxiety and physical complaint disorders.

TABLE 26.1. Major groups of disorders, based on ICD-10 V(F) and DSM-III-R.

| A | B | C |
|---|---|---|
| 1. Dementias<br>2. Delirium and other symptomatic disorders | 1. Organic disorders<br>a. Dementia<br>b. Delirium | 1. Organic mental disorders |
| 3. Alcohol } Acute intoxication<br>4. Drugs } and dependence | 2. Alcohol and drug intoxication and dependence | 2. Alcohol and drug intoxication and dependence |
| 5. Schizophrenic disorders<br>6. Paranoid, acute and other psychotic disorders | 3. Schizophrenia and paranoid disorders | |
| 7. Affective (mood) disorders | 4. Severe affective disorders<br>a. Mania<br>b. Psychotic depression | 3. Severe (psychotic mental disorder) |
| 8. Neurotic (anxiety) disorders<br>9. Somatoform disorders<br>10. Psychophysiological disorders<br>11. Stress and adjustment disorders | 5. Neurotic disorders<br>a. Neurotic depression<br>b. Anxiety and phobic disorders<br>c. Physical complaint disorders<br>d. Adjustment and stress disorders<br>e. Eating disorders | |
| 12. Adult personality disorders<br>13. Other behavior and impulse disorders of adults | 6. Adult personality disorders | 4. Neurotic, stress-related and personality disorders |
| 14. Disorders of childhood and adolescence<br>15. Developmental disorders | 7. Disorders of childhood, adolescence and development | 5. Disorders of childhood, adolescence and development |
| 16. Mental retardation | 8. Mental retardation | 6. Mental Retardation |
| 17. No psychiatric disorder | 9. No psychiatric disorder | 7. No psychiatric disorder |

TABLE 26.2. Short classification.

| | |
|---|---|
| 1. Disorders of childhood, adolescence and development | |
| 2. Mental retardation | child<br>adult |
| 3. Acute intoxication with | alcohol<br>drugs |
| 4. Organic mental disorder | dementia<br>delirium |
| 5. Severe (psychotic) mental disorder | |
| 6. Dependence on | alcohol<br>drugs |
| 7. Neurotic personality and stress disorders | |
| 8. No psychiatric diagnosis: Go to problem list | |

## The Short Classification

Table 26.2 shows the categories in the short classification, derived from column C of Table 26.1 with only slight modifications, and Table 26.3 shows the questions that are required to arrive at them. Figure 26.1 shows part of the decision tree on which the classification is based. It is necessary to develop a decision tree, to give the best sequence of questions for the management charts, and to form the basis of any computer programs that may be developed as an aid to data analysis. Because of the importance of problems related to alcohol and drugs as a public health problem in many countries, both intoxication and dependence have been highlighted even in this short classification.

For some of the more important decision points, a summary of guidelines and especially important clinical observations is required and can be provided most conveniently for the primary health care worker in the form of a series of charts. Figure 26.2 is an example of such a chart; it is of convenient A4 size, with clear and simple statements that cover both the likely diagnosis from the short classification and important reminders.

TABLE 26.3. Questions for short classification.

1. Child, adolescent, or adult?
2. Have current problems occurred after a period
    1. of normal development in childhood?
    2. of normal adult behavior and activities?
3. Is there a cognitive disturbance? (see Figure 26.1)
4. Is there evidence of recent excess alcohol or drugs (see Figure 26.1)
5. Does patient hold incredible beliefs, or see or hear things others cannot, or have persistent strange acts?
6. Is patient distressed, weepy, anxious, or are there persistent physical complaints without physical disorder?

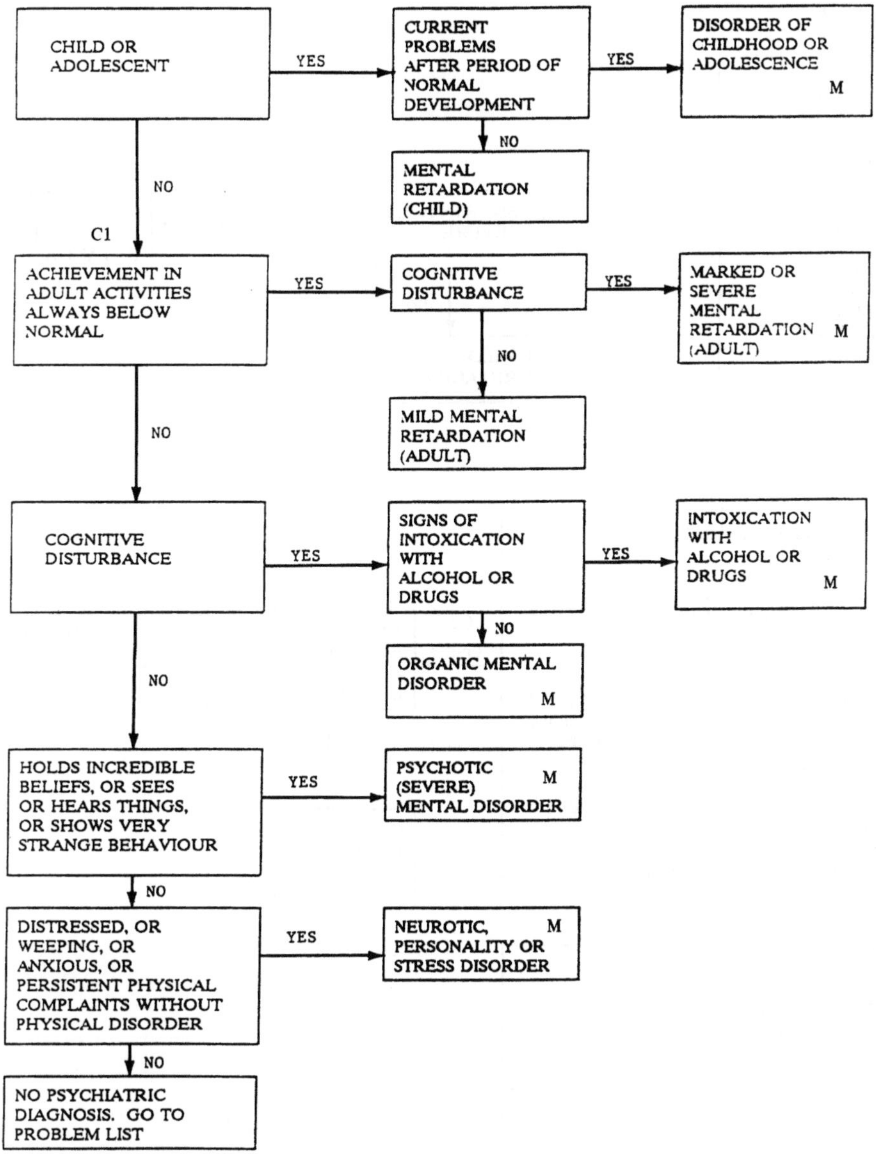


FIGURE 26.1. Decision tree for use with short classification.

For instance, the chart shown in Figure 26.2 labelled as C1 is used at the decision point marked C1 on Figure 26.1 to assess the presence of a cognitive disturbance. If the decision is that a cognitive disturbance is present, then chart C2, shown in Figure 26.3, gives further guidance about the assessment of intoxication by drugs or alcohol.

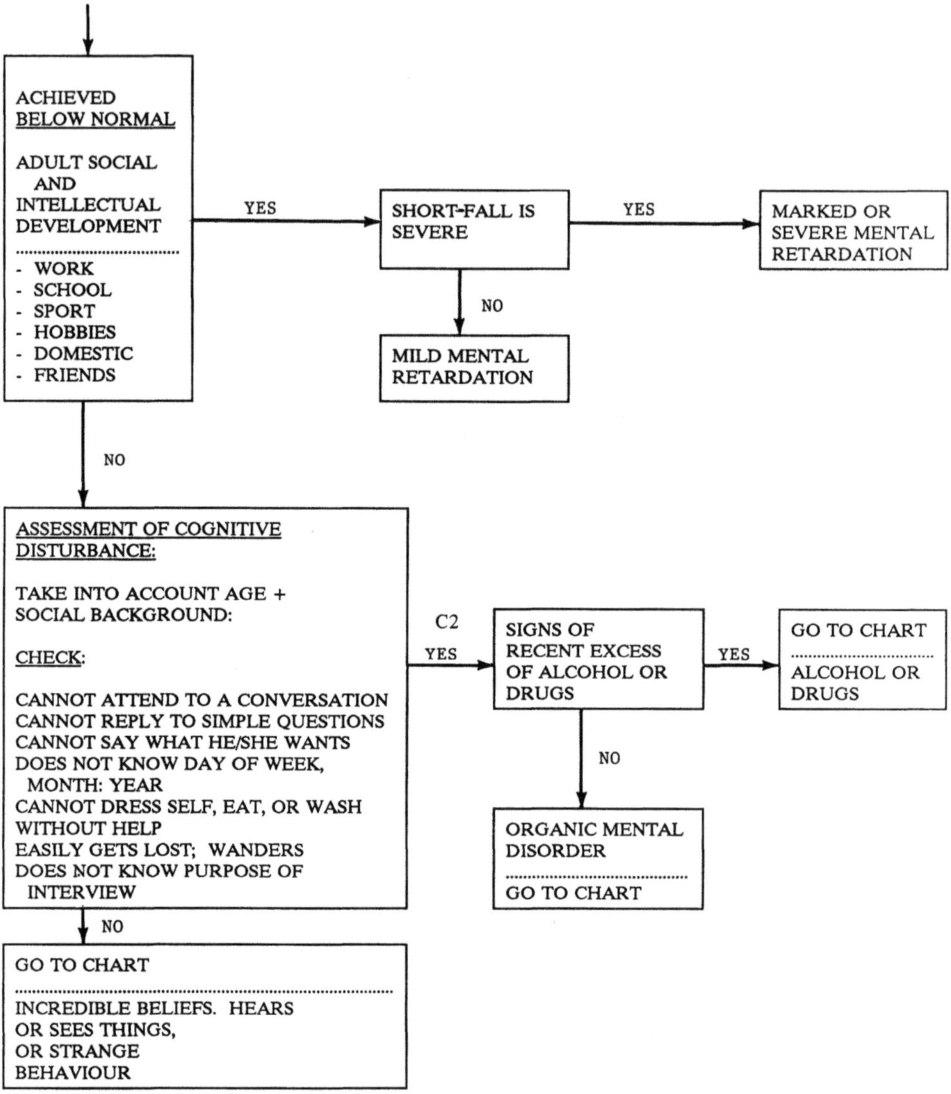


FIGURE 26.2. Example of flowchart (C1).

Depending on the amount of detailed guidance required by the health worker in a particular work setting in which this system is being used, a further set of more detailed management charts could also be provided at points marked M on Figure 26.1.

To cover the main decision points in this short classification, a total of six charts is needed. The number of additional management charts that come into use after a diagnostic decision has been made is optional, and

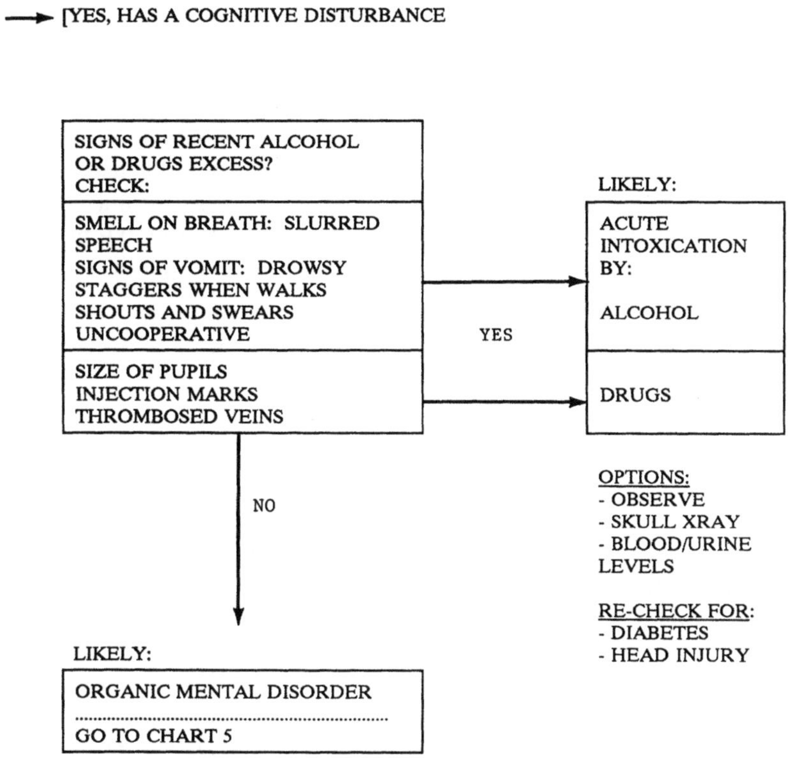


FIGURE 26.3. Flowchart for use in assessment of intoxication (C2).

so is the level of detail at which they can be provided. It is worth noting again that this whole approach is designed with health workers in mind who may have comparatively little detailed information available and only a short time with each patient. Psychiatrists who are accustomed to being provided with a great deal of information and plenty of time in which to interview and decide about the patient are likely to be unfamiliar with this way of working.

The use of management flowcharts or decision trees as guidance for primary health care workers is, of course, not a new suggestion. A similar approach to the one described here was adopted by Essex and Gosling (1982) in their collaborative work with the WHO, where their main aim was to work toward management from "mode of presentation." The eight types of presentation that are the starting point for their management charts are (1) violence to others, (2) violence to self, (3) delusions and hallucinations, (4) withdrawal, (5) abnormal speech, (6) overactivity or unusual behavior, (7) anxiousness, and (8) depression.

However, there is a difference of emphasis in that the decision trees of Essex and Gosling give greater emphasis to the presentation of physical disorders than those described here. In spite of this, an examination of the charts of Essex and Gosling shows that a statement about the likely diagnosis on the short classification can be inserted quite easily at a number of decision points.

At this stage in the development of the short classification, it remains to be seen which of the two approaches will be the more useful. It may well be advantageous to develop two options because primary care and general health care work settings vary considerably in the extent to which the health workers can assume that important physical disorders have already been identified and treated.

## An Intermediate Classification

The seven-category short classification derived from ICD-10 and DSM-III-R is envisaged as suitable for use by primary health care workers who are not qualified as doctors or clinical psychologists. For health professionals with an extensive medical or psychological training, although not a specifically psychiatric one, a classification somewhere between the 16 major categories of the full classification and the 7 of the short one would be appropriate.

Table 26.4 shows such an intermediate classification, which is likely to be suitable for general practitioners. It has 9 major categories, and with some obvious subdivisions, gives a total of 15 categories. However, five of these are subcategories of the most notoriously difficult group of diagnoses, called here Neurotic, Stress-related and Physical Complaint Disorders, Category 8. These subdivisions are (1) neurotic depression, (2) anxiety and phobic disorders, (3) physical complaint disorders, (4) adjustment and stress disorders, and (5) eating disorders.

The term Somatization Disorder has not been used here because, although it is becoming familiar to psychiatrists, many general practitioners are more at home with the term physical complaint disorder or something similar.

Figure 26.4 shows part of the decision tree for differentiating this group. Only testing out the scheme with accompanying charts and management options, as already illustrated, shows how many general practitioners will want to go to that level of detail, and how much training and experience is required to make these subdivisions reliable and fairly quickly.

To a psychiatrist, there are obvious implications for different treatments and managements in these subdivisions, but not all general practitioners are convinced that it is useful to make such distinctions themselves. Nevertheless, a substantial minority of general practitioners feel that it is their responsibility to make psychiatric diagnoses at this level, so it is well worthwhile pursuing. There is also an obvious educative spinoff from the

TABLE 26.4. Intermediate classification.

1. Disorders of childhood, adolescence and development
2. Mental retardation (child or adult)
3. Acute intoxication by alcohol and drugs
4. Dependence on alcohol and drugs
5. Organic mental disorders
    a. Symptomatic delirium and dementia
    b. Primary dementia
6. Schizophrenic and paranoid disorders
7. Severe affective (mood) disorders
    a. Mania
    b. Severe (psychotic) depressive illness
8. Neurotic, stress related and physical complaint disorders
    a. Depression
    b. Anxiety and phobias
    c. Physical complaints disorder
    d. Adjustment and stress disorders
    e. Eating disorders
9. Adult personality and behavior disorders
10. No psychiatric diagnosis: Go to problems list (continue investigations/assessments)

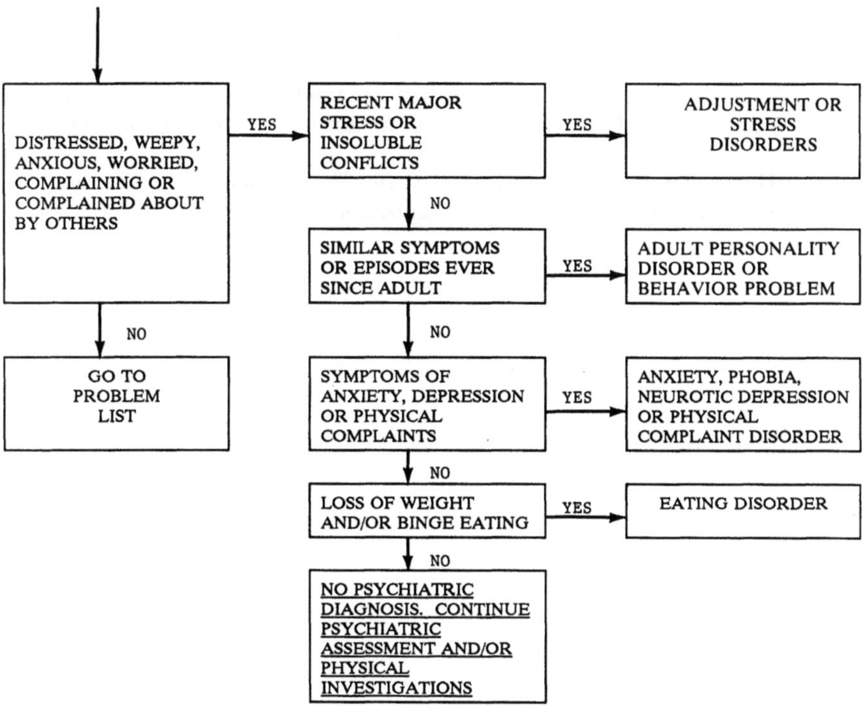


FIGURE 26.4. Decision tree differentiating neurotic, stress-related, and physical complaint disorders.

use of these diagrams and charts, so several motives exist for further work and development of this intermediate classification.

## Conclusion

What has been outlined is only the first stage in the development of short and simple versions of ICD-10 V(F) for primary and general health professionals. Up until now, the work has been done by psychiatrists; this is not surprising, because the chosen starting point was a classification designed for use by psychiatrists. But now that a start has been made, it is both appropriate and necessary to involve primary and general health care professionals in the subsequent stages of development and field trials. The main problems to be faced are likely to be practical rather than theoretical, and solutions are most likely to be found by those with direct and practical experience of the working conditions in which it is hoped that these versions of ICD-10 V(F) will be used.

## *References*

American Psychiatric Association (1987). *Diagnostic and Statistical Manual of Mental Disorders* (3rd ed, rev). American Psychiatric Association, Washington, DC.

Essex B, Gosling H (1982). An algorithmic method for management of mental health problems in developing countries. *British Journal of Psychiatry* 143:451–459.

World Health Organization (1992). *ICD-10 Classification of Mental and Behavioral Disorders*. World Health Organization, Geneva.

# 27 North American Perspectives: Toward a DSM for Primary Care

Allen Frances, Kelly McKinney, Willa Hall, Myriam Kline, Helen Stayna, and Nina Rosenthal

The issue of how best to expand psychiatric classification to meet the challenges of primary care is one of the most interesting and innovative aspects of psychiatric classification at this time. The development of modern systems of classification in the last 150 years initially began with a focus on severely ill inpatients, which led to classification of psychotic disorders. Then, largely under the influence of Freud, and changes in practice habits that resulted from the development of psychoanalysis, psychiatrists became increasingly interested in outpatients and the classification of the less severe conditions. This has been the most important development in psychiatric diagnosis during the last 80 years. We are now finding that our classification is not working very well in primary care settings, a situation that has important theoretical and practical implications.

One basic problem has been the lack of a widely accepted definition of what constitutes a mental disorder, of where one draws the line between normality and pathology. This is particularly pertinent in primary care settings in which one must ascertain whether the degree of discomfort experienced by a patient is sufficient to qualify for a diagnosis of a mental disorder. Unfortunately, definitions of mental disorders work least well in delineating the boundary between normality and pathology. Moreover, this boundary is likely to vary greatly from culture to culture and the definition is also likely to depend on the availability of practitioners to treat the disorders that have been defined. When there is a scarcity of practitioners to provide care, it becomes a luxury to define the less severely ill people as having a mental disorder.

The difficult theoretical issue about the boundary between mental disorder and normality in the primary care situation also raises an enormous practical question. If we add new and milder diagnoses (eg, mixed anxiety depression, minor depression, brief recurrent depression, or milder forms of age-appropriate cognitive impairment), these are likely to be more common in the general population than the disorders that we have already described within the classificatory system. The overall prevalence of mental disorder will skyrocket if these new disorders are created, perhaps with the effect of trivializing the concept of mental disorders and resulting in the possible provision of unnecessary treatment. If, on the other hand, we limit the definition of mental disorder to more severe cases, many people who could benefit (especially perhaps in a primary care setting) will not receive a diagnosis and may miss out on a potentially effective treatment.

Mindful of these issues, we discuss the three-stage process applied in the development of the *Diagnostic and Statistical Manual of Mental Disorders*, 4th edition (DSM-IV) (Frances et al 1990) as a way of exploring our method of deciding when to create new diagnoses that might be particularly useful in primary care settings. A summary of the work done in depression illustrates how literature reviews, data reanalyses, and field trials help to inform the decisions that will be made in this area.

The first stage, a literature review, has shown several studies suggesting that patients present with less severe depression (either less severe symptomatology or shorter duration) than is required in the third revised edition of the DSM (DSM-III-R) (American Psychiatric Association, 1987) definition but that this depression may nonetheless be clinically significant. There are two different types of spectrum subthreshold depression: one, often called minor depression, has the duration of major depression but a lower level of symptomatic severity; and the second, called brief recurrent depression, has the symptomatic severity of major depression, but a duration that lasts only a few days with recurrences 10 or 12 times a year. The evidence available suggests that patients with these subthreshold types of depression indeed have a degree of impairment that is appreciable, although less than those who have full threshold depression. Clearly, depression presents with continuously distributed severities and whatever threshold is set has tremendous implications for case findings and treatment in primary care settings.

Encouraged by the findings from the literature review, we used funding provided by the John C. and Catherine T. MacArthur Foundation to support a data reanalysis of the Epidemiological Catchment Area study to see whether patients with minor depression identified in the community have a degree of impairment that is consonant with the definition of a mental disorder. The results indeed suggest that patients with depressive symptoms who did not meet the threshold for major depression were at increased risk for various types of impairment (such as days missed at work, hospitalization, and suicide attempts). The rate of depression depends on where the threshold is set. These findings confirmed our interest in minor depression and in primary care applications.

The third stage, was a field trial studying minor depression and brief recurrent depression. First, we wanted to determine the reliability of these (perhaps very difficult to diagnose) subthreshold conditions. Second, we wanted to determine the best diagnostic set of items and how they should be joined in developing a threshold. Finally, we studied the degree of impairment occassioned by these proposed conditions and their course and relation to other disorders.

One issue raised by opponents of minor depression is the possibility that patients fail to reach thresholds for major depression in primary care settings because of brevity of assessment or lack of experience with psychiatric diagnoses that may occur in such settings. Did the patient fail to meet the threshold for major depression because the evaluation conducted was by physicians not experienced in depression who performed an evaluation of only 5 or 10 minutes? If the evaluation were done by a clinician experienced in psychiatry with more time and skill, it is argued that so-called minor depression might indeed be diagnosed as major depression (of mild severity). In the field trials, we compared diagnoses made by primary care physicians with those made by mental health clinicians.

Another issue that requires attention is one of prevalence. If the definition of minor depression results in a prevalence rate of 20% for the general population, we will worry that we are expanding the definition to allow too many individuals to qualify for a mental disorder. One of our greatest dilemmas is that we will not have evidence on the treatment implications (risks, advantages, and disadvantages) of including these subthreshold diagnoses in time to inform decisions about whether they belong in the official nomenclature. Those who support the diagnoses worry that failure to include these subthreshold forms of depression will produce false negatives and disadvantage those who could benefit from early effective treatment for their conditions. Those who oppose these diagnoses are concerned about false positives, which may lead to inappropriate diagnosis and provision of inappropriate or unnecessary treatment.

If it is decided that minor depression or brief recurrent depression should not enter the official nomenclature of DSM-IV, neither will be included in an appendix for new and interesting diagnoses requiring further study. Another possibility is to indicate these proposed diagnoses much more clearly as examples in the Not Otherwise Specificed (NOS) categories for mood disorders. In one or several of these ways, the DSM-IV system will likely emphasize the milder disorders that tend to present particularly in primary care settings.

## Conclusion

We are working with representatives of various primary care settings to develop a DSM-IV primary care version. This version will emphasize those disorders most commonly encountered in primary care settings and should also be available around 1994.

## *References*

American Psychiatric Association (1987). *Diagnostic and Statistical Manual of Mental Disorders* (3rd ed, rev). American Psychiatric Association, Washington, DC.

Frances A, Pincus HA, Widiger TA, Davis WW, First MB (1990). DSM-IV: Work in progress. *American Journal of Psychiatry* 147:1439–1448.

# 28
# Latin American Contributions to Psychiatric Classification in Primary Care

DANTE E. WARTHON, TALYA LANDMANN, AND ENRIQUE BERNAL

When the International Conference on Primary Care was held in Alma Ata, Soviet Union, in 1978 and the slogan, Health for all by the Year 2000 was coined, the WHO Collaborative Study on Strategies for Extending Mental Health Care in developing countries had already been in progress for three years (Climent and Plutchik 1980, Harding et al 1983). Mental health care was to be offered by primary health care workers in the areas of the pilot study, which were distributed in seven countries, among them two Latin American ones.

In the five years that the WHO project lasted, innovative new methods of investigation were drawn up, but their use demanded a series of previous steps, such as decentralization and integration with general medical services, and motivation of the community to become aware of its own mental health care needs. From the WHO experience, a series of concepts were clearly delimited, the most important of which was the appearance of a new idea of community psychiatry for developing countries. At the same time, a series of questions and necessities for future investigation were postulated. Among these were to "determine the effectiveness of psychosocial interventions at the primary care level and in the community, establish the factors that influence whether individuals with mental disorders will appear for help at primary health care facilities, and devise adequate systems of classifying, recording, and reporting mental disorders and psychosocial problems encountered in primary health care" (Sartorius and Harding 1983).

We show that the development of classification systems in mental health for use in primary care is a necessity that has emerged not only from this WHO study but also from different attempts to put into practice similar strategies in other Latin American countries.

In the pioneering WHO study, it was necessary to assume that diagnostic classification is one of the cornerstones of the exercise of medicine as a science, and to conceptualize this process as the reduction of the characteristics of an individual problem to a group phenomenon that permits "first, discovery of the characteristics sick people share and which can be linked statistically to possible etiological factors; second, prediction of the most likely outcome of the problem, and third, selection of therapeutic interventions which change or enhance the predictable outcome" (Giel et al 1981).

While the WHO project was being developed, a disagreement about the theoretical basis for diagnosis was taking place between practitioners who adhered to the medical model in their manner of conceiving mental disorder and those who thought that mental disorder was a human phenomenon that emerges from sociocultural experience. There were even some who emphasized the interactional aspect of mental disorder, and those who considered it an expression of family or social pathology. In accordance with these conceptions it would have been necessary to invent an appropriate classification system for each theoretical approach. As this was impossible, the WHO investigators used the 9th Revision of the *International Classification of Diseases* (ICD-9) for all stages of the project: resulting in the use of the same classification system that is used in the hospital environment for work in primary care; nowadays this would be conceptually controversial.

The development of classification systems in primary care practice is by nature linked to the design of instruments that facilitate the labor of detecting, diagnosing, and recording mental disorders. We should mention in Latin America the Self Reporting Questionnaire for Adults, whose reliability, validity, and sensibility were tested in Cali, Colombia (Climent and Plutchik 1980). For this and other instruments, a series of appropriate methodological steps for transcultural studies has been developed.

Medina Mora et al (1985) in Mexico validated and standardized the General Health Questionnaire as an instrument for early detection of cases, and the Standardized Psychiatric Interview as an instrument to determine the prevalence of psychiatric disorders among outpatients in a general hospital. In this study researchers used the following major categories of the ICD-9: Psychosis, Major Affective Disorders, Neurosis, Personality Disorders, Alcoholism and Drug Dependence, Psychophysiological Disorders, Transitory Situations, and Organic Mental Syndromes. As will be noticed, they did not diagnose specific categories. This approach permits the epidemiological verification of what is occurring in a population but is not useful for the development of individual treatment strategies in primary care.

One important aspect of this study was the global assessment of the severity of psychiatric pathology that the Standardized Psychiatric Interview permitted, using the following scale: 0, subject is totally asymptomatic; 1, some emotional complaints, but these do not merit treatment or they blend in with the personality of the subject; 2, presenting complaints determine the necessity of help as a general medical or psychiatric outpatient; 3, subject definitely needs psychiatric help, and even hospitalization could be of benefit; 4, subject definitely requires psychiatric hospitalization.

This scale would be directly applicable to the management of patients in primary care as it permits an optimal selection of cases based on the severity of pathology. The relatively greater importance of differentiating severity of pathology versus making an exact nosological diagnosis, in primary care as opposed to specialized psychiatric consultation, was also mentioned in the Second National Institute of Mental Health Research Workshop on Classification of Mental Disorders in General Health Care Settings on January 8, 1990, in Washington, DC.

Kraudy et al (1987) in Nicaragua reported the results of a study on 342 consecutive patients who received primary care from the health system that had been reformed after the Sandinista revolution in 1979. They designed an instrument that used the ICD-9 at the level of major categories, even though they did diagnose more prevalent specific categories, as can be seen in Table 28.1.

In this study, two other interesting contributions were made, one referring to the symptomatological evaluation and the other to the reasons for the consultation. These results are presented in Tables 28.2 and 28.3.

Penayo (1989), also in Nicaragua, presented the experiences of the first psychiatric primary care team in that country with a sample of 198 consecutive patients who received diagnoses from 19 ICD-9 categories. The evaluation was made with a semistructured clinical interview that the team developed and it included, in addition to the classical clinical

TABLE 28.1. Mental disorders in primary care, Nicaragua, 1986.

| Diagnoses | % ($N = 342$) |
|---|---|
| Neurotic depression | 20 |
| Neurotic disorders | 10 |
| Ajustment reaction | 11 |
| Depressive reaction | 10 |
| Alcoholism | 9 |
| Schizophrenia | 7 |
| Personality disorders | 7 |
| Psychosomatic disorders | 5 |
| Mental retardation | 5 |
| Epilepsy | 5 |
| Organic psychosis | 3 |
| Major depression | 3 |
| Schizoaffective disorder | 2 |
| Other | 3 |

Modified from Kraudy et al 1987.

TABLE 28.2. Presenting psychiatric symptoms in primary care, Nicaragua, 1986.

| Symptoms | % ($N = 342$) |
|---|---|
| Anxiety and depression | 28 |
| Anxiety only | 22 |
| Delusion/hallucination | 11 |
| Depression | 8 |
| Mental retardation | 8 |
| Somatization | 6 |
| Manic disorders | 3 |
| Agitation | 2 |
| Excitement | 2 |
| Other | 8 |

Modified from Kraudy et al 1987.

history, a list of symptoms and a questionnaire about the influence of war, bereavement, other catastrophes, and the social situation, as Table 28.4 shows.

It can be appreciated that this is an attempt at classification using an axis of psychosocial stressors and adapting it to primary psychiatric care in Nicaragua, resulting in an approach close to reality in Latin American countries, where the family often has greater importance as a social support system than it does in the industrialized world. The US NIMH 1990 workshop previously mentioned emphasized the necessity of conceptualizing the problems encountered in primary care according to different levels of complexity, that is to say, as symptoms, conditions, and disorders.

In 1987 in Brazil, Mari evaluated the prevalence of psychiatric disorders in three centers of primary attention of the national health plan and classified psychiatric morbidity into two categories: Minor psychiatric disorders and severe psychiatric disorders. For this study as well, the Self Reporting Questionnaire (Climent et al 1978, Mari 1987) and the Clinical Interview Schedule (Goldberg et al 1970) were used. Once again, the

TABLE 28.3. Reasons for primary care visit, Nicaragua, 1986.

| Reasons for visit | % ($N = 342$) |
|---|---|
| Psychiatric reasons | 36 |
| Family conflicts | 15 |
| War-related problems | 14 |
| Alcoholism | 9 |
| Psychiatric reasons and family conflicts | 7 |
| Nonpsychiatric reasons | 5 |
| Other | 7 |
| None | 7 |

Modified from Kraudy et al 1987.

TABLE 28.4. Problems that cause the consultation.

| Problem | % ($N$ = 198) |
|---|---|
| Conflict with spouse | 16.7 |
| Conflict with children | 8.6 |
| Conflict with parents | 15.2 |
| Conflict with other relatives | 8.1 |
| Conflict with work | 15.7 |
| Conflict with neighbors | 2.5 |
| Conflict relating to the economic situation | 2.0 |
| Conflict relating to war | 3.5 |
| Conflict relating to natural catastrophes | 2.5 |
| Mourning | 2.0 |
| None | 23.2 |

Modified from Penayo 1989.

global severity of illness was evaluated according to the following levels: no psychiatric disturbance; mild subclinical psychiatric disturbance; clinically significant, mild; clinically significant, moderate; and clinically significant, marked.

All of these efforts have given rise to the question of whether the diagnostic and classification necessities of the professionals who work in primary care are satisfied by standard international classifications, which historically have had a fundamentally clinical content, based on a hospital-oriented, specialized medicine with an emphasis on illness as a severe, potentially lethal process, whereas primary care must fight against conditions that usually do not threaten life. Lima and Busnello (1986) questioned both ICD-9 and DSM-III because they do not have "adequate classificatory space for the recording of the psychosocial problems seen in primary care." Lima and Busnello attribute this, first, to the fact that the conditions encountered in primary care are qualitatively different from those that benefit from hospital care. These are not less severe forms but rather, entities that require new theoretical constructs for their description; as these do not exist, their present-day classification is deficient and vague. Second, the psychiatric conditions found in primary care are colored by local culture. When one designs a worldwide classification, this local essence is lost, with a consequent exaggeration of the similarities and a subestimation of the differences of the clinical picture. As a result, the description or classification becomes imprecise here, too. Finally, there is a notable gap between the relatively homogeneous and stable culture of those who classify (physicians with a Western education) and their primary care patients who are often poor and in transition from rural to urban cultures. This difference of perspective is another factor that separates actual reality, object of the classification, from the classification itself.

In Peru, the National Institute of Mental Health (Honorio Delgado–Hideyo Noguchi) has a Department of Community Mental Health that attends to mental health needs in general medical primary care centers located in its geographical area. A permanently stationed psychiatric nurse in each of these centers attends to the new patients and follows them up through repeat visits. A psychiatrist visits the primary care center once or twice a week for supervision and conducting assessments and consultations. The location of the primary care centers near to patients' dwellings opens up a series of possibilities for the practical management of mental disorders seen, in primary care, and permits, for example, performing home visits to schizophrenic patients or stimulating the motivation of patients who would never get to the hospital to receive treatment.

In these centers, the diagnostic system used is the ICD-9, because the psychiatrists are responsible for consolidating the clinical history and assigning a diagnostic category to each patient. However, as we have already discussed, it is not possible to diagnose a large part of important social, psychological, and clinical conditions using this system.

For all of these reasons, primary care psychiatric workers in Latin America wait with great expectation for ICD-10 that is being developed by the WHO and that proposes a special adaptation for use in primary care. There is hope that the special classification will serve well in this area, in developed as well as in developing countries, and that it will be useful for primary health care workers with different levels of training.

In spite of the experiences that have been described that attempt to extend mental health coverage by resorting to primary care, we are still very far from reaching the desired goals in the majority of Latin American countries. One of the crucial responsible factors is the sociocultural characteristics of a large sector of the population. The clash of two worlds, which began 500 years ago with the arrival of the Genoese Christopher Columbus in America, has not yet created a homogeneous culture. Among a large part of the rural population, above all in the countries where major pre-Columbian cultures existed, traditional beliefs that explain sickness in general as due to supernatural causes still persist. This obviously affects belief systems in regards to illnesses of the mind and behavior. It not only hinders the recognition of psychiatry and medicine as culturally sanctioned institutions but also interferes with good communication between the population with official health services, which coexist with a rich traditional folklore that has never been adequately studied and certainly not taken into account in official health plans.

Akerele (1987), recognizing the vast reserves of human power constituted by traditional medical practitioners, be they called exorcists, witch doctors, traditional healers, or the like, said, "The improvement of health for all underserved populations, through the full utilization at community level of available resources, both human and material, is fundamental to the primary health care approach. By securing the co-operation of traditional practitioners, Member States are utilizing one of the most abundant and valuable health resources that they have to extend health coverage. Traditional practitioners are, as a rule, important, and influential members of their communities, and they should be associated with any move to develop health services at the local level."

In the same vein, the integration of traditional medicine into official health systems requires designing a well-planned policy with appropriate strategies for its implementation, and the adoption of a totally different attitude, setting aside our medical and world ethnocentric perspectives.

In this context, we would like to present a study conducted by the third author in the town of Salas, on the northern coast of Peru. In this town, witchcraft (a form of traditional healing) together with agriculture, constitute the principal occupations of the population. It has become a well-known healing center for people from the whole northern Peruvian coast as well as from Lima, the capital, where one-third of the country's population live.

The town has an urban population of 2000 and a rural population of 6000 distributed among 25 outposts. Although the traditional healers live in town, their healing practices take place in the countryside. These consist of group séances that are usually held at midnight around a special table on which there is a collection of amulets, religious images, and symbolic artifacts. The healer and the clients consume alcohol and a hallucinogenic substance, San Pedro (*Trichocereus pachanoi*), among other substances. In the trance state produced, the healer interprets the sufferings of the clients in light of the psychosocial forces that cause them according to the healer's own system of beliefs and values.

When the sociodemographic and psychopathological aspects of these healers are studied, we find that they are usually male, illiterate, over 50 years of age, and married or living with a partner (Table 28.5).

Traditional healers begin to take San Pedro at around 18 years of age. Ten years later, often coinciding with the appearance of permanent suspiciousness and paranoid ideas (even without taking drugs), they begin to work as witch doctors.

From a psychopathological viewpoint, chronic organic brain or substance-induced syndromes are found in almost all of them, probably due, among other things, to their chronic alcohol and hallucinogenic consumption. There are also depression and other symptoms, as Table 28.6 shows.

What about the clients of these traditional healers? What are the reasons that motivate them to ask for help? There are three kinds of problems: First, there are specific mental disorders, mainly those that can benefit from suggestive procedures that the healers use. Among them, in order of importance, we found hysteria, conversive or dissociative disorders, and hypocondriasis. A second category is that of specific physical

TABLE 28.5. Characteristics of traditional healers from Salas, Peru.

| Demographic information | % ($N = 24$) |
|---|---|
| Sex | |
| Masculine | 91 |
| Feminine | 9 |
| Age | |
| Older than 50 years | 83 |
| Younger than 50 years | 17 |
| Marital status | |
| Common-law union | 50 |
| Married | 42 |
| Single | 8 |
| Education | |
| Illiterate | 83 |
| Can read and write | 17 |
| Language | |
| Spanish | 100 |
| Quechua and Spanish | 4 |
| Part-time job | |
| Agriculture | 29 |
| Agriculture and livestock | 46 |
| Other | 25 |
| Religion | |
| Catholic | 96 |
| Buddhist | 4 |
| Characteristics of their dwellings | |
| Mud bricks-tin roof | 100 |
| Running water | 62 |
| No water | 38 |
| No sewage disposal or electricity | 100 |

disorders that have not yet been treated or that cannot be treated by official medicine. A third group is formed by the so-called culture-bound syndromes. These are important for their significance in primary care and they have been the object of a large number of scientific studies refering to their medical, sociological, and anthropological aspects.

TABLE 28.6. Principal symptoms of mental exam in traditional healers from Salas, Peru.

| Symptom | % ($N = 24$) |
|---|---|
| Suspiciousness and paranoid ideas | 100 |
| Deficits in orientation, memory, mathematical ability, intelligence, comprehension, and reasoning | 92 |
| Excessive ingestion of alcoholic beverages | 50 |
| Depressive symptoms | 17 |

In Peru, the following cultural syndromes have been described: *el daño* (harm), *el susto* (fright), *la nevada* (irritability), *el chucaque* (ataque *de nervios*), and *el mal de ojo* (evil eye). According to our viewpoint, these need appropriate conceptualization and should be incorporated into a classification of mental disorders for primary care.

# Conclusion

A number of clinical and epidemiological contributions to psychiatric concepts and procedures for primary care have been made in Latin America in recent decades. These are reviewed along with illustrating issues on folkloric psychiatry and culture-bound syndromes of relevance to primary care.

## *References*


Akerele O (1987). The best of both worlds: Bringing traditional medicine up to date. *Social Science and Medicine* 24:177–181.

Climent CE, de Arango MV, Plutchik R, et al (1978). Development of an alternative, efficient, low-cost mental health delivery system in Cali, Colombia. I: The auxiliary nurse. *Social Psychiatry* 13:29–35.

Climent CE, Plutchik R (1980). Confiabilidad, validez y sensibilidad de los items de una escala de auto-reportaje de sintomas de enfermedad mental. *Revista Colombiana de Psiquiatria* 8.

Giel R, de'Arrigo Busnello E, Climent CE, et al (1981). A reliability study in the WHO collaborative study on strategies for extending mental health care. *Acta Psychiatrica Scandinavica* 63:61–74.

Harding TW, Climent CE, Giel R, et al (1983). The WHO collaborative study on strategies for extending mental health care, II: The development of new research methods. *American Journal of Psychiatry* 140:1474–1480.

Kraudy E, Liberati A, Asioli F, et al (1987). Organization of services and pattern of psychiatric care in Nicaragua: Results of a survey in 1986. *Acta Psychiatrica Scandinavica* 76:545–551.

Lima B, Busnello E (1986). The psychosocial components of health problems in primary care: A report on the Brazilian experience. *BPA Quarterly* 15(1):2–8.

Mari JJ (1987). Psychiatric morbidity in three primary medical care clinics in the city of São Paulo—Issues on the mental health of the urban poor. *Social Psychiatry* 22:129–138.

Medina-Mora ME, Padilla GP, Mas CC (1985). Prevalencia de trastornos mentales y factores de riesgo en una poblacion de practica medica general. *Acta Psiquiátrica y Psicológica de América Latina* 31:53–61.

Penayo U (1989). Experiences of psychiatric outpatient team in Nicaragua mental health problems seen in a primary care setting. *Social Psychiatry and Psychiatric Epidemiology* 24:151–155.

Sartorius N, Harding TW (1983). The WHO collaborative study on strategies for extending mental health care, I: The genesis of the study. *American Journal of Psychiatry* 140:1470–1473.

# 29 European Viewpoints on Identifying and Classifying Psychiatric Cases in General Medical Settings

Charles B. Pull and Gilles Chaillet

In Europe, most work on mental disorders in primary care has been done in only a few countries, with Britain at the forefront of research endeavors. Although epidemiological research and quantitative approaches to public health problems find more and more acceptance in other European countries, especially in northern European countries—Germany, Switzerland, and France—investigations in this field have remained scarce outside of the United Kingdom and have been restricted to a small number of studies carried out in only a few individual centers. In contrast, Great Britain has a long tradition of major interest and investment in this field, with a number of important investigations dating back as far as the early 1960s. As such, the present report on European experiences with psychiatric classifications in primary care deals essentially with work done in the United Kingdom during the last three decades.

## Basic Concepts of Psychological Disorders in Primary Care

The basic concepts of psychological disorders in primary care have been elaborated by psychiatrists in Great Britain. In 1960, Kessel coined the concept of conspicuous psychiatric morbidity to described psychiatric disorder as it is perceived by the primary care physician. In 1970, Goldberg and Blackwell introduced the term hidden psychiatric morbidity to refer to a psychiatric disorder that remains unrecognized by the patient's family physician. The most established screening instrument for psychological disorders in general practice studies still is the General Health Questionnaire (GHQ), which was specifically designed for this use by Goldberg in 1972.

## The Prevalence of Psychological Disorders in General Practice

A number of European (in particular, British) studies have demonstrated that general practitioners are confronted with large numbers of patients presenting with psychological disorders. As early as 1960, Kessel, in one practice in south London, estimated a prevalence rate of psychiatric morbidity of 50 per 1000, using only terms in the *International Classification of Diseases* (ICD) chapter dealing specifically with psychiatric disorders; of 90 per 1000 when patients with well-defined psychological disturbances were included, and of 380 per 1000 when patients with physical complaints without detectable organic cause were added (Kessel 1960). Shepherd et al (1966) established more than 20 years ago that it is general practitioners who come in contact with and are responsible for treating the bulk of psychological disorders, and that only a small proportion of the mentally ill who consult them reach the attention of psychiatrists. According to Jenkins and Shepherd (1983), general practice consultations for identified psychiatric disorders outnumber psychiatric outpatient attendances by roughly 10 to 1. In 1973, a report of a working party convened by the Regional Office for Europe of the World Health Organization (WHO) estimated that between 10 and 20% of the general population present to general practitioners in any year as psychiatric patients. More recently, large epidemiological studies such as the Munich Follow-Up Study (Wittchen and von Zerssen 1988) have confirmed that patients with all forms of mental disorders have about 100% more general medical consultations than people without mental disorders, and that a large proportion of patients with mental disorders are not seen by psychiatrists or psychologists, but exclusively by their general practitioners.

## Variation of Prevalence Rates

During the same period, a number of surveys in the United Kingdom have demonstrated great variations in prevalence rates of psychiatric morbidity as reported by individual general practitioners. In 1966, Shepherd et al showed a ninefold variation between general practitioners in London. In the early 1970s, data from National Morbidity Surveys in Great Britain demonstrated enormous interpractices variation in consultation rates for the different mental disorders, indicating that general practitioners could not possibly be diagnosing clinical problems in any standardized way (Crombie 1986). More specific investigations have shown that much of the general practitioner's ability to detect psychiatric morbidity can be attributed to physician practice style and personality (Marks et al 1979), physician attitudes and experience (Goldberg and Huxley

1980) and physician training and hence, skill in diagnosing mental disorders (Goldberg 1978).

## Special Features of Psychological Disorders in Primary Care

General practitioners' attributes are, however, but one of many special features that influence the detection of psychological disorders in primary care. According to Jenkins and coworkers (1988), there is a high incidence of transient disorders at this level of health care, disorders are often seen in their early stages, before the full clinical picture has been developed, and they often comprise a complex mixture of physical, emotional, and social elements. Numerous studies have convincingly argued that many patients find it difficult to express their problems in psychological terms, and either somatize their complaints or describe it in terms of social problems (Jenkins et al 1988, Goldberg and Bridges 1987). In addition, it has been shown that many patients who consult their general practitioner present with relatively mild psychiatric symptoms, or with ill-defined psychological problems, that are often seen in the presence of other disease states (Weyerer 1990), and that become a disorder only in the presence of other social, economic, or health problems (Sartorius and Goldberg 1990).

On the whole, at least three views have been expressed regarding the nature of psychological disorders commonly seen in general practice. One is that these disorders are essentially the same as those seen by psychiatrists, but less severe. A second view is that many of the psychological disorders seen in general practice are not discrete entities but largely consist of various mixtures of different syndromes. Finally, a more recent view emphasizes the fact that many of the psychological problems seen in primary care are ill-defined disorders for which diagnostic criteria would still have to be drafted before they can be investigated in a reliable way.

## Classification of Psychological Disorders in Primary Care

A significant obstacle to the study of psychological disorder in primary care is the lack of agreement about the best way of classifying these problems. There has been no general consensus up to now on what type of classification should be used, by whom, or for what purpose. It is not possible to discuss this extensive subject in any detail here. Some examples of classifications used in the study of psychological disorders in primary care will be discussed briefly, with an indication of how they cope with those disorders.

## Classifications Designed by General Practitioners

According to Cooper (1990), classifications designed by general practitioners are the result of energetic attempts to modify and even to extend already existing psychiatric classifications. As a consequence, they are often more detailed and lengthy than those designed by research psychiatrists.

The 1984 psychiatric classification of the UK Royal College of General Practitioners is based on the 9th revision of ICD (ICD-9), Chapter V, but the number of rubrics have been increased and categories additional to those found in the ICD have been added.

The International Classification of Health Problems in Primary Care (ICHPPC) (WONCA 1979) is also an adaptation of the ICD for use in primary care. It is designed to represent a consensus on the content of primary care derived from a wide practical experience of many different doctors from many different countries and covers various aspects of the consultation (including site and duration of service, clinical laboratory investigations, diagnostic imaging, therapeutic procedures, clinical and administrative services), in addition to simply recording the diagnostic and associated problems. In Europe, the ICHPPC has hardly ever been used outside of Great Britain. In a study by the General Practice Research Unit of the Institute of Psychiatry in London, Jenkins and coworkers (1988) concluded that the ICHPPC could not be applied consistently by general practitioners and that the diagnostic agreement achieved with the ICHPPC were only slightly more satisfactory than those obtained with the ICD.

## Classifications Designed by Psychiatrists

Classifications designed by psychiatrists for the study of psychological disorders in primary care have as a rule been comparatively brief, and consist in broad and inclusive categories. In the United Kingdom, several classifications of this type have been developed during the last decades.

According to Cooper (1990), the classification developed by Shepherd in 1966 for surveys of psychiatric illness in general practice in the United Kingdom is still one of the most acceptable and useful and can be used quickly and without serious difficulties by most general practitioners. It divides psychiatric disorders into the two main groups: Formal Psychiatric Illness, and Psychiatric-Associated Conditions, using 10 categories in all (Table 29.1).

Goldberg and Blackwell (1970) have proposed a simple classification that views psychiatric disturbances in relation to the overall spectrum

TABLE 29.1. Classification of mental disorders in primary care.

| Formal psychiatric illness | Psychiatric-associated conditions |
|---|---|
| 1. Psychosis (schizophrenia, manic–depressive psychosis, organic psychosis) | 6. Physical illnesses (where psychological mechanisms have been important in the development of the condition) |
| 2. Mental subnormality | 7. Physical symptoms |
| 3. Dementia (deterioration of mental powers in excess of normal aging process) | 8. Physical illnesses (that have been elaborated or prolonged for psychological reasons) |
| 4. Neurosis (anxiety state, depressive, hysterical, phobic or asthenic reactions; others) | 9. Physical symptoms |
| 5. Personality disorder | 10. Other psychological or social problems |

Note. Shepherd et al 1966.

of complaints and disorders presented by patients in general medical settings. The classification uses eight categories (Table 29.2).

More recently, Goldberg and Bridges (1987) have proposed a classification of four possible types of psychological disorders frequently encountered in primary care and of their relationship to physical disorders (Table 29.3).

Examination of the process by which general practitioners make their diagnoses has led Jenkins and her group to the conclusion that a multidimensional approach is the most appropriate system of classification in general care. The classification rests upon four axes or dimensions (Table 29.4).

Axis I is the psychological dimension; Axis II consists of a classification of social problems and supports; Axis III is a classification of personality; and Axis IV is one of physical disorder. Within each dimension, duration and severity are recorded, making 12 subcategories in all. The psychological axis is so constructed as to enable general practitioners to make a broad diagnosis without requiring specialist knowledge and to

TABLE 29.2. Classification of mental disorders in primary care.

| | |
|---|---|
| A. | Entirely physical complaint or illness |
| B. | Physical illness in a neurotic personality |
| C. | Physical illness with associated psychiatric disturbance |
| D. | Psychiatric illness with somatic symptoms |
| E. | Unrelated physical illness and psychiatric illness |
| F. | Entirely psychiatric illness |
| G. | Miscellaneous, not ill, unclassifiable |
| H. | Parents of sick children |

Note. Goldberg and Blackwell, 1970.

TABLE 29.3. Classification of mental disorders in primary care.

| Classification | Diagnostic criteria |
|---|---|
| 1. Physical illness with secondary psychiatric illness | 1. All somatic symptoms can be attributed to physical illness<br>2. Treatment of the psychiatric illness will not remove the physical symptoms<br>3. The psychiatric illness would not have occurred without the physical illness |
| 2. Physical illness with unrelated psychiatric illness | No etiological link exists between the two; treatment of one would not affect the other |
| 3. Somatized psychiatric illness | 1. Consultation is for physical symptoms<br>2. Patient attributes all problems to a physical illness, or thinks symptoms constitute the problem<br>3. A psychiatric illness (DSM-III) is present<br>4. Treatment of the psychiatric illness would alleviate or remove the physical symptom (all four must be satisfied) |
| 4. Entirely psychiatric illness | Either no somatic symptoms are present, or patient considers somatic symptoms to be part of psychiatric illness |

Note. Goldberg and Bridges 1987.

TABLE 29.4. Classification of psychiatric disorders in primary care.

| | |
|---|---|
| I. | Psychological axis |
| II. | Social axis |
| | A. Antecedent and consequential problem |
| | B. Social supports |
| III. | Personality axis |
| IV. | Physical axis |
| Psychological axis | |
| 00 | Asymptomatic |
| 01 | Symptoms present but no diagnosis made |
| 02 | Depression |
| 03 | Depression with prominent anxiety |
| 04 | Anxiety state, phobias |
| 05 | Other neuroses |
| 06 | Psychoses |
| 07 | Dementia |
| 08 | Alcohol abuse |
| 09 | Drug abuse |
| 10 | Eating disorders |
| 11 | Sexual disorders |
| 12 | Mental handicap |

Jenkins et al 1988.

allow the single presence of individual symptoms to be recorded even when they are not sufficiently severe or numerous to warrant a diagnosis.

## The Future of Psychiatric Classifications in Primary Care

Psychiatric classifications, whether designed by general practitioners or by psychiatrists can be said to have had only limited use and success so far in the study of psychological disorders encountered in primary care settings. Investigations in this field have confirmed that psychological problems are frequently seen in primary health care, but just what the nature of the different types of problems is and how they can be classified remains uncertain.

For the future, Jenkins et al (1988) recommend the development of simple forms of multiaspect systems of classification for use in primary care. Sartorius and Goldberg (1990) emphasize the need for drafting diagnostic criteria for disorders that are often characterized by relatively mild symptoms or those that have remained ill-defined up to now, such as neurasthenia, fatigue syndromes, pain syndromes, and somatoform disorders. For Cooper (1990), the outstanding classificatory and diagnostic problem for psychiatry in primary care will be how best to conceptualize and to describe mixed states of anxiety and depression, at mild and moderate levels of intensity. For Angst (1990), future research on general practice and community samples should focus more on operationalized subgroups of depression and anxiety.

In the past, and even more so in recent years, WHO has shown a major interest in the study of psychiatric classifications in primary care. In the development of ICD-10, special attention has been paid to those psychiatric disorders that are of particular importance to professionals working in general medical settings, for example: mixed anxiety and depressive disorder. A multiaspect version of ICD-10, for the classification of patients, disorders, and problems in primary care is currently in preparation as part of the ICD-10 family of instruments. Finally, WHO has launched a major investigation of the psychological disorders seen in general health care facilities. An impressive number of centers from all European countries are participating in these endeavors.

## Conclusion

Thus, on the whole it would appear that there is a growing interest in Europe for psychiatric classification in primary care and that many European countries, in addition to Great Britain, can be expected to contribute to enhance our knowledge about psychological disorders seen in general medical settings.

## *References*

Angst J (1990). Depression and anxiety: A review of studies in the community and in primary health care, pp 60–68. In N Sartorius, DP Goldberg, G de Girolamo, JA Costa de Silva, Y Lecrubier, HU Wittchen (eds), *Psychological Disorders in General Medical Settings*. Hogrefe & Huber, New York.

Cooper JE (1990). The classification of mental disorders for use in general medical settings, pp 49–59. In N Sartorius, DP Goldberg, G de Girolamo, JA Costa de Silva, Y Lecrubier, HU Wittchen HU (eds), *Psychological Disorders in General Medical Settings*. Hogrefe & Huber, New York.

Crombie DL (1986). Classification of mental illness for primary care. In M Shepherd, G Wilkinson, P Williams (eds), *Mental Illness in Primary Care Settings*. Tavistock, London.

Goldberg DP (1972). *The Detection of Psychiatric Illness by Questionnaire*. Oxford University Press, London.

Goldberg DP (1978). Mental health priorities in a primary care setting. *Annals of the New York Academy of Science* 310:65–68.

Goldberg DP, Blackwell B (1970). Psychiatric illness in general practice: A detailed study using a new method of case identification. *British Medical Journal* 2:439–443.

Goldberg DP, Bridges K (1987). Screening for psychiatric illness in general practice: The general practitioner versus the screening questionnaire. *Journal of the Royal College of General Practice* 37:15–18.

Goldberg DP, Huxley P (1980). *Mental Illness in the Community: The Pathway to Psychiatric Care*. Tavistock, London.

Jenkins R, Shepherd M (1983). Mental illness and general practice, pp 379–409. In P Bean (ed), *Key Issues in Mental Illness*. Wiley and Sons, London.

Jenkins R, Smeeton N, Shepherd M (1988). Classification of mental disorder in primary care. *Psychological Medicine* (suppl 12).

Kessel WIN (1960). Psychiatric morbidity in a London general practice. *British Journal of Preventive and Social Medicine* 14:16–23.

Marks JN, Goldberg DP, Hillier VF (1979). Determinants of the ability of general practitioners to detect psychiatric illness. *Psychological Medicine* 9: 337–353.

Royal College of General Practitioners (1984). *Classification of Diseases, Problems and Procedures* (Occasional Paper No. 26). Royal College of General Practitioners, London, UK.

Sartorius N, Goldberg DP (1990) Conclusions, pp 171–175. In N Sartorius, DP Goldberg, G de Girolamo, JA Costa de Silva, Y Lecrubier, HU Wittchen (eds), *Psychological Disorders in General Medical Settings*. Hogrefe & Huber, New York.

Shepherd M, Cooper B, Brown AC, Kalton GW (1966). *Psychiatric Illness in General Practice*. Oxford University Press, London.

Weyerer S (1990). Relationships between physical and psychological disorders, pp 34–46. In N Sartorius, DP Goldberg, G de Girolamo, JA Costa de Silva, Y Lecrubier, HU Wittchen (eds), *Psychological Disorders in General Medical Settings*. Hogrefe & Huber, New York.

Wittchen HU, von Zerssen D (eds) (1988). *Verläufe behandelter und unbehandelter Depressionen und Angststörungen*. Springer-Verlag, Berlin.

World Health Organization (1973). *Psychiatry and Primary Medical Care*. Lyseba, Oslo.

World Organization of National Colleges, Academies and Academic Associations of General Practitioners/Family Physicians (1979). *International Classification of Health Problems in Primary Care* (2nd ed). Oxford University Press, Oxford.

# 30
# Psychopathology Explorations and Findings in African Primary Care Settings

AYO BINITIE

In a previous report, Binitie (1988) pointed out that psychiatric diagnosis in its present form enabled scientists to view the African world through Western eyes. The reverse of viewing the Western world through African eyes, so that a universal ethos emerges, is yet to be considered. Consider the scenario in Benin City, Nigeria, where I live. In each one of the better areas lives a traditional healer, who receives two or three clients a day, and sometimes more. The client usually comes with a number of relatives. A healer gave examples of the patients seen prior to my visit.

## Case Studies

### *Case 1*

A woman in her late thirties was accompanied by her husband, her mother, and a sister of the husband. The husband spoke for the family. He complained that they had no surviving children in spite of six live deliveries. He further complained that the wife was not marking progress in life. Her business never had "head or tail," meaning that she always failed in whatever business enterprise she had engaged. The woman was once again pregnant and the consultation was begun to prevent another death of offspring after delivery.

The diviner played the oracle and divined that there was some trouble within the family and that the patient was made to sacrifice her children by these family witches. The treatment was to appease the witches with a goat and shift the burden from the patient. The technique used for doing this was to make an image and put it on, with parcels symbolizing the burdens of the patient, and then bury the image with the burden. As the image was buried, the goat was slaughtered while appropriate incantations and prayers were said. The client was yet to deliver but the healer was absolutely convinced that the problem was over for the client: "I have dealt with many more serious cases of witchcraft in the family."

## *Case 2*

The patient was brought in by her mother and an aunt. These elder women knew of the skills of the healer and so they had recommended him to their daughter. The 29-year-old daughter, an educated girl, had graduated and was a teacher in a secondary school. Her husband was a senior civil servant in one of the ministries.

The consultation was considered necessary by the observation that the girl had been married for 7 years and had not had a baby. She had been to several hospitals and was told after examinations that her tubes were blocked.

The healer cast his *oguega* and divined that the girl's womb had been "borrowed" by an older woman. The result was the observed infertility. He treated the young woman with special herbs. In addition, she sacrificed a male goat to the witches so they would return her womb. At the time of the last visit the lady was over three months pregnant. The healer explained that caution was required to prevent the loss of the baby. There was the need for frequent visits so as to continually monitor the activities of the witches and prevent harm.

## *Case 3*

A young lady in her late twenties who complained of abdominal pains was brought in by her parents and an aunt. The young woman had been to three different hospitals within the city, including the teaching hospital, at which she had been examined. Nothing was found to be wrong with her, thus the relatives had brought her to this traditional pactitioner.

The healer cast his *oguega* and divined that the client attended a witch's conclave where she had been elected as treasurer. It was the function of the treasurer to store the witch's money in the "stomach." As long as she was treasurer her abdominal pain would continue.

The healer, looking straight in the eyes of the aunt who had accompanied her said, "Next time you go to the meeting, make sure you let the treasury (place where money is kept) go to someone else. Vote her out again." According to the healer the patient was better within a month of the consultation.

## *Case 4*

An older well-to-do man had married a new young wife. Within two years the wife was having an affair with a particular young man. The affair appeared to be growing stronger. The man was afraid the younger man would take his wife from him.

He consulted the healer. "I want you to stop his prick (penis) so he cannot seduce my wife". The healer explained that he normally did not undertake such tasks. In this instance, he decided to help the man because the man had rights and justice on his side. No one should take another's wife; there are enough women in the world for every man. In fact, women are in surplus. A tortoise was obtained, and then a black thread was tied around the penis of the tortoise. Incantations were chanted and then the tortoise was taken into the forest and left there. It is very difficult to reverse the process once done; that is, it is not easy to make the penis work again.

## *Case 5*

The entire family came: a husband and his wife, his mother, the wife's mother and father, the husband's sister, and many other relatives. The problem was that the husband's mother was accused of being a witch, following the death of two children in the family. The husband's mother was indignant and called on the family to take her wherever they would, because she had not had anything to do with the death of the children. They came to the healer for consultation. The traditional healer was prepared for this kind of business. He had special powder which changed color in the hands of anyone who was guilty of such offence. The powder was placed on the open palms of all the clients, after which they were all asked to close their palms and clench their fists. At the end of the given period, during which incantations were chanted, the witch would be identified by the change in color of the powder. On this particular occasion, the healer announced that not only would the powder ferret out the witch but the witch would come out and behave in a strange manner and would confess. It was the mother of the children herself who first got up, said the place was very hot, became restless and then began to shout, tearing her own clothes and stripping herself naked. The healer said, "You remember I told you the witch would show herself." She then confessed she was a witch.

## *Case 6*

The client was a well-to-do businessman who wanted to produce charms to prevent thieves from entering his house. The healer described the procedure he adopted in dealing with this particular request. He went to the forest, picked the leaves that had been shown to him by his father who was also a healer and from whom he had learned. He burnt these with an egg. He pulverized the residue into a black powder. It was this black powder that he spread round the premises of the client. As he spread the powder he recited suitable incantations from the main body of the *oguega* tradition. He charges reasonable fees for this kind of consultation. He explained that if thieves approached the house and got over the threshold, something would happen to make the thieves quarrel among themselves. They would continue quarrelling until it was light and then disperse without achieving their objective.

## Case 7

"I want to be strong so that witches and wizards or any evil-minded person cannot touch me." The speaker of these words was a 35-year-old businessman who is getting on in his business. He is worried because he feared that envious neighbours, witches, and wizards may wish to drag him down and bring him to ruin.

The healer precribed a bath, with special herbs, which has an antiwitch quality. He was to serve his ancestors and his own head. In addition, the healer made some cuts on his forehead and rubbed these with some black powder as a protective charm. The ceremonies were duly performed, and all the parties concerned were satisfied that a good job had been done.

## Case 8

A 60-year-old man brought his 3-year-old daughter. The little girl was accompanied by her mother. The little girl had previously been able to walk and then suddenly lost the capacity to stand.

The healer's explanation was that the people of the night were responsible for the girl's ailment. She was destined to be a great woman and travel to many places. She would return and be master over many people. The witches, knowing her destiny, were anxious to prevent this. Clearly, if she were paralyzed she would not be able to run her business. Indeed, she would be so preoccupied with her ailment that she would have no time for anything else. The healer cleansed her legs with a specially prepared medicinal broom which by tradition is part of his healing tools. This had the effect of sweeping away all the little stringlike cobwebs the people of the night had used in binding her legs. In addition, she was given special herbal medicines. The girl is now walking.

## Case 9

A 32-year-old farmer with three wives and seven children was brought in by the senior wife when she observed the condition of the husband. She was sure he was going to die unless something was done immediately. Consequently, she rushed the husband to the native doctor at about midnight to save the husband from catastrophe. The husband complained of chest pain. It all started suddenly; within a few minutes the husband's breathing was heavy and his breath was very hot. He felt something clutching the front of his chest and then hooking up in his back as though someone was trying to tear out his heart through his back. Shortly after, he fainted and water was poured on him. This revived him somewhat but the wife was sure something serious was amiss and unless something was done, he would die.

The healer was aroused from his sleep. He saw the condition was critical and, therefore, cast his oracle that very night to find out what was amiss. He learned that the man was troubled by witches within the family. He sent for all the wives. In the meantime, he applied a medicated bath and gave some herbal preparation to the patient. This settled the patient, and he continued the bath and medicines. In the meantime, the wives arrived. He got in the bath, rubbed his face with special preparations and asked the wives to look at the healer direct in the eye.

One of the wives, on catching the eye of the healer, confessed to being a witch. The husband who after a week was feeling well and determined to send away the wife. The healer would not agree to this plan of the husband. According to the healer, the wife had confessed openly to being a witch, and as a result, could no longer function as a witch. The healer was determined not to leave the patient alone until he agreed to let the wife stay.

## *Case 10*

This patient was brought in by his mother who knew of the reputation of the healer. She brought two sons whom she was convinced were plagued by witches who were trying to kill them.

The elder of the two patients complained of heaviness in the legs and a sensation as though air was being blown into the brain. In addition, he had no energy. He went to a hospital and was examined but nothing was found. He also visited many chemists who gave him drugs but to no avail. While the mother was battling trying to think what to do, a similar illness started in the younger brother.

## *Case 11*

The younger brother complained of dizziness, fearfulness accompanied by palpitations, weakness and body pains, and very bad frightful dreams of people pressing him down and trying to choke him or chasing him with a cutlass.

The mother again took him to the hospital where blood and urine tests were found to be normal. Nothing was found on physical examination.

The mother was now definitely convinced that witches were at work. She had to be up and doing before the witches could kill her two sons. Fortunately, she knew this powerful native doctor and asked for his help to fight the witches. The doctor confirmed that indeed her children were made ill by witches. He gave antiwitch baths and drinks and also prescribed sacrifice to their guardian angels and the ancestors.

After a 1-week stay at the therapeutic center, the brothers were much improved, and were prepared to go home with their mother.

### *Case 12*

This man in his midfifties had a disagreement over a piece of land. He had apparently usurped the rights of this individual and built a house on their land. At least, the healer was not convinced he had any better claims over the land. The other party had sued and the case was in court. The client of the traditional healer did not want the case heard and so consulted the traditional healer. The traditional healer prepared charms and applied them to the tips of a specially constructed fork (*aban*). Then he carried the *aban* into the distant forest and secured it with the help of nails to an Iroko tree in the forest. The case, the healer told me, has been in court for four years but no pleadings had been taken. He assured me that as long as the tree was standing and the *aban* was on the tree, the case would not be heard.

## Using the International Classification of Disease, 10th Revision

The following comments reflect the vicissitudes of trying to use the ICD-10 with these case summaries.

### *Case 1*

This does not fit well into any of the existing classificatory system. It can conceivably be characterized using the broadest categories available as F4, Neurotic, Stress-Related and Somatoform Disorders. The reason for inclusion is connected only to the word stress-related; it is not possible to go further.

### *Case 2*

Infertility is a common ground for diagnosis. However, as reported by the healer, the woman has since become pregnant, thus the diagnosis cannot be sustained.

### *Case 3*

Nonspecific abdominal pain successfully treated by psychological means could conceivably be classified as F45.3 or 4, Somatoform Disorder under the rubric psychogenic autonomic dysfunction or pain syndrome without organic cause.

### *Case 4*

There is clearly no provision for this kind of disorder in the ICD (ie, stopping a rival's penis from functioning).

### *Case 5*

There is clearly no provision for this kind of disorder in ICD (ie, a family consultation about who was responsible for children's death in the family).

### *Case 6*

There is clearly no provision in ICD for preventing thieves from entry.

### *Case 7*

"I want to be strong" has no place in ICD classificatory system.

### *Case 8*

Inability to walk could be a physical disorder or could be a psychological disorder under the rubric F44.5, Dissociative Disorder in the category of psychogenic disorders of voluntary movement.

### *Case 9*

Difficulty in breathing accompanied by fainting could be from the description conversion reaction F44.5, Panic Attack or F41.0, Asthmatic Attack.

### *Case 10*

Heaviness in legs and sensation as though air was being blown into the brain could be classified as Somatoform Disorder, F45.0. Our experience, however, shows this type of disorder to be a Mild Depressive Disorder F31.1.

### *Case 11*

This is similar to Case 10.

### *Case 12*

There is no clear provision for this kind of disorder in ICD.

## Reports from Western-Type African Institutions

There are reports from Western-type institutions in Africa about the kinds of patients seen in secondary and tertiary institutions. Such reports have come from Carothers (1953), Lament and Blignault (1953), Moffson (1955), Smartt (1956), Vyncke (1958), Forster (1958, 1972, 1974), German (1969, 1987), Kagwa (1965), Orley et al (1979), Onyeama and Onuora (1980), and Copeland (1968).

In addition to these, there are some reports about psychiatric disorders in a primary care setting. These reports have come from Tooth (1950), Field (1958), both reporting from Ghana, Leighton et al (1963), and Binitie (1981a, 1981b). Field's study and Laubsher's study are similar to the studies reported earlier in that they have come from traditional healers. The reports from Tooth, Field, Leighton et al, and Binitie are reviewed next in some detail.

### *Tooth's Study*

Tooth (1950) used counters and laypeople, and made inquiries among heads of communities to conduct his census. In the 2-year period of the study, 400 patients were contacted; 173 of them had detailed records as from the north, and 75 from the south. Tooth found a male-to-female ratio of 2 to 1, similar to the finding of Carothers in East Africa (see Table 30.1). In Accra Assylum, there were 1833 admissions in which 184 were females, a sex ratio of approximately 9 to 1.

The study suffered from a number of methodological problems. Particularly relevant was the method of case finding that would only bring out the more severe forms of disorders (ie, mainly psychoses). Tooth in this study commented on the rarity of depression having found only 6 of 34 affective states.

### *Field's Study*

Field (1958, 1960) is a psychiatrist who was also trained as an anthropologist. She offered many useful insights not only into Ghanian cul-

TABLE 30.1. Diagnoses present in Tooth's study (1950).

| Diagnoses | No. (%) |
|---|---|
| Organic | 36 (20.8) |
| Delusional state | 38 (22.0) |
| Schizophrenia | 33 (19.1) |
| Affective state | 34 (19.7) |
| Mental defect | 6 (3.5) |
| Psychopathy | 4 (2.3) |
| Neurosis | 15 (8.7) |
| Unclassified psychotic | 7 (4.0) |

ture but, in fact, to African culture in general when she wrote "The great majority are healthy people supplicating for protection." Financially successful men are full of fear lest envious kinsmen should by means of bad magic or witchcraft bring about their doom. The statement could equally well apply all over Africa. Field found that in rural Ghana, involutional depression is (as in our own society) one of the commonest and most defined mental illnesses.

Field's findings concerning depressions have been criticized. Murphy and Lubis (1962) believed that the findings were situationally determined and showed that the symptoms of guilt distinguished only between depression and schizophrenia statistically but not between anxiety and depression.

Further work was done to clarify these problems. Binitie has studied (1971, 1981a, 1981b, 1983) and more recently (1987) has reopened the issue. Although agreeing that guilt was not common, he suggested that it (guilt) was not that uncommon.

## *The Studies of Leighton and Lambo et al (1963)*

This study intends two things: First, setting a scene so that international comparisons could be effectively made, and second, trying to take into account local conditions.

However, as pointed out earlier, this is a mere foray into traditional belief systems without really adopting its methods of classification. Thus there was no information about the number of witches seen or the number of persons plagued by the devil if we use the terminology for the transitional group. This is just to indicate that the study is one that uses Western eyes to study African cultural problems. In the study, the following classification of people into categories ABCD was used: D is symptom free, C has only a few symptoms, A is a respondent whom psychiatrists regard as a definite psychiatric case, and B is a probable psychiatric case.

Table 30.2 shows that psychoneurotic disorders were predominant in Abeokuta. Meaningful comparisons of psychotic disorders cannot be made because the numbers are small.

The Leighton survey showed that 21% of village respondents and 31% of town respondents rated A. An additional 19% in villages and 14% in

TABLE 30.2. Diagnostic distribution of psychiatric cases in Nigeria (villages and Abeokuta) and Canada (Sterling County).

| | Villages ($N = 262$) | Abeokuta ($N = 64$) | Sterling County ($N = 1010$) |
|---|---|---|---|
| Psychoneurosis | 71% | 77% | 52% |
| Psychosis | 2% | – | 1% |
| Brain syndrome | 5% | 8% | 3% |

Abeokuta town rated B. The combined findings for A and B were 40% for villages and 45% for Abeokuta town. Even if only the figures of A were used, this represents quite a high proportion of disease rate. As has been pointed out, the method of case finding has a bearing on the results.

## *Binitie's Study*

This study (1981a) looks at the total population of a relatively isolated oil palm plantation where the medical facilities available are the only ones for miles around. Patients, if they feel ill, are obliged to use the services as they have no other choice other than to go to traditional care around the locality. Because the ministrations of the traditional practitioner are not officially acceptable, the patient must see a Western physician to get time off. The result of these social pressures is that the worker who is ill must of necessity see a physician, thus ensuring a complete and total recording of contact. The results are shown in Table 30.3.

There have been other surveys of special populations such as those of drug abuse studied by Odejide and Sanda (1976), Ifabumuyi and Ahmed (1962), and Nevadomsky (1985). They contributed information about the abuse of drugs. There is a need for more studies so that we can get a clearer picture of what is going on in our region.

# Discussion

It is a well-documented observation that mental illness among Africans differs from that held by many Western societies. There is a widespread tendency among Africans to attribute mental illness to intervention of supernatural forces such as gods, spirits, witches, and magicians.

The treatment of mental illness in Africa is quite complex, and there is still widespread division of diseases into those that can be cured by Western medicine, like diabetes and malaria; and those that are not likely to be successfully treated with Western techniques. Mental illness is

TABLE 30.3. Diagnostic distribution of cases in the only medical facility available in an isolated plantation in Nigeria.

| Diagnosis | *N* | Rate/1000 |
|---|---|---|
| Anxiety | 67 | 28.8 |
| Depression | 12 | 5.2 |
| Excitement | 3 | 1.3 |
| Alcoholism | 1 | 0.4 |
| Total | 83 | 35.7 |

normally considered to be immune (cannot be effectively treated and cured) to Western medicine. Largely because of this, the majority of the mentally ill in Africa tend to seek cures from traditional healers at the onset of illnesses. In another report from Claver, the Ivorians' world is peopled by living creatures and spirits that may be beneficial or harmful. Furthermore, large trees, mountains, rocks and rivers are the dwelling places of spirits. One patient claimed that on the way to the hospital one day, she saw her deceased husband standing by her in the bus. She quickly alighted from the bus. However, she claimed the deceased followed her until they came close to the hospital fence. Subsequent discussions with the patient revealed that she had failed to attend the burial ceremony of her previous husband as a result of opposition from her current spouse. In our African culture, therefore, the problem of which heads to count out (ie, those who are not influenced by the African belief) turns out to be complex. Should we adopt the Western model and style of illness and use the instruments familiar to Western trained psychiatrists such as ICD or *Diagnostic and Statistical Manual of Mental Disorders* (DSM), or shall we adopt our own African view of the cosmos and make enquiries about which of our citizens are bothered by Ogbanje, witches, curses, enemies, and envious neighbours? Which one of us has incurred the wrath of the ancestors or the various deities that live in our cosmos? We cannot simply dismiss the idea. The majority of the people (Africans) believe in the African view that traditional doctors are better placed to cure mental illnesses and so they consult with these practitioners in moments of need.

If a majority of people believe that an imaginary situation is real, then the phenomenon becomes real in its consequences; such is the situation with a $100 bill. The paper itself is of little value; however, to the extent that the citizens invest this piece of paper with the value of $100, then the piece of paper acquires the status of a $100 bill.

To further complicate the problem of our head count is the existence of a transitional group (Binitie 1987) whose doctrines are intermediate between those of traditional African and Westernized African. The group has its world peopled by witches, wizards, devils, and saints. The traditional African gods have been removed and have been replaced by Jesus or Jehovah. Living prophets, seers, and priests constitute the intermediary between Jehovah and the worshippers. Their healing sects have in recent years grown considerably, especially in urban areas. Odiase (1981) has studied one such group and came to the conclusion that one-third of the patients brought by the adherents of a sect for healing had mental illnesses and that prayers and holy water were the system of treatment.

In the face of the multifarious forces challenging the African psychiatrist, the response has been to stick to what is known medically (that is the Western training) and to make occasional forays into the traditional and transitional systems.

## Conclusion

A set of case summaries from individuals seen by traditional healers in Nigeria have been reviewed to illustrate the intricacies of the presentations and the multiple informational perspectives needed to understand them. Attempts to inscribe these cases within ICD-10 diagnostic categories are then outlined. Finally, several clinical studies conducted in Sub-Saharan Africa are briefly reviewed; all these materials point out the need for comprehensive culture-sensitive diagnostic approaches.

## *References*

Adomako CC (1972). Mental hospital patients: A Castile Road profile. *Ghana Medical Journal* 2:65–70.

Anumonye A (1975). Psychiatric inpatients in a Nigerian university general hospital: Historical background. *African Journal of Psychiatry* 1:17–23.

Binitie A (1971). *A Study of Depression in Benin City, Nigeria.* MD Thesis, University of London.

Binitie A (1974). Mental health services in developing countries with reference to Africa. WHO/OMN/EC/74/7, Geneva.

Binitie A (1981a). Psychiatric disorders in Bendel, State of Nigeria. *Acta Psychiatrica Scandinavica* 64:273–280.

Binitie A (1981b). The clinical manifestation of depression in Africans. *Psychopathologie Africaine* XVI:(1/2/3)36–40.

Binitie A (1983). The depressed and anxious patient; care and treatment in Africa. *International Journal of Mental Health* vol 12 No. 3,44–57.

Binitie A (1987). The Care of the Mentally Ill in African Traditional and Transitional Societies. In 80th Anniversary Publication of Psychiatric Hospital, Yaba. Ed. Johnson B. Yaba-Lagos Gbajumo Press.

Binitie A (1988). Diagnosis and classification of mental disorders and alcohol and drug-related problems in Nigeria. In JE Mezzich, ME von Cranach (eds), *International Classification in Psychiatry.* Cambridge University Press, Cambridge.

Boroffka (1973). Mental illness in Lagos, history and admission statistics of Yaba Mental Hospital. *Psychopathologie Africaine* IX(3):405–417.

Carothers JC (1953). The African Mind in Health and Disease. Monograph Series No. 17. World Health Organization, Geneva.

Claver B (1968). Concepts of mental illness among the Ivorians. In OA Erinosho, NW Bell (eds), *Mental Health in Africa.* Ibadan University Press, Ibadan.

Copeland JR (1968). Aspects of mental illness in West African students. *Social Psychiatry* 3:7–13.

Crawford BKA (1961). Developing psychiatric services in Kenya. In TA Lambo (ed), *Report of 1st Pan African Congress.* Ibadan Government Press, Ibadan.

Field MJ (1958). Mental disorder in rural Ghana. *Journal of Mental Science* 104:1043–1051.

Field MJ (1960). *Search for Security: An Ethno-Psychiatric Study of Rural Ghana.* Faber & Faber, London.

Forster EFB (1958). *A Psychiatry Review for Ghana.* Publication No. 35, EETA WFMH WHO.
Forster EFB (1966). A longitudinal ecological study of 100 consecutive admissions to the Accra Mental Hospital. *Ghana Medical Journal* 5:123–127.
Geil R, Van Luik JN (1975). Psychiatric morbidity in a small Ethiopian town. *British Journal of Psychiatry* 115:149–162.
German GA (1969). Psychiatric morbidity among Ugandan student population. *British Journal of Psychiatry* 115:132–139.
German GA (1987). Mental health in Africa: The extent of mental health problems in Africa today: An update of epidemiological knowledge. *British Journal of Psychiatry* 151:435–439.
Gordon HL (1936). An inquiry into the correlation of African civilization and mental disorder in the Kenyan native. *East African Medical Journal* 12:327–335.
Ifabumuyi D, Ahmed MH (1962). A survery of alcoholism among out-patients in Kaduna. *Nigerian Journal of Psychiatry* 1:45–49.
Ihenzue UH (1982). Some observations and comments on psychosocial profile of first ever referrals to Psychiatric Hospital Enugu. *Acta Psychiatrica Scandinavica* 789:1–10.
Jegede RO, Adaranijo (1976). In-patient psychiatry in a Nigerian teaching hospital. *African Journal of Psychiatry* 2:311–314.
Kagwa BH (1965). Observation on the prevalence and types of mental diseases in East Africa. *East Africa Medical Journal* 43:673–682.
Lambo TA (1956). Neuro-psychiatric observation in Nigeria. *British Medical Journal* 2:1388–1394.
Lambo TA (1960). Further neuro-psychiatric observations in Nigeria. *British Medical Journal* 2:1696–1704.
Lament A, Blignault W (1953). A Study of male Bantu admissions to Weskoppies during 1952. *South African Medical Journal* 27:637.
Laubacher BFJ (1973). *Sex Customs and Psychopathology: A Study of South African Natives.* Routledge and Kegan Paul, London.
Leighton AH, Lambo TA, Hughes CC, Leighton DC, Murphy JM, Mercklin (1963). *Psychiatric Disorder among the Yoruba.* Cornell University Press, New York.
Margetts EL (1956). Traditional Yoruba healers in Nigeria. *Management* 65:115–118.
Moffson A (1955). A study of 400 consecutive admissions: Male Bantu admissions to Weskoppies. *South African Medicanl Journal* 29:689–692.
Murphy HM, Lubis DB (1962). The materials in "Search for Security." *Transcultural Research in Mental Health Problems* 13:50–54.
Nevadomsky JJ (1985). Drug use among Nigerian university students. *Bulletin of Narcosis* XXXVII:31–42.
Nwanunobi CO (1980). Sects in an Urban Phenomenon in Contemporary Eastern Nigeria. *Anthroposthe International Review of Ethnology and Linguistics* 75:117.
Nwosu VA (1971). *Prayer Houses and Faith Healing.* Tabansi Press, Onitsha, Nigeria.
Odejide AO, Sanda AO (1976). Observations in Drug Abuse in Western Nigeria, *African Journal of Psychiatry* 2:303–309.

Odiase GI (1981). Members and types of illness and relationship between the incidence of bringing sick and disturbed persons for healing among adherents of an Aladura church in Benin City, Nigeria. Presented at the 8th World Congress of Psychiatry, Zagreb.

Onyango P (1982). Concepts of illness among the mentally ill in Kenya. In CA Erinosho, NW Bell (eds), *Mental Health in Africa*. Ibadan University Press, Ibadan.

Onyeama WP, Onuorah AN (1980). A prospective study of 314 new patients referred to psychiatric hospital Enugu, Nigeria. *Psychopathologie Africaine* XVI:321–331.

Orley J, Wing JK (1979). Psychiatric Disorders in two African villages. *Archieves of General Psychiatry* 36:513–520.

Prince RH (1964). Indigenous Yoruba psychiatry. In A Kiev (ed). *Magic, Faith and Healing*. Free Press, New York.

Smartt GFC (1956). Mental maladjustment in the East African. *Journal of Mental Science* 102:441–466.

Tooth C (1950). *Studies in Mental Illness in the Gold Coast*. HMSO Colonial Research Publication No. 6, London.

Vyncke J (1958). *Assistance Psychiatry in Rwanda*, pp 52–55. OCTA/CSA Publication No. 35.

Younis YO (1973). Psychiatric morbidity among Khartoum (Sudan) university students. *Tropical Medicine and Hygiene* 77:200–203.

# 31
# A Japanese Study on Psychiatric Classification in General Medical Care

SABURO ANZAI

In Japan, private outpatient clinics play an important role in keeping local people healthy. Their functions and activities differ from hospitals. Moreover, they are usually located in residential areas, and because they look much like local residences, people feel free to visit them and to ask for help not only for their illnesses but also for many problems of their daily lives. In many of these clinics there are specialists in fields such as psychiatry and neurology, who also work as general practitioners. (Anzai 1982).

Anzai Iin is one of these clinics. Anzai Iin (an outpatient clinic is called Iin in Japanese) is in Yamato, which is a city located about 20 km south of Tokyo and west of Yokohama. Yamato has a population of about 190,000, many of whom commute to Tokyo or Yokohama. Industries in Yamato are mostly related to the daily lives of local residents.

There are three mental health facilities in Yamato. One is local health authority. Another is a traditional "closed" (ie, patients are not allowed to come and go freely) mental hospital that has 280 beds and does not have any rehabilitation facilities. The third is our clinic, Anzai Iin, which has an outpatient clinic, a day care, and a workshop for mental patients. We will start by explaining the clinical circumstances that form the basic framework of our general medical care.

The outpatient clinic consists of a general psychiatrist and a child psychiatric clinic. Each has a day clinic, a night clinic, and a Sunday clinic.

The day clinic is open from 9 am to 3 pm, 5 days a week. On average, about 80 patients come to the day clinic per day. Many are chronic mental patients but about 30% suffer from general physical illnesses such as a cold, hypertension, and diarrhea. A couple of new psychiatric patients come to see us every day. Among these patients we have some whom we cannot classify under diagnostic criteria currently available.

TABLE 31.1. Classification of new patients (January to June 1990).

| Major diagnosis | Male | Female |
|---|---|---|
| Affective disorders | 7 | 25 |
| Schizophrenia | 14 | 13 |
| Mental retardation | 9 | 3 |
| Anxiety disorders | 7 | 10 |
| Eating disorders | | 5 |
| Substance use disorders | 12 | 4 |
| Somatoform disorders | | 1 |
| Dissociative disorders | 1 | 3 |
| Epilepsy | 3 | 4 |
| Autism | 3 | 2 |
| Senile dementia | 2 | |
| Parkinsonism | | 1 |
| Hemicrania | | 1 |
| Unclassified | 36 | 42 |
| Total | 94 | 114 |

Table 31.1 illustrates the classification of new patients at our clinic during a period of 6 months (from January to June 1990). Almost all of them ask for help with various difficulties and problems in their lives. According to statistics in the local health authority (Yamato Local Health Authority 1990) there are about 1000 schizophrenic patients in Yamato. Some of them are living untreated in the community. About 200 of them come to our clinic to get medication and also to ask for help with problems in their daily lives and human relations. The night clinic is open from 7 to 9 pm, 3 nights a week. Patients who work at a workshop or for a company on the same terms as the general population usually come to the night clinic. They get medication and also talk about their social lives with one of the physicians. It is very important that they can talk confidentially with us about subjects that they would not feel comfortable talking about to others, especially with associates at work. This allows them to discharge stress and return to work the next morning. The Sunday clinic is open from 9 am to noon, two Sundays a month. If patients want to come to the Sunday clinic or are thought to need to come to the Sunday clinic, they must make a reservation and specify the duration and the session. Usually, patients come with their families but sometimes only the family or only the patient comes to the Sunday clinic. By talking with the physician, they can learn about their illness, medications, treatments and how to cope with them.

## Day Care

Patients who are thought to require treatment in day care, or who want to join the day care are enrolled as day care members. Usually, we open the day care only to schizophrenic patients. The members can come to day care any time they want, and may select programs in which they wish to participate. They are never forced to join and are always welcomed. If necessary, we sometimes visit patients or families at their home and explain what the day care is or how they are treated in the day care. After several visits we may then take the patients to the day care.

The members of day care programs typically take part in planning their programs, events, or entertainments. We think it is very important to create an environment that does not alienate the members and consider, the staff and the members of the day care program to be partners. We must cooperate to overcome the disabilities of the members. We call our day care an "open system" day care.

Only a small number of day care members can return directly to work situations and earn wages. Most of them must take the workshop as the first step in training towards regular work situations.

## Workshop

The workshop is more like an actual work environment than the day care. Members of the workshop are thought to be able to deal more skillfully with their daily lives and human relations than members of the day care. We call members of the workshop "trainees". The target of the amount of work in the workshop is one-third of that in normal work situations. The wages they get are also one-third as much, usually about 40,000 to 50,000 yen ($300 to $400) a month. They can manage their usual living needs with these wages.

The workshop is open from 9 am to 4 pm. The "trainees" must be at workshop during these times. The workshop is open 5 days (from Monday through Friday) a week and "trainees" come to work regularly at the workshop. It is different from the open system of day care in that in the workshop the "trainees" are requested to come to work regularly. So we call the workshop a "closed system." If members of the day care want to go over to the workshop, they are requested to decide by themselves whether they can or cannot. We think this decision-making process plays an important role in the patients' rehabilitation. There are now 40 trainees in our workshop. Almost all of them have decided to attend by themselves and now take part in workshop every day.

The income from the work in the workshop amount to almost 2 million yen a month, which is about $15,000 and is all paid to the "trainees" according to the assessments done by the assessment team of the workshop.

## Study Aims

The methods and aims of this study were to analyze diagnostically the new psychiatric patients in Japanese general medical care and to survey the practical meaning of the problems that new, unclassified psychiatric patients had in their daily lives. If possible, we wanted to clarify the important relationship between the rehabilitation of severe schizophrenic patients in our clinical situations and problems of daily lives that new patients came to ask for help with in our clinics.

## Method

As illustrated in Table 31.2, the total number of new patients that came to our clinic during the 6-month period (January to June 1990) were 208 (94 males and 114 females). We could classify 130 of them in the first examination, mainly by *Diagnostic and Statistical Manual of Mental Disorders*, 3rd edition, revised (DSM-III-R) diagnostic criteria (American Psychiatric Association, 1987), but 78 patients remained unclassified (36 males and 42 females). Fig. 31.1 shows the age of first visit of patients. Both males and females had two peaks, one at age 20 and another at age 40 to 50 (the peak of the females appeared about 10 years later than that of the males but females had one more peak at age 70).

People visited our clinic desiring consultation on a wide variety of issues, not only questions related directly to the illness, but also about adaptation to school, work, married life, or interpersonal problems, such as quarrels with neighbors. These difficulties and problems that people had in their everyday lives were not necessarily diagnosable under diagnostic criteria currently available. On many occasions we might take care of them on the basis of criteria not directly related to a diagnosis. First of all, we tried to talk with them. Some of them felt relieved of their stressful situation merely by talking with a physician. But others required more concrete means, for example, visiting their homes, or trying many times to achieve targets that had been planned beforehand to cope with their problems.

TABLE 31.2. New patients (January to June 1990).

| | |
|---|---|
| Total number | 208 |
| Male | 94 |
| Female | 114 |
| Diagnosis classified | 130 |
| Male | 58 |
| Female | 72 |
| Diagnosis unclassified | 78 |
| Male | 36 |
| Female | 42 |

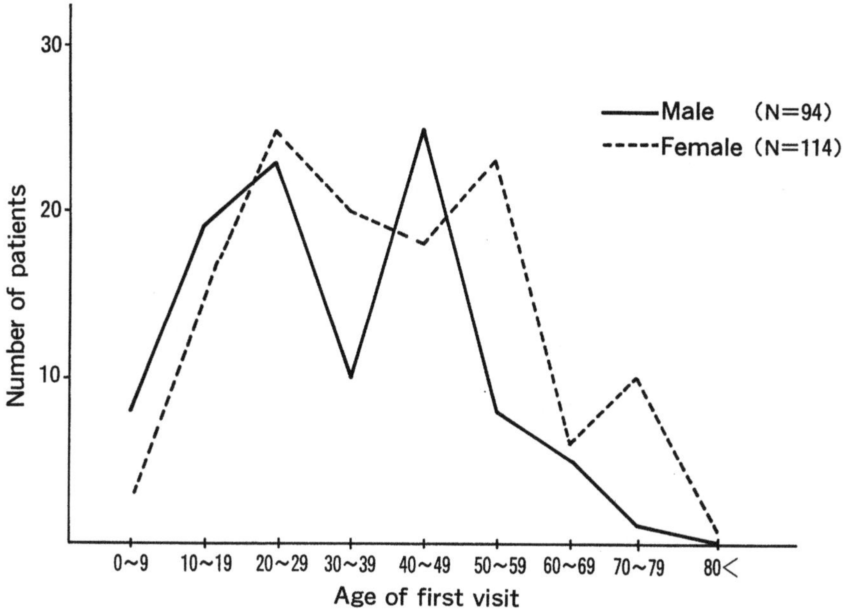


FIGURE 31.1. Age of first visit of patients (January to June).

## Problems of New Patients and Meanings of the Problems

Table 31.3 shows complaints of these unclassified patients (many patients had multiple complaints). The most common complaints in both males and females were insomnia; anxiety, tension and headache; abdominal pain; nausea; and other somatic discomforts. They visited our clinic with these complaints as if they were somatic patients. But in the process of intake many of them began to talk about their daily living problems. Table 31.4 shows these problems and psychosocial states in unclassified patients. Many of the problems are likely to occur in the daily lives of the general population. One important issue was that they visited the clinic as somatic patients with some awareness that their somatic symptoms were coming from problems of their daily lives. They could not directly express their psychological problems. Their problems (shown in Table 31.4) reflected many difficulties and contradictions in the life of modern Japanese society. The problems that were mentioned most frequently in both sexes were changes in social role or situation. Typical problems in males were unemployment, divorce in middle age, job retirement, new business, etc. In females the typical problems were life after a move from a distant place, family life after retirement, living apart from

TABLE 31.3. Complaints of new patients.

| Complaints | Male | Female |
|---|---|---|
| Insomnia | 16 | 17 |
| Anxiety and tension | 10 | 11 |
| Depressive mood | 2 | 5 |
| Nervous and sensitive to others | 3 | 2 |
| Headache, abdominal pain, nausea and other somatic signs | 5 | 7 |
| Spiritlessness, abulia | 1 | 3 |
| Tic | 3 | |
| Thought disturbances | 2 | 2 |
| Bad breath, body odor, sweating | | 3 |
| Fatigue | 2 | |
| Narrow field of vision, impaired hearing | | 2 |
| Unable to get up in the morning | 1 | |
| Feel something wrong in the body | 1 | |
| Trichotillomania | 1 | |
| Nightmares | | 1 |
| Mysophobia | | 1 |
| Wrist-cutting | | 1 |
| Feel onself being called to be crazy | | 1 |

the husband, etc. The last one in females seemed to be a problem specific to Japanese society. Some of the wives must live apart from their husbands who had been transferred to distant places. The next most common problems in males were problems of living behaviors, such as

TABLE 31.4. Daily living problems, psychosocial states in unclassified patients.

| Problem state | Male | Female |
|---|---|---|
| Change in the social role and situation | 13 | 13 |
| Problems of living behavior | 9 | 6 |
| Problems of human relations | 2 | 12 |
| Staying away from work | 3 | 2 |
| Long absence from school | 3 | 3 |
| Living alone (single) | 6 | 2 |
| Not making friends in school | 3 | |
| Staying home and doing nothing | 2 | 2 |
| Overwork | | 2 |
| Drinking | 2 | |
| Alcoholic problems of husband | | 2 |
| Becoming unable to talk with others | | 2 |
| Irregular life | 2 | |
| Schizophrenia in family member | 2 | |
| Pollakisuria at midnight | 2 | |
| Traffic accident | 2 | |
| Entrance examination | 2 | |
| Excitement, agitation | | 2 |
| Married life of aged couple | | 2 |

bed wetting, lying around the house, violence, frequent job changes, etc. In females the next most common problems were ones relating to human relations, such as quarrels with neighbors, bad relationships at school or at work, noises in the neighborhood, etc.

There were many other problems and psychological situations they asked for help with at our clinic (see Table 31.4). Some of these were more strongly connected to environmental situations (living alone, entrance examinations, etc) or family situations (schizophrenia in the family members, married life of aged couples etc). Other problems were more closely related to the psychological situations of the patients themselves (excitement, agitation, inability to talk with others, staying away from school, etc). We think that these two types of problems (ie, environmental and psychological) derive in part from deficiencies in daily living skills. These deficiencies required more social support on the one hand and psychological or technical training on the other. For example, Yamato has begun to open classes for young mothers to teach them how to play with their babies. There were increasing numbers of young mothers who cannot live with and bring up their babies adequately. These problems that we had in our community were essentially the same living problems that we faced in the rehabilitation of schizophrenia (Liberman 1988).

## Prognosis and Diagnosis of Unclassified Patients

We performed a follow-up diagnostic study on the prognosis of our unclassified patients. We selected 49 patients under 15 years of age from the new patients during a period of 10 years (1978–1987) whom we could not diagnose at their first visits. Table 31.5 shows their prognosis in 1990 when 27 patients (55%) led their daily lives normally. Only 16 patients (33%) were diagnosed as suffering from schizophrenia, affective disorders, and learning disorders. The diagnosis of six patients still remained unclassified. Table 31.5 shows that over half of the patients who were unclassified at their first visit have overcome their problems within 10 years. About 12% were still facing problems in spite of our efforts and were not classifiable. Among the 16 patients diagnosed as suffering from psychiatric disorders, 75% had schizophrenia.

We had little knowledge about the signs and problems specific to schizophrenia that occurred before the outbreak of schizophrenic symptoms. Usually we could not distinguish them from the complaints of the general population. Table 31.6 shows complaints and daily living problems of 14 new patients later classified as having major psychosis. In contrast to anxiety, tension, and insomnia observed in all other unclassified patients, Table 31.7 shows that somatic symptoms and absence from school characterized these patients. However, we do not think these

TABLE 31.5. Diagnostic outcome after 10 years (1978–1987) of 49 patients under 15 years of age (30 males, 19 females).

| Outcome after 10 years | No. of patients (%) |
|---|---|
| Healthy | 27 (55) |
| Male | 16 |
| Female | 11 |
| Mental ill | 16 (33) |
| Schizophrenia | 12 |
| Affective disorders | 2 |
| Learning disorders | 2 |
| Still unclassified | 6 (12) |
| Male | 5 |
| Female | 1 |

symptoms were specific to schizophrenia because the children suffering from the so-called school phobia might be absent from school or complain of somatic symptoms (Anthony 1975). As shown in Table 31.6, patients later classified as suffering from major psychosis complained of many symptoms that did not distinguish them from the other unclassified patients (see Table 31.4). However, if we change our perspective and examine the progress of these patients, we find clear differences between those who developed major psychosis and those who returned to normality. Table 31.7 shows these differences very clearly.

Symptoms and problems in new patients who later developed major psychosis continued to exist during these 10 years. We were usually able

TABLE 31.6. Daily live problems, psychosocial states and complaints of patients who later developed major psychosis.

| Problems, states, and complaints | Male | Female |
|---|---|---|
| Headache, abdominal pain, other somatic complaints | 4 | 3 |
| Absent from school | 3 | 4 |
| Insomnia | 1 | 2 |
| Refuse to go to school | | 1 |
| Shaking head | 1 | |
| Spiritlessness | 1 | |
| Not talking with others | 1 | 1 |
| Delayed speech | 1 | |
| Depressive mood | | 1 |
| Nervous and sensitive to others | | 1 |
| Cannot swallow | | 1 |
| Being bullied in the school | | 1 |
| Anxiety and tension | | 1 |
| Eating disorders | | 1 |
| Cannot get up in the morning | 1 | |
| Enuresis | | 1 |

TABLE 31.7. Differences in initial daily live problems, psychosocial states and complaints between patients who developed psychoses and those who returned to normality.

| Category | Developed psychoses | Returned to normality |
|---|---|---|
| Living problems and complaints | Continue or extend to other living area with advent of new life events | Usually transient |
| Response to helping intervention | Responds temporarily but intervention makes the situations more complex and difficult | Good response |
| Response to medication | Unsatisfactory and often discontinued | Good response |

to find transient symptoms and problems through careful examination, even when they seemed to have disappeared. Moreover, when patients happened to encounter new life events, these symptoms and problems appeared again to the extent of disturbing their daily lives (relapse-liability) (Utena 1974) or extended to other life areas. In healthy people, these symptoms and problems were usually transient or even if they appeared occasionally, they never disturbed their daily lives.

In regard to the responses to helpful interventions in patients of later major psychosis, it was very difficult for us to get good responses. The responses were usually only temporary or partial. There seemed to exist in very complex situations that involved problems of human relations, disabilities, family problems, and other psychological handicaps. Because of these complexities, our interventions often tended to make situations more complex and difficult. Accordingly, we were only able to observe. The responses to medications in patients of later major psychosis were also usually unsatisfactory. The medications could not eliminate their complex problems but often tended to reinforce negative tendencies such as depressive mood or side effects. Moreover, not only patients but also family members often did not like taking medicines.

## Discussion

First of all, we must recognize that we have many cases in our community that we cannot classify by using established diagnostic criteria. The cases we showed in method are only part of all the living cases in our community. There are a wide variety of symptoms and problems (see Tables 31.3 and 31.4), but about half of the patients are thought to be able to return to normal life through psychotherapeutic education, medication, management, and human services which are becoming more important methods of general medical care (Anderson et al 1986, Liberman 1988, Anzai 1989, Fujita 1987). It is important in our clinic to treat them with these methods until we are able to determine their diagnosis. The important point is that the process of diagnosis is at the same time the therapeutic process. About 33% of 49 unclassified patients were diagnosed as having major psychosis, mainly schizophrenia (see Table 31.5). But we cannot find any difference in the daily living problems between the patients of later major psychosis and general unclassified patients (see Tables 31.4 and 31.6). We think that these problems in both cases are fundamentally the same, because they occur in the complex interactions between environment and biological existence. We think it is necessary to offer some therapeutic approaches such as human services and psychotherapeutic education, in addition to medical treatments such as medication. These therapeutic approaches should also be useful for diagnosis.

As mentioned earlier, we offer several sorts of services such as night clinic, Sunday clinic, day care, workshop, etc. We think that these facilities are very effective in coping with the problems of people living in our community. If patients want to take part in these services, they will be allowed to do so at any time. For example, we tried to rehabilitate a 28-year-old male schizophrenic patient who stayed home doing nothing for 10 years (Table 31.8). When treating the problems of patients we set stepwise targets that meet mutual, attainable, and specific goals of treatment for each problem (Anderson et al 1986). The first target was the creation of an intimate relationship with the family. This was usually done in the Sunday clinic. At that time, we could collect much information about the patient and his family. Sessions in the Sunday clinic also enabled both patient and family to learn about the illness, coping techniques, and how to reduce stress. The second target was to get the patient out of his home. The target was satisfied when the patient left his home with a therapist. The third target was to take the patient to day care. As shown in Table 31.8, we made many targets with the patient, one after another. If a patient is able to achieve these various goals he will overcome his disabilities and be able to return to the actual society.

TABLE 31.8. An example of rehabilitation approach to a 28-year-old male schizophrenic patient who stayed home for 10 years.

| | |
|---|---|
| 1. Family meeting for 2 years | Target: To make contact with family members |
| 2. Therapist visits patient's home once a week for a month | Target: To get the patient out of home |
| 3. Therapist visits patient's home and takes him to day care once a week | Target: To go to day care; it is good for patient to be in day care; therapist takes care of him only in the therapy room |
| 4. Therapist takes patient to day care once a week | Target: To engage in simple craft only by himself in the therapy room with a therapist. |
| 5. Therapist takes patient to day care once a week | Target: To engage in simple craft in a small group. |

The target goal must be set to fit to the specific problems of the patients, and the problems will have to be divided into small items in order to facilitate stepwise achievement by both patient and therapist. We are using targets to treat the problems of outpatients in our clinic. We think the target concept is more applicable to people who want to have some help with their daily living problems than to schizophrenic patients. Diagnosis is a long process, but individual targets should be achievable within a short period of time. The attaining processes involve psychotherapy, training, education, and other therapeutic processes. We think that the processes to attain each target will give us much information to apply diagnostic criteria. Thus, the process of attaining targets becomes a diagnostic process. We think that the process of attaining targets is more important for our daily practice of general medical care than the diagnostic process. We should remember that the aim of our general medical care is not only diagnosis of the patient but also support, psychologically and socially, to enable them to lead fruitful lives.

## Conclusion

In the practical situations of Japanese general medical care we come across many patients whom we cannot classify by the diagnostic criteria currently available. These patients have many living problems that can be treated effectively by setting stepwise targets that should be planned in advance and in accordance with the specific problems being experienced.

In the follow-up study of unclassified patients under 15 years of age, we found that about half of them were back to normal living situations by using target techniques but about 33% of them developed schizophrenic symptoms within 10 years.

From these experiences we have reached the conclusion that it is very useful and important for the unclassified patients to be treated with attainable short-term goals until a diagnosis can be made. This target technique usually gives us much information about the patients and helps us diagnose them as well.

## *References*

American Psychiatric Association (1987). *Diagnostic and Statistical Manual of Mental Disorders* (3rd ed, rev). American Psychiatric Association, Washington, DC.

Anderson C, Reiss DJ, Hogarty GE (1986). *Schizophrenia and the Family*, Guilford, New York.

Anthony EJ (1975). School phobia, pp 2150–2151. In AM Freedman, HI Kaplan, (eds), *Comprehensive Textbook of Psychiatry*, II. Williams & Wilkins, Baltimore.

Anzai S (1982). Mental health care in the general medical care of private outpatient clinic in Japan, pp 262–293. In H Masno, K Kondo (eds), *The Practices of Community Mental Health Care*. Kongo, Tokyo (in Japanese).
Anzai S (1989). Psychiatric rehabilitation in the private outpatient clinic in Japan, pp 166–186. In H Hachiya, N Murata (eds), *Community Rehabilitation of Chronic Psychiatric Patients*. Igaku-Schoin, Tokyo (in Japanese).
Fujita M (1987). *Human Service*. Budousha, Tokyo (in Japanese).
Liberman RP (1988). *Psychiatric Rehabilitation of Chronic Mental Patients*. American Psychiatric Press, Washington, DC.
Utena H (1974). On relapse-liability: Schizophrenia, amphetamine psychosis and animal model, pp 285–287. In H Mitsuda, T Fukuda (eds), *Biological Mechanisms of Schizophrenia and Schizophrenia-Like Psychoses*. Igaku-Shoin, Tokyo (in Japanese).
Yamato Local Health Authority (1990). *Year Book of Yamato Local Health Authority*, pp 59–62. Yamato, Japan (in Japanese).

# 32 Experiences on Psychiatric Classification in South Asia Primary Care Facilities

R. SRINIVASA MURTHY

Focus on the mental health needs at primary care is a recent phenomenon both in developed and developing countries. In the developed countries, the stimulus came from the studies of the General Practice Unit (Shepherd et al 1966) and the Royal College of General Practitioners in the United Kingdom in the 1960s and 1970s. Goldberg's (1970, 1972, 1984) efforts have provided a continuous new flow of information regarding this area as seen in the Western countries.

## Mental Health Care in Developing Countries

In the developing countries, the movement for the organization of mental health services is of recent origin (less than 2 decades old). The beginnings, for an approach to this area came from the WHO efforts in the 1970s. The Sixteenth Expert Committee Report on Organization of Mental Health Services in Developing Countries (WHO 1975) provided a new framework for mental health care programmes. One of the chief recommendations was to integrate mental health care with primary care.

"In the developing countries, trained mental health professionals are very scarce indeed—often they number less than one per million of the population. Clearly, if basic mental health care is to be brought within reach of the mass of the population, this will have to be done by non-specialized health workers—of all levels, from the primary health worker to the nurse or doctor—working in collaboration with, and supported by, more specialized personnel. This will require changes in the roles and training of both general health workers and mental health professionals" (WHO 1990). In the last 15 years, there has been substantial progress in this area.

The progress in the National Programmes of Mental Health since 1975 has been the result of a number of interacting factors namely, (1) national identities, (2) focus on primary care since 1978, (3) increasing number of mental health professionals, (4) growing public demand for services, (5) advances in the area of mental health, and (6) community mental health care movement of the West. The most significant aspect of this movement relevant to psychiatric classification is that mental health care is organized using a public health approach. In other words, in the West, focus on mental health programs at primary care occurred against the background of well-established mental health care systems. In developing countries, community mental health care is the direct and focused effort to provide services by integrating mental health with primary care, especially with primary health care (PHC) services (Harding et al 1980, Wig et al 1981, Srinivasa Murthy and Wig 1983, WHO 1990).

The essential aspects of this approach are to identify priorities, provide task-oriented training, and develop continuous support and supervision to the PHC personnel. This method of organizing care is in progress in the following countries of southeast Asia: Afghanistan, Bangladesh, Burma, India, Indonesia, Nepal, Pakistan, Sri Lanka, and Thailand. Similar efforts are in progress in Africa. Based on personal experience of visits to some of these countries and literature relating to the developments in most of these countries, it can be said to be a major revolution in the field of mental health care. The most important point is the initial success of integration utilizing primary care personnel of health, education, and welfare sectors for the care of the severely ill and for mental health promotion and for prevention of mental disorders (Srinivasa Murthy 1983, 1989).

## Psychiatric Classification and Primary Care

The need of psychiatric classification for primary care arises from three areas: (1) the needs of PHC personnel to identify, diagnosis, record, and report periodic statistics as part of the general health services; (2) the requirements of mental health professionals working with PHC personnel to support and supervise mental health care and to link it with the larger mental health classificatory development; and (3) classification of conditions currently not clearly identified as mental health problems but seen frequently by PHC personnel.

### *Needs of Primary Health Care Personnel*

The focus on PHC personnel as first-contact care providers means that they can only provide care for a limited range of problems. This also means identification of priorities and a limited list of classificatory conditions.

In the last 15 years, data have been available from a number of countries to demonstrate the feasibility of this approach. The manuals developed identify only 6 or 7 major diagnostic groups. The care provided by PHC personnel also covers about six conditions (WHO 1987). In India, a number of centers have examined this issue and the classification used included acute psychosis, chronic psychosis, depression, mental handicap, neurosis, and drug dependence (Srinivasa Murthy 1987). Wig and Parhee (1988) have focused on the place of acute and transient psychoses from the perspective of developing countries, and urged the need of putting them in a new category in the international classification.

These observations are in contrast to the experience of developed countries, where the focus is on minor psychiatric problems (Sartorius et al 1990, Shepherd 1983). This difference in emphasis is a reflection of the PHC structure.

## *Mental Health Professionals Working with Primary Health Care Personnel*

Support and supervision form an essential part of the process of mental health care at primary care. A psychiatrist working at this level meets a number of problems: (1) the need to condense the large number of diagnostic categories into a few for use by PHC personnel as outlined above; (2) the limitations of time and available information to reach a specific diagnosis; (3) the unclear nature of the complaints with greater somatization, and lastly; (4) the need to simplify the experience and draw conclusions based on the experience for wider professional communication. There is no answer as yet for all of these. Most of us working in this area recognize these needs and hope to find solutions. The danger that public health mental health professionals might lose professional specificity is a real one, often resulting in a consequential inference to consider the primary care mental health as "rough and dirty" or "second rate." This is an area for future work, and a classification system is an important area in this development.

## *Nature of Conditions at Primary Care*

The majority of mental health problems seen in primary care are not traditional psychiatric problems. A psychiatrist working at this level may observe the following: "Only about 10% of the total cases seen fell into any one of the categories ordinarily seen in public mental hospitals."

This will be illustrated using data from a rural health facility (Sriram et al 1987), where 1853 persons seeking help were screened for mental health problems. It was found that 10% of them were found to have functional complaints. What was striking was that the majority presented

TABLE 32.1. Mental health problems in primary health care.

| Category | No. (%) |
|---|---|
| Physical problems | 1635 (90) |
| Psychosocial problems | 193 (10) |
| Symptoms | |
| Sleep disturbance | 103 (3) |
| Tiredness | 89 (46) |
| Body ache | 84 (44) |
| Poor appetite | 82 (43) |
| Headache | 68 (35) |
| Backache | 57 (30) |
| Sadness | 56 (29) |

Note. Modified from Sriram TB et al 1987.

diagnostic problems. Most of them did not fit into a known category and presented with wide and varying somatic symptoms (Table 32.1).

This has led to the consideration of them with terms such as functional complaints, psychosocial distress syndrome, emotional distress syndrome, and descriptive terms psychalgia, myalgia, sexual neurosis, etc. A classification system for this group has to be different from that for mental health professionals.

A good approach suggesting such a linkage between health worker, physician and specialist has been presented by Cooper (1988). This need is all the more urgent in developing countries where the beginnings of mental health care occur primarily at this level. In a way, the larger acceptance of mental health program could depend on an appropriate classification system.

Recent biological studies of individuals presenting culture-bound syndromes such as *Latah*, *trance* (Simons and Hughes 1985, Simons et al 1988, Ervin et al 1988) have opened many new possibilities for studying these syndromes from a biological viewpoint and not only from a psychosocial perspective.

## Conclusion

Psychiatric classification in primary care settings is an important need of developing countries. Emphasis should be placed on the immediate basic mental health services and subsequent widening of the range of conditions to be included in primary care. Similar are the needs in the areas of school mental health and preschool child care, as they also need to start providing basic mental health care. The challenges for mental health professionals in the developing countries are many in this area, as pointed out by Sartorius et al (1990): "The challenge of the next decade will be to complement our knowledge about psychological disorders seen in general medical settings in different parts of the world in order to devise effective interventions for their treatment, and to find ways to ensure the training of all general medical staff in their use."

## References


Cooper JE (1988). The structure and presentation of contemporary psychiatric classifications with special reference to ICD-9 and 10. *British Journal of Psychiatry* 152:21–28 (suppl).

Ervin FR, Palmour RM, Pearson BE, Prince RA, Simons RC (1988). The psychobiology of trance-II. *Transcultural Psychiatric Research Review* 25: 267–284.

Harding TW, de Arango MV, Baltazar J, Climent CE, Ibrahim AHA, Ignacio LL, Srinivasa Murthy R, Wig NN (1980). Mental disorders in primary health care: A study of their frequency and diagnosis in four developing countries. *Psychological Medicine* 10:231–241.

Goldberg DP (1972). *The Detection of Psychiatric Illness by a Questionnaire.* Maudsley Monograph No. 21. Oxford University Press, London.

Goldberg DP (1984). The recognition of psychiatric illness by non-psychiatrists. *Australian and New Zealand Journal of Psychiatry* 18:128–134.

Goldberg DP, Blackwell B (1970). Psychiatric illness in general practice: A detailed study using a new method of case detection. *British Medical Journal* 2:439–442.

Sartorius N, Goldberg D, de Girolamo GO, Costa de Silva JA, Lecrubier Y, Wittchan HU (eds) (1990). *Psychological disorders in general medical settings.* Hogrefe & Huber, Toronto.

Shepherd M (1983). Mental disorders and primary care in the United Kingdom. *Journal of Public Health Policy* 4:83–88.

Shepherd M, Cooper B, Brown AC, Katton GW (1966). *Psychiatric Illness in General Practice.* Oxford University Press, London.

Simons RC, Ervin FR, Prince RH (1988). The psychobiology of trance-I. *Transcultural Psychiatric Research Review* 25:249–266.

Simons RC, Hughes CC (1985). *Culture-Bound Syndromes.* Reidel, Boston.

Srinivasa Murthy R (1983). Treatment and rehabilitation of the severely mentally ill in developing countries: Experiences of South East Asia. *International Journal of Mental Health* 12(3):16–29.

Srinivasa Murthy R (1987). Recent developments in community mental health care in India, pp 37–40. In *Collaborative Studies on Severe Mental Morbidity.* Indian Council of Medical Research, New Delhi.

Srinivasa Murthy R (1989). Mental health care in developing countries. *Community Mental Health News* (NIMHANS, India) 2:13–14.

Srinivasa Murthy R, Wig NN (1983). A training approach to enhancing the availability of mental health manpower in a developing country. *American Journal of Psychiatry* 140:1486–1490.

Sriram TB, Kumar K, Moily S, Chandrasekhar CR, Isaac MK, Srinivasa Murthy RS (1987). Minor psychiatric disturbances in primary health care: A study of their prevalence and characteristics using a simple case detection technique. *Indian Journal of Social Psychiatry* 3:212–226.

World Health Organization (1975). Organization of mental health services in developing countries. Technical Report Series No. 564. World Health Organization, Geneva.

World Health Organization (1987). *Annotated Directory of Mental Health Training Manuals*. World Health Organization, Geneva.

World Health Organization (1990). *The Introduction of Mental Health Component into Primary Health Care*. World Health Organization, Geneva.

Wig NN, Parhee R (1988). Acute and transient psychosis: A view from developing countries. In JE Mezzich, M von Cranach (eds), *International Classification in Psychiatry—Unity and Diversity*. Cambridge University Press, New York.

Wig NN, Srinivasa Murthy R, Harding TW (1981). A model for rural psychiatric services—Raipur Rani experience. *Indian Journal of Psychiatry* 23:275–290.

# Epilogue: A Universal Approach to Psychiatric Diagnosis

Horacio Fabrega

There is no more basic and important task in psychiatry than diagnosis. Traditionally, diagnosis has involved identifying and naming the disorder or disorders that underlie and explain a patient's clinical condition which, in turn, can be thought of as the totality of clinically relevant manifestations of the patient. In recent decades, as the complexity of how psychiatric disorders unfold and respond to treatment has been clarified, the idea of diagnosis has expanded to include the codification of additional clinical information beyond merely the identity of a disorder or disorders. The outcome has been the concept of multiaxiality (Mezzich 1979, and Chapter 17).

Diagnosis is basic to the therapeutic enterprise because it crystallizes for the clinician the direction that needs to be charted in order to restore well-being and social functioning. Diagnosis is also basic to the research enterprise because in standardizing the focus of inquiry and experimentation it promises to produce information that helps clarify the nature of a disorder in a way that is reproducible and allows for the accumulation of knowledge.

Intrinsic to any scientific enterprise such as biomedicine and psychiatry, as a component within it, is organization and systematization. It is thus natural that in addition to naming and categorizing information about psychiatric disorders there should evolve a system of classification. Such a system enables categorizing the full range of disorders that are likely to be encountered as well as the relations that they have to each other. Systems of diagnostic classification are basic features of all literate medical traditions. In the contemporary nation states, one finds medical bodies or subdisciplines that almost literally articulate and validate their clinical pursuits via clearly specified systems of diagnostic classification. Such systems, in effect, mark the maturity of a medical discipline.

It is understandable that because biomedical psychiatry, as a variety of the universal science of medicine, aims for generalizability it should develop a need for a universal system of psychiatric diagnosis. Such a system should in theory be applicable in all societies.

The authors of this book can all be viewed as responding to this need for a universal, scientific standardization in psychiatry. They report on their efforts to advance a universal system of psychiatric diagnosis. Their dedication and achievements cannot but be applauded, for the material of the chapters are rich documents that carefully describe thought-out protocols of investigation and scholarship aimed at achieving a universal science of psychiatric diagnosis. Indeed, the range of clinical information reviewed in this volume that pertains to the details of psychiatric diagnosis and classification of disorders is little short of astonishing considering the variety of settings in which these efforts have been carried out.

As articulated in the Preface, the organization and content of this book recognize the complexity of the theory of clinical reality that diagnostic systems represent. Both the need to consider the historical context and cultural framework of psychiatric classification as well as the requirements imposed by the various aspects of clinical care are attended to through the chapters of this volume. This epilogue pays particular attention to universal issues in the conceptualization of psychiatric classification.

Any realistic achievement of an ambitious goal such as that of a universalist schema of psychiatric diagnosis encounters a number of impediments that need to be overcome. All psychiatric scientists cannot be expected to share the same perspective regarding the nature of psychiatric disorders, including their typology and characteristics. Furthermore, they all are members of distinguished national traditions of medicine and psychiatry that, of necessity, frame the task of diagnosis and practice in different ways. The kinds of disorders that occupy a discipline as well as the rationale for identifying them (including in particular the purposes and end point of therapy) cannot but be different given the variety of medical and cultural traditions. Thus, it cannot but be anticipated that there will be manifest in a compendium such as this one considerable variety of approaches and philosophies as well as fundamental differences in the definition, interpretation, and assessment of accomplishable goals attendant with respect to a universal system of psychiatric diagnosis.

In this epilogue I attempt to summarize some of the problems associated with what I will term the universalist agenda of psychiatric diagnosis. I pursue this goal by illustrating how the authors have described and handled these problems and obstacles.

## On the Nature of a Psychiatric Disorder

Any system of psychiatric diagnosis must confront the basic problem of the essential nature of entities or objects that it deals with. In this light, one is allowed to ask: What indeed is a psychiatric disorder or "the psychiatric"? In an attempt to answer this question meaningfully, one quickly becomes mired in theoretical quandaries that involve the biological, psychological, and social sciences as well as history and philosophy. Entailed in the idea of psychiatric disorders are behavioral problems (and sometimes frank behavioral breakdowns), and modes of adapting or maladapting that often depend on disturbances in physiological systems but that exist in cultural and historical space (Fabrega 1993a, 1993b). Because of this specificity, such disorders are interpretable only with respect to symbolic conventions about ordered behavior or normality that are specific to the societies in question (Devereux 1956).

With few exceptions (eg, Mezzich 1989), clinicians and researchers in psychiatry leave the concept of psychiatric disorder unexamined, taken for granted, a "primitive given" as the philosophers of science would say. Yet, it is basic to the enterprise of this book, which deals with a classification of such "disorders" that aspires to universality (Kendell 1989).

Although the theoretical problem of what constitutes a psychiatric disorder was acknowledged by many researchers (explicitly so in Chapter 2 by Frances et al), no serious attempt to define this or at least to provide a frame of reference for understanding was undertaken by any of the authors of this book. It can be assumed that, by and large, the authors hold that this problem is crucial to the full realization of a science of psychiatric practice, and that in the interim progress needs to be made in areas that are more empirically tractable and no less vital. Nevertheless, such authors as Pull and Chaillet (Chapter 29), Binitie (Chapter 30) and Anzai (Chapter 31) as well as Frances et al (Chapter 27) who reported on the experiences of using psychiatric categories in a primary medical care setting richly illustrate in a direct way the quandaries of establishing exactly what constitutes a psychiatric disorder. Moreover, an indirect yet equally compelling illustration of differences regarding the essential nature of a psychiatric disorder was provided in the chapters that reported on the experiences of accommodating national psychiatric classification systems with the international ones, most explicitly, the chapters by Shen (Chapter 8) and Fujinawa (Chapter 10A) on the People's Republic of China, and on Japan, respectively.

## The Idea of Psychiatric Classification in Antiquity

It can be argued that 2500 years ago, even if there had existed an awareness of a global world, the idea of a universal approach to psychiatric diagnosis would have seemed nonsensical (Fabrega 1990, 1992). For one, a concept of the psychiatric or of psychiatric disorders had not evolved. In fact, this concept continues to change and evolve up to the present, even if it is rarely defined or entertained in a serious way as was mentioned above (Kendell 1989).

One is able to say that a concept pertaining to Human Behavioral Breakdowns (HBB), roughly analogous in meaning to madness or insanity, has commanded attention in all of the literate traditions of medicine of which we have any record (Chiu 1985, 1986, Dube 1988, Halipur 1984, Tseng 1973, Unschuld 1983, Weiss 1977, Yanchi 1988a, 1988b). Each literate tradition of medicine, specifically those of China, India, and of Europe of the classical era, contains descriptions of conditions that conform to HBB. Analogous categories are also found among peoples that fall outside of the sway of the civilizations that gave life to the literate medical traditions, such as Africa, Oceania and Meso America. An idea such as HBB most probably constitutes a human or cultural universal. Thus, that people were vulnerable to conditions that today we call "psychiatric disorders" were a part of the experiences of all people.

An awareness that HBB were likely to constitute a part of the medical experiences of all people was thus a theoretical possibility in antiquity given their likely personal experiences with them and the capacity of the human mind to generalize and imagine alternative groups or societies and the problems they might have encountered. However, as mentioned, the idea of a universal classification would have appeared nonsensical because such disorders (HBB) would have been accorded very specific meanings that could not easily have been abstracted from meaningful social contexts, much less equated across geographic boundaries.

Although possibly identifiable in the descriptive texts of the literate traditions of medicine as well as among the understandings of contemporary descendants of people outside the sway of the respective civilizations (Chiu 1985, 1986, Dube 1988, Halipur 1984, Tseng 1973, Unschuld 1983, Weiss 1977, Yanchi 1988a, 1988b), the "disorders" in question grew out of complex epistemologies based on the cultures that were integral to these traditions of medicine. Each tradition constituted a comprehensive approach to health and sickness and the "disorders" or, more properly, the symptom complexes identified in them (some of which would have included psychiatric-like descriptors), carried an amalgam of meanings that incorporated spiritual, moral, as well as bodily and behavioral/psychological sorts of things that connected in an individual in a special and unique way (Temkin 1963).

The chapter by Binitie (Chapter 30) provides a rich contemporary illustration of the social, cultural, and spiritual rootedness of problems of behavior that are thought of as medical by a traditional people but that simply could not easily be abstracted out of their specific context. The idea that these (holistic, person bound) sicknesses constituted objective, ontological "things" pertaining to a "psyche" that could, moreover, be equated in a universal system of classification would scarcely have been entertainable. What today with hindsight one might term psychiatric disorders were simply too bound up in the exigencies of individual's lives and the associated web of meanings about health and sickness to be conceptualized as generic entities common to all people and hence, classifiable across societies.

In a much more muted and subtle way, the difficulties that users of evolved national traditions of psychiatric diagnosis have today in accommodating to the categories of *International Classification of Diseases*, 10th revision (ICD-10) and the *Diagnosis and Statistical Manual of Mental Disorders* (DSM) system that spring from different national traditions, can be seen as illustrations of how cultural differences regarding the nature of disorders make it difficult to equate categories across national boundaries. The chapters by Wig (Chapter 1), Stromgren (Chapter 4), Johnson (Chapter 7), Shen (Chapter 8), Fujinawa (Chapter 10A) and Okazaki (Chapter 10H) all illustrate this point.

## The Agenda of a Universal Classification of Psychiatric Diagnosis: Cultural and Historical Aspects

One should begin by stressing at the outset that an agenda of a universal classification of psychiatric diagnosis entails pairing two seemingly inconsistent tenets: (1) all persons are creatures of enormous variation when viewed in the light of genetic structures, cultural characteristics, and historical circumstances; and (2) all persons are vulnerable to developing a finite, common set of behavioral manifestations of disorders that are in the process of being identified and described by the science of psychiatry (Fabrega 1993a, 1993b). Implications of the first point are taken up in the following section. Let us emphasize the second point first.

A sustained impetus towards a conception of psychiatric disorders as naturalistic, scientific "objects" is largely a development of the 19th century (Fabrega 1989). This development, as indicated above, continues to evolve in a concrete and most vivid sense whenever the agenda of national or international psychiatric diagnostic systems is proposed and seriously pursued, as it most assuredly has as evidenced by the chapters of this book. Initially centered on madness and insanity, forms of melancholia that included mood and somatic symptoms, and a variety of chronic and degenerative neurological conditions, a concept of the psychiatric has evolved to encompass neurotic conflicts and symptoms (emotional, psychological, bodily) as well as disturbances of social behavior attributable to personality disorders (Jackson 1986).

Thus, an agenda of a universal system of psychiatric diagnosis is based on a historically and culturally bound (ontological) concept about disorders of behavior as medical objects. In addition, the agenda presupposes a reasonably well-demarcated conceptual and empirical description of the kinds of human problems of behavior and adaptation that should qualify as instanciations of such disorders. These basic presuppositions are part of the scientific, biomedical epistemology and of the enterprise of a medical taxonomy that is integral to it.

The preceding ideas would probably be shared by most, if not all, contributors to this important volume, although researchers who reported on their experiences in primary care settings would be aware of the limitation of these ideas. However, not elaborated in any of the chapters of the book, are the historical, political, economic, and cultural foundations of what can, for the sake of convenience, be termed the universalist's agenda for psychiatric diagnosis (ie, that psychiatric disorders are naturalistic, scientific objects common to *homo sapiens* and capable of being defined, diagnosed, and classified). Special social problems intrinsic to the late 18th and 19th century in European societies stemming from industrialization, urbanization, intra- and international migration and a capitalist economy created conditions that alerted government representatives, religious leaders, members of charitable organizations and physicians to the plight of the marginal, the impoverished and the mentally ill (Fabrega 1989, Scull 1979). This, of course, complemented efforts already expended in the private trade involving the seriously psychiatrically ill as well as in medical settings more generally, where varieties of the psychiatric disorders were to be found. Widespread appreciation of these social psychiatric problems and the necessity of dealing with them in a prudent and humane way created the conditions that facilitated the growth of the asylum and with this opportunity to care for and study the psychiatric disorders that increasingly came to be identified and described.

Thus, what one could term a Western European social agenda about the complex assortment of social problems posed by the seeming, if not actual, increased prevalence of the psychiatric disorders gave impetus to the science of psychiatry, including the science of psychiatric diagnosis and eventually, of classification. This was a correctionist agenda that was anchored in an awareness that these disorders were rooted in social problems and had an impact on them in special ways. In other words, in addition to what one could term a medical agenda pertaining to sickness and healing that is intrinsic to the medical enterprise everywhere, there was also found during the pivotal early stages of the growth of the scientific appreciation of psychiatric disorders an orientation that these disorders grew out of and fed into social relations and activities vital to the maintenance of social order. The workplace, the schools and universities, the conduct of religious services, and the integrity of the family all were connected to these psychiatric disorders in special ways.

Not only was a distinct historical and political economic setting the birthplace of the psychiatric as we understand this today, but also a distinct cultural tradition that gave meaning to ideas basic to the psychiatric enterprise (Fabrega 1993a, 1993b). Ideas about the nature of persons, the self and behavior more generally were an integral part of the culture that made possible a definition of the psychiatric (Fabrega 1992). These ideas involved voluntarism, individuality, responsibility, autonomy, as well as more basic notions having to do with the nature of subjectivity, the mind as compared to the body and what behavior consisted of, including its rationales and purposes and how it came to be produced (Fabrega in press).

In short, a highly specific culture about persons, medicine, and social order shaped the meaning of the psychiatric and psychiatric disorders, what these disorders meant from a social standpoint, and how they should be dealt with from a sociomedical policy standpoint. It should, of course, come as no surprise that the idea of an international classification of psychiatric diagnosis is quintessentially a Western European cultural idea. That this highly culture-bound idea, together with its culturally specific social correctionist agenda, now serves to galvanize the efforts of representatives of diverse national and cultural traditions is itself an astonishing and highly interesting fact that cannot be fully explored here but which, it can be appreciated, would prove profoundly interesting to critical theorists and philosophers of science more generally (Geuss 1981).

## Why There Should Be Points of Tension in the Universalist's Agenda

That there should exist tensions in an agenda for a universal system of psychiatric diagnosis is to be expected given the considerations reviewed above. Stated in a bold way, the agenda by definition implies that (1) all people develop the same psychiatric disorders; (2) a common way of defining, describing, identifying, naming, and classifying such disorders is possible; and (3) a common system of psychiatric diagnosis constitutes a basic first step towards arranging for a common prudent and humane way of dealing with such disorders. Yet, that agenda is (1) about disorders integrally bound up with human behavioral individuality; (2) to be applied to people of highly diverse populational/genetic, national, and cultural traditions; (3) by people (ie, psychiatrists) who themselves are of diverse cultural origin; (4) in settings (ie, societies, communities) with highly variable cultural traditions about sickness and healing. The relevance of this last point needs some elaboration.

Sickness and healing, we should all be reminded, constitute the basic, underlying categories of the medical, including the psychiatric, and these categories, although themselves in some way universal, are also realized (ie, instanciated) in culturally distinctive ways. In other words, the universalist agenda is to be applied in societies with very different cultural traditions about sickness and healing. This gives rise to a number of problems tied to the following question: How is a universalist agenda pertaining to psychiatric diagnosis and classification to be applied in societies where there exist highly discrepant ways of conceptualizing sickness and dealing with the sick for purposes of helping, curing, treating, and dealing with them? An attempt to answer this question is beyond the scope of this epilogue (Edgerton 1969), but the question nonetheless serves to make explicit some of the quandaries implicit in the universalist agenda for psychiatric diagnosis.

## Some Examples of How Researchers Deal with the Tensions Implicit in the Universalist's Agenda

Having identified the inevitability of points of tension in the universalist's agenda, it is worth reviewing briefly the ways in which these are sometimes acknowledged and sometimes ignored by the contributors to this volume. Primary emphasis is given to material that reflects difficulty of accomplishing a universal system of psychiatric diagnosis in light of social and cultural considerations. The strict limitations of the current system from the standpoint of treatment was superbly summarized in Chapter 23 by Helmchen and need not be discussed further. The potential value of such a system for spotting psychiatric disorders in primary care settings were covered in several of the chapters and will also not be discussed.

A very specific acknowledgment of the tensions in the universalist's agenda was expressed by Rhi (Chapter 25) and Kitamura (Chapter 13). Rhi referred to much data pertaining to Korea of how the international system has been received in light of that country's ancient medical tradition. He made an explicit plea for broadness of information in diagnosis and indicated that, in the realm of care provision, problems result not from the system of diagnosis (whatever it might be) but from the attitudes and philosophical orientations of the treating physicians. Kitamura, on the other hand, discussed differences between the ICD-10 and the Japanese Conventional Diagnostic System. He drew attention to categories difficult to categorize in the ICD-10 that are much relied on in the Japanese schema: Atypical Psychosis, Anthrophobia, Olfactory Reference Syndrome, Dysmorphophobia, and Coenesthopathic Disorder. Clearly, many of the latter syndromes can be conceptualized as varieties of somatization, but it is important to preserve the content of these since they may well result from genetic, psychophysiologic differences or emphases of the culture having to do with bodily experience. Here the quandary is whether somatization is the important, universal "fact" about these disorders or whether instead, the form that somatization takes is important enough to preserve for purposes of understanding the nature of psychiatric disorders or approaches to treatment.

No demands were made for the need to include new basic categories of disorders, save the concern of some of how to incorporate the so-called culture-bound syndromes. Thus, basic categories such as those of psychosis (or schizophrenia), mood disturbances, anxiety, somatoform, etc seem to be judged as adequate for accounting for disorders in human populations regardless of national or cultural tradition. Srinivasa Murthy (Chapter 9) raised the question of whether concepts of hysteria and or dissociation were sufficient to deal with the complexity inherent in trance (and by extension, in possession). An implication here is the great variety in the content and meaning associated with trance phenomena. This point, merely alluded to in Srinivasa Murthy's chapter, is important for understanding the implications of any nonorganic "disorder" that entails alterations in consciousness and that, moreover, is not usually regarded as pathological or deviant in many traditional societies.

The chapter by Warthon et al (Chapter 15) raised the interesting question (attributed to Wig) of whether disorders of other "morbid emotions" should perhaps be accorded the status of separate basic categories in a universal schema of diagnosis. This question is fundamental to any criticism of a universalist agenda because it underscores the role that cultural biases associated with sadness and despondency have played in rendering Depression an important (indeed, dominating) basic category in the current international schema. Depression is tied to such things as happiness and optimism and, partly because of its devaluation in Western history and culture, has attracted enormous social and medical concern and attention. Indeed, to attempt to understand why and how this particular emotional complex has been valued (really, devalued) the way it has been in European societies (where the universalist agenda had its roots) and raised to a basic category of disorder, is immediately to plunge into an exegesis that leads to an appreciation of the large amount of cultural baggage about emotions intrinsic to Western culture and history. Other dominating emotional experiences are undoubtedly associated with somatic symptoms and equally likely to impair social functioning. Yet such emotions, whether viewed as "morbid" or not (eg, involving envy, sexuality, love, anger), have either not attracted medical/psychiatric attention or have been reduced to melancholia and depression (eg, love sickness) or the personality disorders (Berrios 1984, 1985, 1987a, 1987b, Jackson 1986). The behavioral problems that such emotions can cause are represented in the universalist schema of diagnosis in a variety of other categories (as adjustment disorders, anxiety, somatic problems, paranoia, explosive disorders, etc) but not as separate, basic categories, and the reasons for this are undoubtedly partly based on cultural conventions and biases. The same point of tension inherent in the universalist schema, namely, that of the role played by Western cultural conventions and biases in the definition of basic categories of psychiatric disorder, operates in the Personality Disorders (Fabrega in press) but a full discussion of the implications of this problem is beyond the scope of this epilogue.

Surprisingly few problems appear to be posed by the idea of operational criteria for diagnosis. In other words, a common positive vote seems to be cast for the idea of operational criteria and most authors appear to endorse this feature of the third edition of the DSM (DSM-III) and the new ICD-10; moreover, few problems were raised about specific operational criteria. Many authors proposed additional operational criteria that basically served to enhance the generalizability of the schema for diagnosis. Thus, the idea that it is possible to operationalize the descriptive material or manifestations that make up psychiatric disorders seems to be unproblematic. This is surprising because it is commonly assumed by cultural anthropologists that the basic ingredients of thinking, feeling, and behaving are culture-bound (Kleinman 1988). Presumably, the proponents of universalist operational criteria have stipulated these in a sufficiently abstract language so as to avoid subtleties of local meanings.

A dissenting vote about the problems associated with the idea of operational criteria was cast by Okazaki (Chapter 10H) of Japan. He acknowledged that although diagnostic criteria may be clearly understood and spelled out, they still might be applied differently and lead to differences in diagnosis because of national or even regional cultural traditions. This was amply illustrated in the results reported by Qin Yan, Nakane, and Lee (Chapter 14).

The idea of psychosis appears solidly supported by all authors although there exist many reservations about whether this category is properly partitioned (eg, Schizophreniform, Atypical, Psychogenic). In short, whether there exist third, fourth, etc psychoses appears controversial. Problems were raised about whether somatization problems should be separately classified, regardless of the structural nature of the symptoms, or whether they should be allowed to enter into other categories (eg, as a form of psychosis based on somatic delusions).

The need to connect with the specific cultural and social circumstances of people, a key reminder of the origins and purposes of diagnosis and classification, was an implicit concern of those who argued for psychogenic psychoses. This category may be thought to echo a concern about the context specific component of a psychiatric disorder. A similar concern for contextuality is seen in those who promote the idea of multiaxiality, with incorporation of stress and social supports, for the latter constitutes ways in which cultural and social realities attach to psychiatric disorders. A concern for cultural considerations was explicit in the case of Mezzich (Chapter 17) who outlined the development of guidelines for a cultural formulation to complement standard diagnostic ratings, as part of a project to enhance the cultural suitability of DSM-IV (Mezzich et al in press).

In addition to the powerful statement provided by Binitie (Chapter 30), a sensitive awareness of the tensions implicit in the universalist's agenda was demonstrated by Yamazaki (Chapter 10G) in his discussion of dilemmas associated with the diagnosis of childhood disorders. He drew attention to problems of diagnosis stemming from a child's developmental stage and the role of parent–child relations. Even more directly, his discussion pertaining to quandaries about how to handle school refusal and violence in the family made explicit the tension between abstract, "scientific," behavioral criteria and realities linked to social behavior and its evaluation in culturally specific circumstances. Yamazaki's appreciation of the problems implicit in the universalist's agenda did not, however, distract him from arguing for the value of this agenda. He included in his discussion an explicit awareness of how to use a universalist approach to diagnosis for purposes of establishing the validity of these disorders. Despite, or perhaps because of, an awareness of theoretical tensions in the universalist agenda for diagnosis, Yamazaki expects future systems of diagnosis to reflect "a more biological and scientific orientation," which implies a conception of the limitations in the way the agenda can be actualized at present.

## Conclusion

Differences exist in the degree of optimism expressed implicitly and explicitly by proponents of a universalist agenda for psychiatric diagnosis and classification. Some of the reservations about such an enterprise have been discussed, along with their implications. The case for optimism in the realization of the agenda was most directly expressed by Cooper (Chapter 16), "One of the main conclusions arrived at by the large number of international experts that helped to develop the ICD-10 chapter on mental disorders is that there is a surprising amount of agreement and compatibility among schools of psychiatric thought across countries. The remaining differences are comparatively small, and require to be dealt with by research rather than by attempts to set up special classifications that are incompatible with ICD-10 Chapter V(F) in its international role." Although Cooper was most explicit and eloquent in the prospects for a universalist agenda, it would appear that many, perhaps most, researchers reflect optimism about the agenda. Clearly, no one can object to the need for more research into the empirical intricacies of developing a universal schema, and it is hoped that the deployment of such a schema will lead to a culturally informed, prudent, and humane way of dealing with the human problems and sicknesses currently conceptualized as "psychiatric disorders."

In summary, this volume presents the state of the art in the development of psychiatric diagnostic systems as universal languages, with an emerging recognition of the importance of cultural framework in such development. What is at stake is not only a matter of high theoretical interest but the actual effectiveness of psychiatric diagnosis to potentiate clinical care.

## *References*


Berrios GE (1984). The psychopathology of affectivity: Conceptual and historical aspects. *Psychological Medicine* 14:303–313.

Berrios GE (1985). Descriptive psychopathology: Conceptual and historical aspects. *Psychological Medicine* 15:745–758.

Berrios GE (1987a). Dementia during the seventeenth and eighteenth centuries: A conceptual history. *Psychological Medicine* 17:829–837.

Berrios GE (1987b). Historical aspects of psychoses: 19th century issues. *British Medical Bulletin* 43(3):484–498.

Chiu ML (1985). Insanity in Imperial China, pp 75–94. In A Kleinman, TY Lin (eds), *Normal and Abnormal Behavior in Chinese Culture*. Reidel, Dordrecht.

Chiu ML (1986). Mind, body and illness in a Chinese medical tradition. (PhD dissertation). Harvard University Press, Cambridge, MA.

Devereux G (1956). Normal and abnormal, pp 23–48. In J Casagrande, T Gladwin (eds), *Some Uses of Anthropology, Theoretical and Applied*. Anthropological Society of Washington, Washington, DC.

Dube KC (1988). Nosology and therapy of medical illness in Ayurveda. *Comparative Medicine East and West* 6(3):209–228.

Edgerton R (1969). On the "recognition" of mental illness, pp 49–72. In R Edgerton, SC Ploy (eds), *Changing Perspectives in Mental Illness*. Holt, Rinehart and Winston, New York.

Fabrega H Jr (1989). An ethnomedical perspective of Anglo-American psychiatry. *American Journal of Psychiatry* 146(5):588–596.

Fabrega H Jr (1990). The concept of somatization as a cultural and historical product of Western Medicine. *Psychosomatic Medicine*, 52(6):653–672.

Fabrega H Jr (1992). The role of culture in a theory of psychiatric illness. *Social Science and Medicine* 35(1):91–103.

Fabrega H Jr (1993a). A cultural analysis of human behavioral breakdowns: An approach to the ontology and epistemology of psychiatric phenomena. *Culture, Medicine and Psychiatry* 17:99–132.

Fabrega H Jr (1993b). Towards a social theory of psychiatric phenomena. *Behavioral Science* 38:75–100.

Fabrega H Jr (in press). Personality disorders as medical entities: A bio-historical anthropological perspective. *Journal of Personality Disorders*.

Geuss R (1981). *The Idea of a Critical Theory*. Cambridge University Press, Cambridge.

Halipur CV (1984). Madness in ancient India: Concept of insanity in Charaka Samhita (1st Century AD). *Comprehensive Psychiatry* 25(3):335–344.

Jackson SW (1986). *Melancholia and Depression*. Yale University Press, New Haven, CT.

Kendell RE (1989). Clinical validity. *Psychological Medicine* 19:45–55.

Kleinman AM (1988). *Rethinking Psychiatry: From Cultural Category to Personal Experience*. Free Press, New York.

Mezzich JE (1979). Patterns and issues in multiaxial psychiatric diagnosis. *Psychological Medicine* 9:125–137.

Mezzich JE (1989). An empirical approach to the definition of mental disorder. *British Journal of Psychiatry* 154:42–46 (suppl 4).

Mezzich JE, Kleinman A, Fabrega J Jr, Parron D (in press). *Culture and Psychiatric Diagnosis*. American Psychiatric Press, Washington DC.
Scull A (1979) *Museums of Madness*. Allen Lane and St. Martins Press, New York.
Temkin O (1963). The scientific approach to disease: Specific entity and individual sickness, pp 629–647. In AC Clembie (ed), *Scientific Change*. Basic Books, New York.
Tseng WS (1973). The development of psychiatric concepts in traditional Chinese medicine. *Archives of General Psychiatry* 29:569–575.
Unschuld PU (1983). Medicine in China: A History of Pharmaceutics. University of California Press, Berkeley.
Weiss M (1977). Critical Study of Unmada in the Early Sanskrit Medical Literature. (PhD dissertation, University of Pennsylvania, Philadelphia.)
Yanchi L (1988a). *The Essential Book of Traditional Chinese Medicine, Volume I: Theory*. Columbia University Press, New York.
Yanchi L (1988b). *The Essential Book of Traditional Chinese Medicine. Volume II: Clinical Practice*. Columbia University Press, New York.

# Index

## J



## K



## L



## M

9 780387 942216

MIX
Papier aus verantwortungsvollen Quellen
Paper from responsible sources
FSC® C105338
FSC
www.fsc.org

If you have any concerns about our products,
you can contact us on
**ProductSafety@springernature.com**

In case Publisher is established outside the EU,
the EU authorized representative is:
**Springer Nature Customer Service Center GmbH**
**Europaplatz 3, 69115 Heidelberg, Germany**

Printed by Libri Plureos GmbH
in Hamburg, Germany